Auditory Competence
in Early Life

Auditory Competence in Early Life

The Roots of Communicative Behavior

Rita B. Eisenberg, Sc.D.
Director, Bioacoustic Laboratory
Research Institute
St. Joseph Hospital
Lancaster, Pennsylvania

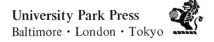

University Park Press
Baltimore · London · Tokyo

UNIVERSITY PARK PRESS
International Publishers in Science and Medicine
Chamber of Commerce Building
Baltimore, Maryland 21202

Typeset by The Composing Room of Michigan, Inc.

Manufactured in the United States of America by
Universal Lithographers, Inc. and The Maple Press Co.

Library of Congress Cataloging in Publication Data
Eisenberg, Rita B
Auditory competence in early life.
Bibliography: p.
Includes index
  1. Auditory perception. 2. Infants (Newborn) 3. Psychoacoustics.
4. Developmental psychobiology. I. Title. [DNLM: 1. Auditory per-
ception — In infancy and childhood. WV270 E36a]   BF 251.E37
612'.85   75–37782
ISBN 0-8391-0773-0

Contents

Figures

Tables

Abbreviations

AER, auditory (or acoustic) evoked responses
ANS, autonomic nervous system
CN, cochlear nucleus
CNS, central nervous system
CNV, contingent negative variation
COCB, crossed olivocochlear bundle
CPR, cochleopalpebral reflex
CV, consonant-vowel
DAF, delayed auditory feedback
EEG, electroencephalogram
EKG, electrocardiogram
EMG, electromyography
EOG, electrooculography
ERG, electroretinography
HR, heart rate
IC, inferior colliculus
ISI, intersignal (or interstimulus) interval
K-S test, Kolmogorov-Smirnov test
LIV, law of initial values
MFB, medial forebrain bundle
MG, medial geniculate body
NP, negative preception
OQ, orienting quiet
OR, orienting response
RAS, reticular activating system
SON, superior olivary nucleus
SLP, sound pressure level
t, time intervals
T_{hab}, speed of habituation
T_o, stimulus onset
VER, visual evoked response
VOT, voice onset time
V potential, vertex potential

Preface

In everyday life, the ability to perceive different sounds in different ways at the same time is taken for granted, and there is perhaps no clearer example of this than the course of events associated with a telephone call. First of all, the telephone rings and—provided we are within earshot—we are "alerted." This alerting serves to trigger some chain of adaptive behavior that varies with circumstance. If we are very close to the phone, for instance, the initial event may be a startle reflex or perhaps a blink; if we are farther away, it will differ according to whether we are sitting or standing or engaged in an activity. In any event, we perform a series of preparatory, or "orienting," actions, both voluntary and involuntary, during which the communicative exchange is anticipated. Furthermore, from the moment we pick up the telephone receiver, we proceed, almost instantaneously and usually without conscious thought, to make a good many judgments about the sounds we hear. The connection is classified as clear or noisy. The voice at the other end of the telephone line is recognized as familiar or unfamiliar, male or female, soft or loud, pleasant or unpleasant, and so forth. If background sounds are audible, they automatically are sorted out as voices, music, or any number of mechanical noises.

These different kinds and levels of auditory behavior constitute functional properties of sound during adult life. They testify to man's extraordinary auditory competence and reflect the fact that hearing is not a unitary function. It is, in fact, a hierarchy of functions having different kinds and degrees of adaptive significance; and it reflects a hierarchy of mechanisms for processing physical properties of sound.

The question of how these processing mechanisms become organized during development is central to an understanding of language learning and perhaps even of "intelligent" human behavior. What sensory specializations underlie man's use of verbal codes? Are they present at birth or acquired during the course of development? What properties of the central nervous system permit organisms to hear different things in different ways at the same time?

These are some of the questions currently under investigation at the Bioacoustic Laboratory, and this book is concerned with why and how the questions evolved. It discusses both the thinking that dictated given inquiries and the thinking that grew out of answers to those inquiries. It deals specifically with methods for obtaining infant data on audition and with the substantive information such methods have yielded. It considers methodologic problems that remain to be resolved and presents recent data that remain to be confirmed.

Research programs are like organisms in that they increase in complexity as they mature. Moreover, their rates of growth, the activities engaged in, and the means by which goals are pursued are conditioned by internal and external forces. In the case of the Bioacoustic Laboratory program, it seems only proper to note at the outset that the prime determinants were my notions about the nature of auditory competence and National Institutes of Health funds (Special Fellowship NBI-EP; BT-929 from NINDS; Grant No. R 01 HD 00732 from NICHHD) that permitted their exploration and testing. The program, which has grown fairly complex in the years since it was initiated, consequently reflects influences that have shaped my professional and personal growth. In this volume, therefore, the methods of approach toward research questions, the data to be reviewed, and the manner in which these data are interpreted are biased by my background as a professional person and, to some extent, by an innate skepticism of what is parochial or doctrinaire.

In terms of my own development, I am inclined to think this book premature, though I daresay any investigator who has spent enough time working in a particular area to recognize how little he knows feels similarly. In any case, I am hoist with my own petard. Having noted in a 1966 report to the NINDS Subcommittee on Human Communication and Its Disorders (Eisenberg, 1970a) that "A basic, up-to-date text or manual, bringing together under one cover all of the information germane to developmental auditory processes, is very urgently needed," I finally have been persuaded to accept a task that others, perhaps wiser than I, have avoided. Whether this volume covers all of the information that is germane is a moot question. However, calling upon personal experience, I have tried to include in it the kinds of material for which I would have been grateful when I first became involved in studies of communicative behavior during early life.

It has proved a difficult book to organize, partly because, over the years, Bioacoustic Laboratory studies have covered so much ground. Questions have become increasingly sophisticated during the progression from total to relative ignorance. Specific indices for measuring auditory behavior have increased in number and complexity. The nature and age range of the study population have expanded. Nonetheless, despite such changes and in the face of expanding information on infant performance and its determinants, our views about the nature of communicative development have been clarified rather than altered, and basic methodologic strategies developed during our earliest years remain serviceable.

The book, as it has evolved, can be considered part memoire and part textbook—a kind of chronologically arranged, annotated journal detailing the highlights in a research program devoted entirely to systematic studies in the ontogeny of auditory competence. Thus, this volume begins with a section on our first explorations, and, since the sequence of laboratory interests is inextricable from personal history, it includes some minor consideration of my background and biases. For the most part, the Introduction discusses preliminary observations not previously reported in the literature. Although some of the material perhaps may be viewed as anecdotal, this earliest work is reviewed for several reasons: it offers a perspective on an area of inquiry that has bourgeoned only within the past decade; it provides insights into the kinds of knowledge and skills required for studies in communicative development; and it affords an orientation for those clinicians who still regard basic research as "ivory tower" activity.

Part I of the text proper is concerned with basic information that has conditioned both concepts and practical efforts at the Bioacoustic Laboratory. Determinants of human development are reviewed briefly and related to communicative functions, and methods of studying auditory behavior during early life are detailed. Part II considers representative laboratory inquiries illustrating how the methods detailed can be applied to particular experimental paradigms and varied measurement techniques. Part III, which reviews current information on auditory processing in early life and relates it to various correlates in the performance of lower animals and adult humans, proposes a tentative model for the organization of intrinsic hearing mechanisms and discusses its implications for clinical practice and for basic research.

The book is directed toward specialists and nonspecialists alike, but, since a good bit of the material covered is inherently complex, some portions may prove hard going for those with limited background. Therefore, in providing facts, I have sought not only to integrate information pertinent to the development of auditory competence but also to present it in the simplest possible fashion. However, productive infant work requires considerable cross-disciplinary knowledge, and meeting the needs of readers at various levels of expertise in the several areas considered has meant striking a balance between telling some people more than they want to know and telling others less than they want to know. I accordingly have resorted to certain expedients which, it is hoped, will increase the utility of this book for all readers.

First, the very extensive reference list is designed to provide resource material at various levels of difficulty. The focus, for the most part, is on articles or books published within the past few years. However, a distinct effort has been made to include "landmark" papers in all areas and all papers, published or unpublished, that have special relevance for the study of auditory behavior during infancy. To compensate for necessarily restricted discussion of material peripheral to the major concerns of this volume, citations include both general reviews that can fill in the gaps for nonspecialists and technical reports that may be useful to specialists in given areas.

Second, extensive ancillary material is provided. Appendix A consists of a glossary which either defines or amplifies discipline-specific terms and concepts and which affords detail on anatomic structures or physiologic mechanisms that are covered only briefly in the text. Appendix B is an up-to-date compendium that lists, in alphabetic and chronologic order, studies that have been concerned, in one way or another, with responses to sound by human subjects under the age of 3 years. Derived largely from Bioacoustic Laboratory files, it provides a badly needed resource whereby investigators in any discipline can seek out specific studies that are relevant either to their research interests or their chosen measurement techniques. Appendix C is a technical section designed to meet the needs of investigators who may be interested in specific Bioacoustic Laboratory procedures. It shows how single-trial information on behavioral and EEG responses to sound can be coded for computer treatment and contains diagrams of our research circuitry as well as discussion material on special-purpose equipment.

Whatever practical purposes this book may serve—and I hope they will be many—I trust that it reflects a little of my enthusiasm for the subject matter. At least part of that enthusiasm is rooted in a long and happy association at St. Joseph Hospital, and I wish to acknowledge the cooperation of staff personnel there, particularly at the Research Institute. I especially want to thank Anthony Marmarou of the Bioacoustic Laboratory staff for his short-term effort in contributing to Appendix C and for his long-term efforts in putting together a sophisticated research system that has met the heavy demands placed upon it. Next, I would like to note the assistance of at least a few of the people who labored along with me in the tasks of data collection and analysis—specifically, Jane Baker, Patricia Giovachino, Mary Alice Hunter, Marguerite Ochs, Elizabeth Griffin Reus, Nancy Rupp, and Sally Smith. In addition, thanks are due Carol Winicki and Perla Kirchner, who somehow managed to translate my manuscript draft and arrange it for the publisher. Everybody at University Park Press was helpful, but I am especially grateful to Janet S. Hankin for bearing up under a deluge of corrections and addenda. Finally, I would like to express my respect and affection for Ernest Glen Wever, who listened to my ideas when they were still nebulous, sometimes corrected my facts, and always encouraged my efforts.

Introduction

"Science is simply common sense at its best. . . ."

T. H. Huxley, *Evolution and Ethics* (1896)

Studies of infant hearing are so commonplace now that it is difficult to believe that such investigations were viewed as pioneer efforts not long ago. However, in 1961, when the Bioacoustic Laboratory program was initiated, very few studies with neonates had been undertaken and almost no reliable data on hearing capacities in early life were available. Thus, in thinking about how to start this book, it seemed to me it might be useful to provide some perspective on current efforts in this area, and, along the way, to show by example that the gap between clinic and laboratory is not quite as great as it sometimes seems: clinical problems can and do lead to research programs, and complex research programs often evolve from very simple beginnings.

SOME PERSONAL NOTES

My particular interest in developmental matters grew out of long-term participation in so-called "exemplary" diagnostic settings where I was simply one of many clinical specialists charged with the task of "differential diagnosis" (Eisenberg, 1963*a*, 1966*a*, 1970*c*, and 1971). Over a period of some years, I was exposed to a massive population of preschoolers, a few of whom were younger than 1 year and a majority of whom were somewhere between 2 and 4 years old. Some of these young patients were retarded in all areas of growth and development; a smaller number represented clear-cut clinical entities such as adventitious deafness; a few presented obvious physical or psychologic abnormalities. In many cases, however, and particularly in those where communicative problems played a part, differential diagnosis was something of an exercise in futility. The older the children were, the more impossible it seemed to isolate a salient etiologic factor. Whatever age they were, it was difficult to fit them with a diagnostic label one could be sure of and impossible to recommend therapies guaranteed to work. Moreover, since I was exposed not only to these youngsters but also to the disparate ideas of other specialists about their problems, I began to question my own frame of reference. Indeed, as time progressed, I found myself increasingly dissatisfied with test procedures that failed to address critical questions, and with labeling procedures that failed to define either specific sources of dysfunction or rational methods of intervention. In the end, I came to feel that many developmental disorders of communication would remain unresolved until something was learned of normal maturational processes in hearing (Eisenberg, 1964, 1971, 1972, and 1974a).

Situations in which to learn were almost nonexistent in 1961, however. Specialties devoted to human communication were fragmented into three groups, none of which was especially concerned with normal developmental processes in hearing: audiology was geared to study deafness rather than hearing; speech pathology was focused on speech disorders and mechanisms of human utterance; that segment of linguistics interested in sound-encoding processes was wedded to a "motor" theory of speech perception. Psychology was directed toward the study of almost any aspect of perceptual development except hearing, while psychoacoustics, though concerned with hearing, was directed toward the study of adult functions. Neurophysiology was structured for the study of single neurons or populations of neurons, and otology for the management of hearing pathologies. Ethology had not reached a point of extending its inquiries on auditory-vocal relations to the human species. Pediatrics had neither programs nor facilities to train speech and hearing people for basic research with infants. The fact is there would have been no learning opportunity at all save for a special situation at St. Joseph Hospital[1] and a special fellowship from the National Institutes of Health that permitted me to take advantage of it.

THE LEARNING SITUATION

What St. Joseph had to offer in 1961 was a small research institute directed by a pediatrician[2] who was interested in communicative functions because he was interested in the biochemistry of brain function. The Institute had an electroencephalographic laboratory with a first-rate technician who had been trained to do hearing tests. It had a sound-treated test chamber and equipment for routine audiometric studies. It had cordial relations with local professional personnel and with other hospital departments. It had a good-sized research program in biochemistry. Best of all, the biochemistry folks, who were studying the effects of dietary intake on developing humans, had a population ready and waiting. The group consisted of infants whose mothers had been followed prenatally and who had been delivered at St. Joseph Hospital. Moreover, the infants were being followed, pediatrically and biochemically, at 3- to 6-week intervals during their entire first year of life. In effect, then, a ready made "practicum" in which to acquire information on developmental patterns in speech and hearing was available (Eisenberg, 1963b).

Putting this practicum to use posed a number of problems, most of which eventually turned out to be blessings in disguise. First, since none of

[1] Found for me by William G. Hardy, who, in a long and distinguished career, has shown a remarkable capacity for selecting and supporting "young iconoclasts."

[2] David Baird Coursin, to whom I am everlastingly grateful.

us involved in initiating a Bioacoustic Laboratory program had all of the information and skills required for concerted effort, we were forced to learn from each other. Second, since there was some information on prelinguistic patterns of vocal utterance back in 1961, but no useful data on infant hearing, we had no preconceived notions about what babies *ought* to do with their ears: we were forced to look at them carefully and then to think about what they *did* do when presented with different kinds of sounds. Third, since we had no hardware of consequence, and no immediate prospects of any, we were forced to develop general methods of approach, many of which stand us in good stead today.

EXPLORATORY OBSERVATIONS
ON AUDITORY AND VOCAL BEHAVIOR DURING EARLY LIFE

We started with a longitudinal study for several reasons. First, of course, the study group was immediately available. Second, though we started with a premise that the period around the age of 9 months probably was critical for the development of verbal language (Eisenberg, 1964), we had no useful information on antecedent changes in hearing. Third, while we had some vague notion that there was a relation between what went into the ears and what came out of the mouth, we had neither specific concepts nor specific methodologies. We had no idea which speech or hearing functions might be studied most productively, what kinds of problems would have to be dealt with experimentally, or what kinds of procedures best might serve our eventual ends. To put it more explicitly, we knew very little and decided to learn by doing.

On an educational basis, then, most of 1962 was devoted to the collection and analysis of information on communicative behavior during early life. Serial data were obtained on 102 infants randomly selected from the experimental population, and also on some dozen or so of their 12- to 14-month-old siblings who showed up more or less regularly.

Data on spontaneous vocal behavior under varying conditions of ambient noise, social stimulation, comfort, and physical positioning were obtained in all possible hospital settings. Phonetic notations of infant utterance and anecdotal observations on behavior were made in the waiting room, prior to pediatric study. They were made in the examining room, during the course of a physical examination that included collection of blood samples. They were made in our offices while playing with the children alone, and also while watching them with their parents during routine interviews. Ancillary information was obtained from other hospital personnel by briefing them on what we wanted to know, by asking them to fill out standardized report forms when they could or would do so, and by asking them to answer our questions when they could not or would not fill out forms.

Data on communicative behavior at home were obtained in whatever form was feasible. Where parents were literate, we gave them standardized check sheets on which to record how and when their children reacted to environmental sounds and human voices. We also asked them to jot down, in any hieroglyphics of their choice, what sounds the children made and when they made them. When parents were illiterate, as was often the case, we elicited this information during interviews, trying as best we could to remain nondirective in our questioning.

Observational data on responsive behavior to sound were elicited with noisemakers and also with voice. The noisemakers consisted of a supply of onionskin paper culled from hospital stationary supplies as well as a large collection of toys selected from a standardized kit in use at the Speech and Hearing Unit of the State of Pennsylvania Health Department. Acoustical properties of these items were determined by spectrograph and also by artificial ear, with borrowed equipment.[3] Since I was the only staff member with background in psychoacoustics and presumably would be most cautious about maintaining the fixed calibration distance required for a 75-dB stimulus, the job of signal presentation fell to me by default. All of us participated in scoring response behavior.

During the first 2 months of life, live voice stimuli were limited to nonverbal utterances, such as whistling, humming, gurgling, and so on. Starting at 8 weeks, the infant's name was added; and by 12 weeks, an amiable "Hi there" was tacked on. Later additions were unstandardized and introduced pretty much as and when I saw fit.

Since we were interested in developing a "naturalistic" approach to studies in communicative behavior, test sounds were introduced both in isolation and in additive combination with other cues (Rheingold, Gewirtz, and Ross, 1959). To give an example: first the infant's name would be called from some position where the speaker remained unseen; then it would be spoken directly in the subject's line of vision, but without social cues of any kind; following this, smiling and other signs of affability would be included; and finally, tactile cues would be added as the infant was held affectionately. Though the sequence for presenting voiced stimuli was fixed, the mother and I alternated as speaker once a baby passed his 2-month birthday. Conditions for noisemaker presentation were similar, but the mother was not asked to participate. In this case, the signal was presented with and without visual cues, and, at a reasonable age, the infant was given selected noisemaker toys with which to play.

It probably could be said that our most formal test procedures were informal, though there is every reason to suppose they were valid. In any event, much of the information gleaned during this period of exploratory study proved extremely helpful in later experimental planning. Indeed, four of the noisemakers used in the investigation were employed a year and a half later, when we embarked on our first large-scale study with newborns (Eisenberg et al., 1964). Let me, then, consider briefly a few trends that emerged during data analysis. Some of these trends suggested the order in which certain auditory abilities might emerge; some confirmed reports already in the literature; and others suggested potential avenues of developmental research.

What these preliminary observations indicated was that selective "listening" behavior develops rapidly, and in more or less steplike fashion.

---

[3] The Bruel and Kjaer artificial ear, like the noisemakers, was provided by L. Deno Reed (now at The Department of Health, Education, and Welfare) who, at that time, was in charge of the State of Pennsylvania Speech and Hearing Unit; spectrographic analyses were made possible by the cooperation of Robert Millard at the Lancaster Cleft Palate Clinic.

Preferential responsivity to human voice, as opposed to noisemakers, usually was noted between 11 and 12 weeks of age. Preferential sensitivity to maternal voice, as opposed to a stranger's, quite regularly was remarked between 12 and 14 weeks. Anticipatory cessation of crying at the sound of maternal footsteps was reported most frequently between 14 and 16 weeks. There was a sharp decline in responsivity to all noisemakers somewhere between 15 and 17 weeks.

On the whole, findings on vocal utterance were unremarkable. The nature of the developmental sequence was essentially that reported by Irwin and his co-workers back in the 1940's (Bar-Adon and Leopold, 1971; Carmichael, 1960; McNeill, 1970; and Menyuk, 1971), and Lewis' thesis (1941) that place of articulation varies according to whether infants are "comfortable" or "uncomfortable" seemed to be confirmed. In brief, our data were remarkable only in one respect: that is, growth curves for each of the vowel and consonant functions we were able to analyze seemed much steeper than any reported from earlier studies. Moreover, though it seemed possible that slope was affected by selected dietary supplements (Eisenberg, 1963b), these steeper functions were found, to greater or lesser extent, among all groups of our experimental population. In light of the generalized acceleration in growth rates suggested by cross-cultural studies and other recent evidence (Falkner, 1966; and Tanner, 1971), the possibility of accelerating prelinguistic functions seems worth exploring.

A few comments on variables affecting the incidence of spontaneous vocalization also may be in order here. We found, for instance, that the setting in which subjects were observed exerted strong effects. By far the largest proportion of spontaneous utterance was recorded in our least artificial hospital setting—the waiting room, which usually was crowded with mothers, their respective infants, sundry siblings or relatives, and members of the professional staff. In the same way, as has been pointed out in several papers (McNeill, 1970; Rheingold, Gewirtz, and Ross, 1959; and Schwartz, Rosenberg, and Brackbill, 1970), the incidence of evoked utterance, and particularly of "pleasure" sounds, tended to increase as additional sensory and social cues were made available. For the older infants, it increased greatly when subjects were permitted to manipulate noisemakers themselves. It seemed possible, then, that if we could determine what kinds of sounds elicited the greatest number of responses at given ages, the findings might apply to the design of useful auditory study procedures. Obviously we were not alone in our thinking since Friedlander's imaginative work on acoustic preferences during early life (Friedlander, 1968 and 1970; and Friedlander, Silva, and Knight, 1973) constitutes an application of this subject-participation approach.

Whatever the implications of our findings on vocal utterance, we reached the conclusion that our most productive course of action was to focus on hearing rather than on speech, and to limit ourselves to the early months of life. In the first place, prelinguistic patterns of vocal utterance had been studied extensively—even redundantly, in some respects—whereas the entire area of auditory development was a wasteland. Furthermore, we felt that cineradiography, our method of choice for approaching vocal maturation (Truby, 1959), posed hazards relative to X-ray dosage in the developing human that could not be resolved readily. In the second place, there were many hints that infants could actively process sounds long before they could produce any that were meaningful. In the third place, it seemed obvious that a great many important events in auditory development took place before babies got to be 9 months old. Indeed, patterns of response to some of our noisemaker signals changed so radically within the first 4 months of life that it seemed sensible to concentrate follow-up efforts on this period.

FURTHER LEARNING ACTIVITIES

Our new problem then, centered about which age group to start with and how to go about things specifically. The best part of the next 18 months consequently was devoted to a series of small-sample studies with infants under 4 months of age. A large battery of stimuli, ranging from pure tones in the speech-frequency range through noisebands of increasing width, was used in more ways than need be considered at this point (Eisenberg, 1965a).

To determine which stimulus conditions might be most effective, we systematically studied parameter effects. We varied the duration of signals and we varied their intensity. We varied the number of signals used in a single session and we varied the interval between successive signals. We used homogeneous test schedules and heterogeneous test schedules, and we varied the kinds and numbers of signals within each type of schedule.

To determine which methods of evaluating overt response best might tell us most, we systematically tried out different techniques. We asked observers to look at a single behavioral referent and we asked them to look at several behavioral referents. We asked them to make forced-choice "yes-or-no" judgments about response occurrence, and we compared such judgments with others made on a "yes-no-maybe" basis. We approached the problem of bias in human judgments by having four observers (myself, a speech pathologist, a pediatrician, and the nurse in charge of the newborn nursery) simultaneously record their independent response scores for later correlation with each other and with instrumental measures.

To determine which instrumental measures might work, we monitored skin resistance, respiration, heart rate (HR), and EEG. We monitored these patterns individually and in various combinations. We assessed the problems each presented with respect to variability, artifact levels, and the like. We considered whether and how these problems could be controlled, and we evaluated the relative degree of sophistication required for reasonable statistical treatment.

To develop a frame of reference, we exposed ourselves to infants. During the entire 18-month period, we spent countless hours in the newborn and premature nurseries, in the delivery room, and on the pediatric ward. We watched well babies and sick ones, when they were waking and sleeping, hungry and feeding, crying and cooing. We watched individual babies for hours on end, charting their activity cycles and learning to distinguish sleep states from doze states and doze states from waking ones. We learned to distinguish specific reflexes (Dekaban, 1970; Hutt, Lenard, and Prechtl, 1969; and Peiper, 1963) and charted the frequency with which these occurred spontaneously during given states (Wolff, 1959).

Under pediatric supervision, we learned how to score Apgar tests and how to test for neurologic abnormalities. More importantly, we learned to evaluate the pitfalls of such standardized procedures. The critical observer soon discovers, for instance, that the Apgar score varies according to whether ratings are obtained one or more minutes postnatally (Barrie, 1962; Desmond and Rudolph, 1965; and Desmond et al., 1963) and even according to whether individual examiners judge the color of an infant's extremities according to the same criteria. Thus, when we compared ratings scored for 200 infants by trained members of the delivery room staff, we found that the difference between an Apgar score of 9 and an Apgar score of 10 (Lewis et al., 1967) almost invariably turned out to be the difference between one examiner's "pink" and another examiner's "blue." By the same token, the sophisticated investigator gets to know that neurologic screening (Fiorentino, 1963; Prechtl and Beintema, 1964; Rosenblith, 1973; and Yang, 1962) is more informative about gross abnormalities than subtle ones: more than a few babies who pass such screening tests end up with a notation of FLK ("funny looking kid") on their hospital charts.

EXPLORATORY STUDIES
AS A GUIDE TO PROGRAM DEVELOPMENT

I remain firmly convinced that this kind of intensive preliminary exposure is prerequisite to any really productive work with young infants. Indeed, if our laboratory has been productive, it is largely because we did not stint on these early efforts. More than anything else, they taught us to think concretely about the problems of infant study, to set specific goals and design specific procedures to deal with specific variables.

Our first study, which disclosed broad patterns of auditory and prelanguage maturation during early life, showed us that 9 months was too late to start studying the development of hearing. It enabled us to identify and isolate specific aspects of auditory function that might be amenable to analysis under controlled conditions. In the same way, our series of follow-up studies within the restricted age range led us to newborns and provided opportunities to explore alternative measures. They gave us a handle on the variables we would have to deal with and led us to develop methods for specifying or controlling them.

We hardly expected to focus on newborns when we started our explorations: like most investigators now active in the neonatal area, we worked our way back to them. What we did expect, in light of our longitudinal data, was that 3.5–4 months would turn out to be a critical period for the development of hearing skills. This well may be the case since many of the physiologic and behavioral patterns found between 13 and 17 weeks were not present at any earlier stage. However, we also found that many patterns detectable at 1 month were equally detectable within the first 5 days of life. That being the case, and birth being a natural baseline, it seemed sensible to start at the beginning and define baselines against which to measure ontogenetic change.

As we explored alternative measures, we became increasingly aware that the individual differences also remarked by other investigators (Bridger and Birns, 1963; Clifton and Graham, 1968; Escalona, 1968; Korner, 1964 and 1968; Kron, Ibsen, and Goddard, 1968; Lipton, Steinschneider, and Richmond, 1961*b* and 1964; Richmond, Lipton, and Steinschneider, 1962*a* and 1962*b*; Steinschneider and Lipton, 1965) were very substantial. Consequently, we became increasingly skeptical about the validity of small-sample norms and the utility of one or two selected response measures. Therefore, despite our simplistic early notions, and against all of our inclinations, we began to think in terms of how to approach hundreds of subjects and how to obtain multiple, but somehow related, indices of function and organization.

In evaluating alternative measures of auditory behavior, we were at least as concerned with information yield as we were with experimental design. Acquiring a maximum of data in a minimum of time seemed critical because, back in the early 1960's, even the fact that newborns could hear had not been established unequivocally. Therefore, while we felt that the use of electrophysiologic measures such as HR and EEG might prove valuable at a future date, their immediate use was ruled out on specific grounds: they presented technical and analytical problems we could not expect to resolve in a hurry; they would require a laboratory setting and involve time-consuming procedures; and, considering the nature of our immediate needs, the costs would be excessive. We accordingly decided to concentrate on measuring overt behavior, partly because this technique presented the fewest difficulties and partly because it seemed valid. For individual infants, for instance, we found high correlations between responses measured by cardiac acceleration and those reported by independent trained observers using specified indices for judgment (Eisenberg et al., 1964; and Eisenberg, 1965*a*). It seemed likely, then, that behavioral data could be made highly reliable if motion picture techniques were employed to freeze experimental events in time.

Having decided, for better or for worse, that we would study neonatal responses to sound, we were left with the problem of what questions to ask and how to ask them. It seemed clear that our first order of business was to define the abilities present at birth in operational terms, by systematically studying relations between stimulus and response. In order to do so, we had to learn a great deal more in a good many areas. The material considered in this book reflects much of what was learned and some of what remains to be learned.

Auditory Competence
in Early Life

Part I DETERMINANTS OF COMMUNICATIVE BEHAVIOR

CHAPTER 1
The Endowment of The Developing Human Organism

"... man has a nervous system ... and the function of the nervous system is to bring each part into harmonious cooperation with every other."
  William James, *Principles of Psychology* (1890)

Relations between stimulus and response can be considered productively only with reference to mechanisms that govern those relations. Such mechanisms mature at different rates and operate under rules that vary according to an organism's stage of development. Therefore, unless one chooses to make ontogenetic studies in communicative behavior even more difficult than they need be, it is important to have some fund of basic information on the functions of underlying systems and the ways in which these are organized. The basis for selecting experimental stimuli may depend upon the questions to be asked, but it also has to depend upon how sounds are processed in the central nervous system (CNS). In the same way, the conditions under which questions are asked and the methods by which responses are measured may depend upon practical considerations, but they also must depend upon the maturation of CNS mechanisms. This chapter, then, is concerned with specific systems that underlie communicative behavior and also with nonspecific systems that have to do with arousal, attention, and response capacities.

3

The sole intention here is to provide background material that may make subsequent sections of this book more meaningful. To suppose that anything more might be accomplished within the confines of a short review is fatuous since notions about the way the brain functions have changed radically in recent years and even current thinking is in flux. Indeed, the only firm conclusion to be drawn from the latest physiologic data is that discrete sensory or motor events are not related to cortical events in a simple, straightforward way. We are, therefore, far from the point where the train of processes evoked in the CNS by a given acoustic signal can be traced.

THE NERVOUS SYSTEM

Smith (1953), in a dated but beautiful little book, reduces the complexity of the nervous system to four basic operations (p. 176): conduction within cells; conduction within long processes; secretion of biologically active substances; and transmission across synaptic junctions. For the sake of simplicity, then, response can be considered to reflect some combination of these basic operations, the complexity of which relates to the relative standing of an organism on the phylogenetic scale.

Evolutionary Determinants

In metameric organisms such as worms, the nervous system operates very simply, each event having an immediate effect upon the next link in the chain and all events being under control of no more than a few large nerve centers (ganglia) situated at the anterior, or frontal, end of the organism. In species lower on the phylogenetic scale than reptiles, much of the cerebral cortex is occupied by fibers from the olfactory organs. In pro-vertebrates and lower vertebrates, the chain becomes somewhat more complex, with peripheral nerves being connected in segmental fashion to accord with muscle arrangements.

In mammals, where the organization of nervous mechanisms reflects a long evolutionary history (Dethier and Stellar, 1961; and DuBrul, 1967), the cerebral cortex becomes very complex, differentiating into so-called "new" and "old" brain areas (Diamond and Hall, 1969). As the telereceptors, or distance receptors (nose, ears, and eyes), attained increasing importance over the millenia, the reflex centers relating to these organs became much larger, giving rise to massive ganglia which, in man, constitute the structures of the brain stem. As locomotion in one form or another became more prevalent, another large ganglion developed to form the cerebellum. As organisms increased in complexity, primordial centers for sensation and movement became increasingly separated from each other, giving rise to what is known as association cortex.

This association cortex is developed more highly in man than in any other species (Geschwind, 1964, 1965, 1970, and 1972). It occupies the greater part of the surface in each hemisphere and its fibers become myelinated relatively later than do fibers in other brain areas (Conel, 1963; and Dodgson, 1962). From a functional standpoint, this evolutionary development increases the number of operations and synaptic junctions, and, consequently, the time, between stimulus and response. It additionally provides for increasingly flexible response patterns since the intercalation of association cortex between sensory and motor areas permits both cross-modal associations and integration of different types of incoming information.

Embryologic Determinants

These phylogenetic determinants are reflected in the order of human embryologic development (Dodgson, 1962; and Jacobson, 1966). Almost the entire nervous system is derived ontogenetically from a thickened portion of ectoderm, the neural plate, which is transformed into a neural tube during the course of early embryonic life (Arey, 1965; and Strong and Elwyn, 1974). Once this tube has closed, three imperfectly separated expansions, or vesicles, appear (Windle, 1970). These are known as the prosencephalon, or forebrain; the mesencephalon, or midbrain; and the rhombencephalon, or hindbrain. As embryonic development proceeds, the midbrain undergoes relatively few changes in comparison with other vesicles, eventually coming to contain a host of fiber tracts and cellular masses, some of which are considered further in the discussion of neuronal organization. Hindbrain and forebrain vesicles, on the other hand, go through various metamorphases during the course of intrauterine growth.

The hindbrain vesicle divides into two portions. The first of these, termed the metencephalon, eventually is transformed into the structures of the pons and the cerebellum. The second portion, termed the myencephalon, eventually becomes the medulla oblongata. This, together with the pons and midbrain, comprises what is known as the brain stem.

It is the development of the forebrain that is most important for an understanding of brain function in man. It divides first into an anterior, or telencephalic, portion and a posterior, or diencephalic, portion.

The telencephalon forms the hemispheric vesicles and, expanding rapidly in all directions, it comes to overlap all other portions of the brain. As it does so, it forms three main structures: (1) the rhinencephalon, consisting of the olfactory (pyriform) lobe, the archipallium (old brain), and hippocampal formation (Bargmann and Schadé, 1963; Raisman,

Cowan, and Powell, 1965);[1] (2) the corpus striatum, from whence arises the internal capsule, connecting the cortex with the brain stem and spinal cord; (3) the pallium (new brain), or cerebral cortex (Kaas, Axelrod, and Diamond, 1967). By the seventh month of gestation, all cortical neurons are present (Rabinowicz, 1967), all of the main sulci and convolutions of the cortex are defined (Strong and Elwyn, 1974), and the cerebral hemispheres have expanded to form the frontal, occipital, temporal, and parietal lobes. Rhinencephalic structures, together with portions of the corpus striatum, constitute the so-called limbic system, which has extensive connections with lower centers.

The diencephalon, derived from the posterior portion of the forebrain, divides only into two parts. The dorsal portion gives rise to the nuclear masses of the thalamus and metathalamus. The ventral portion gives rise to hypothalamic structures which play an important role in regulating autonomic functions and endocrine activities.

One purpose of this brief outline of evolutionary and embryologic factors that influence development is to suggest that nature is thrifty. Older structures and mechanisms may be added to or changed as organisms become more complex (Gates et al., 1974; and Katsuki, 1965), but they rarely are thrown away. In considering functional relations in the nervous system, then it is important to recognize that, under normal conditions, the new comes to dominate the old. In short, the CNS is a hierarchal system in which the new brain dominates and, to the extent the human organism is unique, the reasons must be sought in new brain mechanisms.

The Organization of Neuronal Mechanisms

The brain stem region is essentially an extension of the spinal cord and the first major convergence area for sensory systems. All of the available evidence shows this region to be completely myelinated and fully functional at birth. The medulla, which constitutes an important center for the regulation of respiration, sucking, and other vital functions of newborn life, contains the dorsal and ventral cochlear nuclei of the auditory nerve. The superior and inferior colliculi, which are major organizational centers for sight and hearing respectively (Wickelgren, 1971), are located in the rostral portion of the brain stem, at the midbrain level. These nuclear groups receive ascending nerve fibers from their respective peripheral receptors and descending ones from widespread regions of both sensory and association cortex. Running throughout the middle of the brain stem

---

[1] There is some disagreement as to whether such structures as the hippocampus and amygdala properly should be considered part of the rhinencephalon (Bargmann and Schadé, 1963, pp. 237–244).

and extending from the lower medulla up to the thalamus is the so-called brain stem reticular formation (Anokhin, 1961; Brodal, 1957; Camacho-Evangelista and Reinoso-Suarez, 1964; French, 1960; Hernández-Péon, 1966; Moruzzi and Magoun, 1949; and Starzl, Taylor, and Magoun, 1951a and 1951b). This system, part of which (the reticular activating system, or RAS) serves in controlling states of arousal (Hyden and Lange, 1965), is so diffuse (Candia, Rossi, and Sekino, 1967; Roffwarg, Muzio, and Dement, 1966) and contains so many nuclei that it frequently is defined as that portion of the brain stem not identified as belonging to some other well-defined system. Since it comprises a variety of cell types, including some that respond to the motivational significance of signals (Phillips and Olds, 1969) and many that typically are activated by almost any kind of sensory stimulation, it is considered to constitute part of what often is termed the "nonspecific sensory system" (Huttenlocher, 1960; and Saunders, 1967).

The cerebellum is connected to the brain stem by three pairs of massive fiber bundles, or peduncles, and is situated above the back of the pons. It receives input not only from all of the sensory systems, but also from the spinal cord and many areas of cortex. It is a primary center for sensorimotor coordination and influences a host of voluntary movements and involuntary reflexes (Eccles, Ito, and Szentágothai, 1967; Lapham and Markesbery, 1971; and Reis, Doba, and Nathan, 1973).

Contiguous with the brain stem is the hypothalamus, containing not only the pituitary gland, (which is the master control mechanism of the endocrine system,) but also a multisynaptic pathway known as the medial forebrain bundle. The hypothalamic area, which is strongly implicated in appetitive and emotional behavior, is characterized by a functional dichotomy such that one portion, controlling sympathetic activity, is associated with autonomic reactions such as increased respiration and heart rate while the other, controlling parasympathetic activity, gives rise to opposite reactions (Gellhorn, 1967; Hess, 1957; and Singer, 1966). Hypothalamic structures are intimately related to those of the limbic system (Feldman, 1962; and Green, 1964) and, since the effects of limbic system stimulation ultimately are reflected in autonomic changes, the hypothalamus in some sense constitutes an effector for that system. Limbic structures, in turn, are intimately related with prefrontal cortical areas (Geschwind, 1964 and 1965; Pribram, 1969; and Van Hoesen, Pandya, and Butters, 1972), and current evidence suggests that those aspects of human behavior related to affect are governed by cortical, limbic, and hypothalamic mechanisms working in concert (Bargman and Schadé, 1963; Douglas, 1967; and Kimble, 1968).

The thalamus is comprised in great part of sensory nuclei which are not merely relay stations, as once thought, but rather synaptic junctions that serve integrative functions. Its dorsal portion, which develops in close association with new brain mechanisms, contains the reticular nucleus as well as the two geniculate bodies and a group of nuclei projecting to the cingulate gyrus, or cortex of the limbic system. The reticular nucleus, together with other cell clusters that are functionally related to the brain stem reticular formation, projects diffusely to several cortical areas and serves in governing brain excitation. The lateral and medial geniculate bodies are higher level counterparts of the superior and inferior colliculi, projecting to their respective visual and auditory areas in the cerebral cortex.

The new brain, or neocortex, is separated into two hemispheres by connecting fiber bundles, the largest of which is the corpus callosum. Each hemisphere has a laminar organization which, with some exceptions, consists of six well-defined cell types and each is characterized by a number of major landmarks, or fissures. Projection areas for major sensory systems are localized, somatosensory centers being found in the parietal lobes, visual centers in the occipital lobes, and auditory centers in the temporal lobes. Motor centers are situated in the frontal lobes and spatially mapped out in proportion to those skeletal areas over which the greatest amount of control is exerted.

Data on premature infants suggest that the final month of gestation is a critical period in neurologic maturation. It is a time when a large number of behavioral reflexes first appear (Flanagan, 1962; Humphrey, 1970; and Robinson, 1966) and when waking and sleeping patterns first can be differentiated in the EEG (Churchill, Grisell, and Darnley, 1966; Clemente, Purpura, and Mayer, 1972; Dreyfus-Brisac, 1964, 1966, and 1970; Ellingson, 1964; Hughes, Ehemann, and Brown, 1948; Monod, Pajot, and Guidasci, 1972; Parmalee et al., 1967, 1968, and 1969; Prechtl, Weinmann, and Akiyama, 1969; and Scheibel and Scheibel, 1964).

In adding these grossly oversimplified data to the developmental information already provided, a major object is to indicate that the nervous system is organized both horizontally and vertically. Every level of the brain is subject to facilitatory and inhibitory controls of many kinds (Gaddum, 1965), and among the most important of these are the controls exerted by the reticular formation (Magoun, 1963). It is the prime mechanism by which attention can be focused upon aspects of the external world that are important in either the long or the short run. It permits the exclusion of irrelevant sensory information and the passage of selected information relating either to a given modality or to different sensory modalities. It controls attention span and, through the RAS, exerts control upon sleeping and waking behavior alike (Aeserinsky and Kleitman, 1955; Kleitman, 1965; and Oswald, 1962). At subcortical levels, it exerts control on processing operations (Rosenblith, 1959); and to the extent that the

cortex is functional, it contributes to conscious perceptions and intellec-
tual activities.

PHYSICAL CHARACTERISTICS OF NEWBORN INFANTS

Before considering further the roots of human behavior, the physical
characteristics of newborn infants warrant at least brief discussion. They
not only testify to some of the evolutionary factors already mentioned,
but also suggest some of the problems inherent in infant research.

Emerging from the womb, the newborn human bears scant resemblance to the dimpled creature depicted in baby food advertisements. His
skin is red and wrinkled, lying in loose folds. Covering the surface of his
body and lining the external canal (meatus) of the ear is vernix caseosa, a
greasy, somewhat waxlike substance.[2] Much of the body, especially in the
back region, may be covered with fine hair (lanugo) that is shed over the
course of a week or so. The amount of hair on the scalp may vary from
almost nothing to a great manelike mass and, since this is not permanent,
it too will be shed shortly. Not uncommonly, small capillary clusters or
hemangiomas may be found on regions of the neck or face, and these
normally vanish within the first year of life (Nelson, 1975).

The head of the baby comprises about a quarter of his total body
length, as compared to about a tenth during adult life, so that the
relatively large skull looks even larger. The skull bones are not fused as yet
and the anterior fontanel easily is palpable.

The face, which is round and very small in comparison with the skull,
has certain distinctly simian characteristics: the forehead is high and rather
bulging; the bridge of the nose is flat and the nostrils (nares) are large; the
palate appears narrow and vaulted; the mandible, or lower jaw, is less well
developed than the maxilla, or upper jaw, and has an underslung appearance; the larynx is situated high with respect to its position in adult life;
the tongue, though only about half the length it attains in adult life, is
large in respect to the size of the oral cavity and the lingual frenum is both
short and tight, effectively restricting tongue movement and, consequently, affecting the degree to which pharyngeal volume can be controlled. However, the muscle architecture of the tongue tip is mature (Bell,

---

[2] In most hospitals, vernix caseosa is removed from surface areas but, if left in
place, it flakes off during the first weeks of life. The amount seen in the external
auditory meatus tends to be variable (Sprunt and Redman, 1964): in a series of 200
infants examined at St. Joseph Hospital, about 40% of the population showed only
negligible residues in the region of the tympanic membrane at the age of 5 days
(unpublished laboratory data): and Keith (1974) has reported that "usually the
vernix clears by the second day."

1970),[3] the masseter muscles strong (Nelson, 1975), and the sucking reflex present at birth. The eyes, which have bluish sclera, are small, although they look large, and no tears are secreted during crying.

The fundamental frequency of the newborn cry is about 400–500 Hz, with overtones that are roughly in the range between 1,000 and 5,500 Hz (Fairbanks, 1942; Fisischelli, 1966; Fisichelli and Karelitz, 1966; Lind, 1965, and Ostwald, Phibbs, and Fox, 1968). The length of the vocal tract accordingly has been estimated to be about half that of the adult value, or 7.5 cm (Lieberman et al., 1971).

The normal newborn is a tense organism (Dotson and Desmond, 1964; and Schulte and Schwenvel, 1965). His extremities are flexed and his legs bowed. He tends toward mass reflexes of one kind or another. He can raise his head while lying prone, but cannot support it when held upright. In the supine position, he has a distinct tendency to turn toward the right side (Turkewitz, Moreau, and Birch, 1966; and unpublished Bioacoustic Laboratory data).

Despite a weight loss during the first few days of life, the baby becomes a good deal more presentable during the lying-in period (usually 4–5 days). The initial redness of his skin disappears, although the extremities tend to be dusky in color and somewhat mottled because peripheral circulation often remains insufficient during this time. Some tremulousness of the extremities normally is seen, particularly during the earliest days.

From a study standpoint, it is critical to recognize that the neonate is a tender creature. This imposes special requirements with respect to medical oversight, the physical environment in which newborns can be properly observed, and the kinds of manipulations to which they can be properly subjected. These and related matters will be considered in the next chapter.

THE AUDITORY SYSTEM

Fetal Development

The precocious development of the human auditory system is documented by anatomic and physiologic studies (Anson, Harper, and Hanson, 1962; Anson and Winch, 1974; Candiollo and Levi, 1969; Dayal, Farkashidy, and Kokshanian, 1973; Kósa and Fazekas, 1973; Kosyagina, 1967;

---

[3] The diameter of muscle fibers in the tongue is only about half that found during adult life (Bell, 1970).

Madonia, Modica and Cali, 1963; Palva, 1970; Ruben, 1969; Smith, 1973; and Vasilu, 1969), by fetal studies, and by information on the performance of premature infants.

Cochlear function is demonstrable as early as the fifth fetal month, by which time both middle and inner ear structures have reached full adult size (Elliott and Elliott, 1964a; and Nakai, 1970). There is evidence to suggest that the size of end-organ receptors may be mathematically predetermined by the frequencies to be reproduced in extrauterine life (Elliott and Elliott, 1964b), and there is some possibility that man is equipped at birth with an oversupply of sensory cells (Bredberg, 1968).[4] Auditory nerve fibers begin to myelinate during the sixth fetal month (Falkner, 1966, pp. 274–275) and, in the full-term baby, even the auditory cortex is medulated. The fetus has been shown responsive to pure tones and other sounds (Barden, Peltzman, and Graham, 1968; Bench, 1968; Bench and Vass, 1970; Bernard and Sontag, 1947; Dwornicka et al., 1964; Forbes and Forbes, 1927; Grimwade et al., 1971; Johansson, Wedenberg, and Westin, 1964; Murphy and Smyth, 1962; Sakabe, Arayama, and Suzuki, 1969; Sontag, Steele, and Lewis, 1969; Sontag and Wallace, 1935; Tanaka and Arayama, 1969). The premature infant responds both behaviorally and electrophysiologically to sound (Eisenberg, 1965a, 1965c, 1966a, 1966b, 1967; Eisenberg et al., 1964; Eisenberg, Coursin, and Rupp, 1966; and Schulman, 1970a and 1970b).

Given these facts, there is good reason to suppose that the full-term baby emerges from the womb with at least some of the mechanisms he will need to organize his auditory world. Given the nature of the auditory system, however, it seems hard to believe he might have all of them.

Neural Mechanisms of Audition

The auditory, or cochlear, nerve emerges from the internal auditory meatus at the level of the medulla. It constitutes one portion of the acoustic, or eighth (cranial) nerve, system and leads to a maze of fearfully complicated channels that, directly or indirectly, course through or connect with all of the brain areas thus far considered. Many of the neuronal groups they include are poorly understood and the ways in which channels interact, both with each other and with other areas of the brain, remain to be clearly delineated. Thus, while it is known that neural impulses initiated

----

[4] The number of sensory cells required for good hearing is unknown. However, if Bredberg's data (1968), showing a continual slow loss of hair cells beginning some time during infancy, are correct, man seems to be born with more than he needs—a happy precaution, since all of the evidence to date indicates that these highly specialized cells, once lost, cannot be replaced.

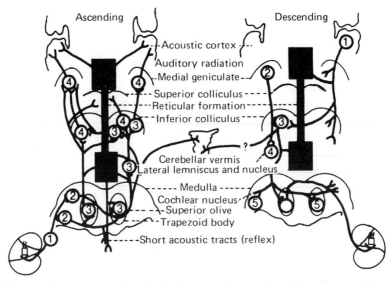

Figure 1. Schematic drawing of eighth nerve pathways. Ascending afferent pathways and nuclei are shown to the left and descending efferent components to the right. Numerals indicate approximate order of neurons, counting from origin of each system. Darkened areas indicate central core of brainstem reticular formation and diencephalic nuclei of generalized thalamocortical system origin. Figure reprinted by permission, from R. Galambros, "Neural mechanisms in audition," *Laryngoscope* 68:388, 1958.

at the cochlea reach the cortex not only by way of the so-called classical auditory pathway (Figure 1), but also by routes lying outside the main line[5], these alternate or recurrent channels will be largely ignored.[6] The focus will be upon a few structural and functional details of the main pathway that afford a reasonably orderly glimpse into the nature of auditory coding operations. Given even these strictures, however, the picture remains unalterably complex.

In man, the snail-shaped cochlea, or receptor organ for hearing, contains about 15,500 hair cells which are differentially, and very intricately, innervated (Darrouzet, 1972) to feed into some 30,000 cells in the spiral ganglion (Wever et al., 1971). These functionally differentiated hair cells (Billone and Raynor, 1973; Dallos et al., 1972; Gleisner, Flock, and Wersäll, 1973; and Spoendlin, 1972), comprising internal and external layers, are distributed along the basilar membrane; and the membrane, as it

[5] Adrian, Goldberg, and Brugge, 1966; Clark and Dunlop, 1971; Desmedt, 1965; Fex, 1965 and 1967; Filogama, Candiollo, and Rossi, 1967; Gacek, 1965; Galambos, 1954; Geniec and Morest, 1971; Kupperman, 1972; Møller, 1973; Rasmussen, 1964; Ross, 1971; and Sachs, 1971.

[6] At least two afferent pathways to the cortex already have been identified clearly (Galambos, Myers, and Sheatz, 1961; Harrison and Irving, 1964 and 1966; Harrison and Warr, 1962; Masterton and Berkley, 1974; and Whitfield, 1971), and there is good evidence for efferent pathways that constitute at least one descending auditory system (Desmedt and Mechelese, 1958; Dunkel and Grubel, 1965; Katsuki and Watanabe, 1966; Nobel and Dewson, 1966; and Rasmussen, 1964).

follows the coil of the cochlea from base to apex, differs in elasticity and other properties (Zwislocki and Sokolich, 1973). The basilar membrane as a whole, then, can be characterized as a short-term analyzer (v. Békésy, 1963): the net result of its differential properties is that areas of maximum vibrations along its length are frequency dependent, high frequency tones producing maximum vibrations at the basal end and low frequency tones producing them at the apical end (Khanna, Sears, and Tondorf, 1968). Electrical responses in the auditory nerve have been found to be synchronous with frequency, suggesting that this parameter can be registered at the periphery (Finck, 1968; Kiang, Sachs, and Peake, 1967; Rupert, Moushegian, and Galambos, 1963; Schwartzkopf, 1967; Suga and Campbell, 1967; and Teas, 1966).

Ascending fibers of the classical eighth nerve pathway, bundled together in the spiral ganglion as they leave the cochlea, follow a main route from their first central way stations in the cochlear nuclei (Dewson, Nobel, and Pribram, 1966; and Greenwood and Goldberg, 1970). They then enter the lateral lemnisci, either directly or, in a fraction of cases, after relaying in the superior olivary complex (Goldberg and Brown, 1968 and 1969; and Harrison and Beecher, 1967). Fibers of the lateral lemniscus, which often relay in scattered nuclei along their paths (Harrison and Warr, 1962; Harrison, Warr, and Irving, 1962), eventually ascend further to the inferior colliculus and medial geniculate body (Watanabe et al., 1966), thence forming the acoustic radiations to primary auditory cortices in the transverse gyri of the temporal lobes. Since all of the way stations are interconnected across the midline, all of them above the level of the cochlear nucleus (midbrain) receive input from both ears.

The ratio of input fibers to subcortical cells is on the order of 1:33 at the medial geniculate (thalamic) level and by the time the primary auditory cortex, with its approximately 100 million neurons is reached, this ratio of input fibers to cells increases to about 1:3,300 (Worden, 1971).

It seems clear from a variety of studies (DeReuck and Knight, 1968; Gersuni, 1971; Møller, 1973; Raab, 1971; Radionova and Popov, 1966; Sachs, 1971; Scheich, Koch, and Langner, 1974; Teas and Henry, 1969; and Whitfield, 1967) that some amount of temporal analysis can be accomplished at the single cell level. Auditory neurons respond differentially to the frequency (Katsuki, Suga, and Kanno, 1962; Møller, 1969; and Whitfield and Evans, 1965) and duration (Gersuni, et al., 1969; Goldberg, Adrian, and Smith, 1964; Goldberg and Greenwood, 1966; and Radionova and Popov, 1966) of acoustic signals, while the spike rates they generate are a function of intensity (Kiang, 1965).

There are extensive differences in structure and organization within individual nuclei of the auditory system (Clark and Dunlop, 1971; Galin, 1964a, 1964b, and 1965; Jane, Yashon, and Diamond, 1968; Ryugo and

Killackey, 1974), and these tend to increase hierarchically (Holstein, Buchwald, and Schwafel, 1969; Radionova and Vartanian, 1971; and Symmes and Anderson, 1967). In general, current data suggest that transmission upward through nuclei in the classical pathway is associated with increasing limitation of neural impulse activities, changes in impulse flow, increases in latency, and other phenomena (Roeder, 1966; and Scheich, 1974) that serve to reduce the degree of correspondence between the signal parameters processed at successive levels. In other words, it would appear that the signal reaching the cortex constitutes something very different from the sound going into the ear and, in all likelihood, something from which various features have been "extracted" (Masterton and Berkeley, 1974).

Neurons are tonotopographically organized; that is, they are arrayed spatially in an orderly fashion according to their frequency characteristics, within most if not all subcortical centers. Moreoever, there are immensely rich synaptic connections within centers (Erulkar and Nelson, 1963; and Nelson and Erulkar, 1963), permitting discrimination of rate, direction, and extent of frequency modulation (Gersuni and Vartanian, 1973; Kelly, 1974; Maruyama et al., 1966; and Neff, 1968), sound source motion (Altman, 1968), and other complex stimulus features (Caspary, Rupert, and Moushegian, 1974; Hind et al., 1963; and Suga, 1973).

Much of the recent neurophysiologic evidence (Masterton and Berkeley, 1974; Møller, 1973; Otellin, 1970 and 1972; Sachs, 1971; and Worden, 1971) indicates that, at the level of primary auditory cortex, where synapses per unit volume are almost double the number postulated for visual cortex, an orderly arrangement of neuronal arrays is lacking (Funkenstein and Winter, 1973). Neurons encountered at given sites may show a wide variety of characteristic, or "best," frequencies; some may be unresponsive to tones of any frequency and react only to complex sounds or even to specific vocalizations (Funkenstein et al., 1971; Goldstein, Hall, and Butterfield, 1968; Newman and Symmes, 1974b; Newman and Wollberg, 1973a and 1973b; Suga, 1972 and 1973; Symmes and Newman, 1974; Winter and Funkenstein, 1973; and Wollberg and Newman, 1972); others respond to moving visual stimuli rather than to sound.[7] Nonethe-

[7] Just as orbitoinsular cortex appears to be less specific than once thought (Loe and Benevento, 1969), recent studies (Colavita, 1974; Colavita, Szeligo, and Zimmer, 1973; Wegener, 1974a and 1974b) suggest that insular-temporal cortex, traditionally considered to be uniquely auditory, in fact may be polysensory. However, auditory cortex remains strongly implicated in the perception of acoustic patterns (Cornwall, 1967; Dewson and Cowey, 1969; Diamond, Goldberg and Neff, 1962; Neff, 1964; Thompson and Smith, 1967; and Wegener, 1964): monkeys, trained preoperatively to discriminate among vowel sounds, cannot be retrained after ablations in the midtemporal area (Dewson, Pribram, and Lynch, 1969).

less, current reports by Gersuni and his co-workers (Baru, 1966; Gersuni, 1971; and personal communications), who employ both behavioral and physiologic techniques, suggest that frequency projection on the surface of auditory cortical areas does indeed exist. Whether or not it can be demonstrated evidently is a function of signal duration since the auditory system is shown to have two mechanisms possessing significantly different attributes. These are designated as "mechanisms which work, respectively, under conditions of a short-" (1–20 msec) "and a long-time constant regime" (Gersuni, 1971, p. 108). The importance of these data for our thinking about communicative functions scarcely can be overemphasized since a basic requirement for any language-coding system is the capacity to detect distinctive features of speech that occur within short time segments (Chomsky and Halle,1968; Corliss,1971; Jakobson, Fant, and Halle, 1967; Kavanagh and Mattingly, 1972; and Mattingly, 1972).

Summing up current neurophysiologic information on hearing mechanisms, one can say not only that the auditory system is enormously complex, but also that it is marvelously well organized for analyzing patterns that vary in the time domain. Cells having the characteristics of feature detectors of one sort or another exist even at relatively low levels of the classical pathway (Møller, 1974), although the weight of current evidence suggests that neurons specialized for the processing of complex signals exist only at the highest levels. The amplification in numbers of neurons as one ascends the classical pathway, together with structural and functional differences among neurons, the myriad possibilities for centrifugal and feedback controls, and the abundance of synaptic connections within and among neuronal aggregates, provide for great flexibility in the coding of acoustic information.

These neurophysiologic data, which stem almost entirely from the study of infrahuman species and very largely from study of lower vertebrates, bear in several ways upon all studies in audition. First, since the findings now available, however confusing and difficult to interpret, show all mammals to have functionally similar auditory systems (Fay, 1974), we can assume the existence of numerous processing mechanisms in man. Some of these have to do with the coding of specific parameters such as frequency and intensity, and others with the coding of multidimensional sounds such as species-specific vocalizations. Second, since many of the newer data suggest that the kinds of operations performed in the auditory system change hierarchically, we must assume that the kinds of signals employed in human studies will determine both the kinds of functions and the levels of neuronal organization under investigation. Third, since communicative behavior differs markedly even among species having apparently identical auditory systems, we must suspect that man's unique patterns of communicative behavior reflect central specializations, that is, those relating to the ways in which acoustic information is utilized and/or controlled by the CNS.

From a practical standpoint, several strategic alternatives for developmental studies in hearing, some already touched upon in the Introduction, present themselves. One can select given parameters or given complex sounds on the basis of available physiologic data and determine whether response activity changes systematically as a function of developmental status. One can select specific stages of development and determine whether that activity changes systematically as a function of signal variables. Or one can try to get an insight into central specializations by posing questions relative to conditioning, habituation, or other general phenomena.

Research Questions

The neural mechanisms just considered so summarily constitute what might be considered the primary input into a human communicative network. Normal hearing for spoken language depends not only upon the integrity of the several decoding channels, but also upon the integrity of external and middle ear structures that serve in transmitting sounds (Curthoys, Markham, and Blanks, 1970). The status of these peripheral mechanisms during newborn life, which is influenced by phylogenetic and embryologic factors (Filogama, Candiollo, and Rossi, 1967, pp. 13–41; Strickland, Hanson, and Anson, 1962; and Webster, 1966), is touched upon elsewhere in this volume. At all stages of development, however, there is reason to suppose that middle ear muscles receive their innervation from a great many sources, including the reticular formation (Carmel and Starr, 1963; Dewson, Dement, and Simmons, 1965; Galin, 1964b; Simmons, 1964; and Simons et al., 1966).

HEARING IN RELATION TO SPEECH AND LANGUAGE

Carrying the network analogy further, neural mechanisms for producing spoken language might be viewed as the primary output source of a human communicative system. Logically, then, one would expect to find certain systematic relations between mechanisms for perceiving sounds and mechanisms for reacting to them (Kent, 1974; Mahaffey, 1970; Mallard and Daniloff, 1973; Mattingly, in press; Ploog and Melnechuk, 1969; Siegel and Pick, 1974; Stark, 1974; Sussman, 1971; and Sussman, MacNeilage, and Lumbley, 1974).

Aural-Oral Relations

The coordinated activities involved in speaking depend upon movement of various respiratory and articulatory muscles. The energy source for utterance is the column of expired air from the lungs while the sound produced at the larynx by the vocal cords is generated in a series of puffs, or bursts. This sound is shaped by resonating cavities of the upper respiratory tract that, during vocal utterance, vary in configuration according to the ways in which the articulatory organs are adjusted.

Given fixed listening conditions, the perceived loudness of an utterance and the stress given to particular portions of it varies as a function of changes in subglottal air pressure[8] and/or laryngeal muscle activity (Lieberman, 1967). The fundamental pitch of the voice, permitting hearers to identify a telephone caller according to sex, or even age, depends largely upon the size of the speaker's vocal apparatus. The overtones, or "quality" of voice, permitting listeners to distinguish among known callers, vary according to individual differences in the conformation of the resonating cavities. The acoustic character of the perceived utterance, allowing hearers to classify vocal output as speech, nonspeech, or some segment of speech, depends upon the manner in which the resonating cavities are modulated over time. This modulation imposes a physical structure upon utterance such that the acoustic energy is concentrated within particular frequency bands, or formants. It is the relation of these formant frequencies to each other that determines the phonetic properties of speech sounds, that is, whether they are discerned as vowels or consonants, or some combination of the two.

Developmental Determinants of Speech Production

Once cherished notions of speech as an "overlaid" function (Karlin, Karlin, and Gurren, 1965), like notions about the specificity of neurons, no longer are tenable. Leiberman and his colleagues (Lieberman, 1968, 1969, and 1971; Lieberman and Crelin, 1971; Lieberman, Crelin, and Klatt, 1972; and Lieberman, Klatt, and Wilson, 1969), in a series of brilliant studies comparing speech structures in today's humans with those found in Neanderthal man and primates, have shown convincingly: (1) that adaptations of supralaryngeal structures have resulted in reduced efficiency for some basic functions; (2) that adult speech patterns depend upon anatomic specializations which are present only partially in neonatal life; and (3) that the supralaryngeal tract of the newborn bears a certain resemblance to the configuration seen in primates and Neanderthal. The resemblance, which has to do with both the proportions of the speech organs and their relative arrangement within the confines of the vocal tract, imposes one set of constraints upon the kinds of sounds an infant

---

[8] The amplitude of vibration of the vocal cords increases directly with the force of expiration.

can make. Still other constraints are imposed by his physiologic immaturity. Although the muscular coordination required for such reflex patterns as crying and sucking is present at birth and, indeed, motor planning for the crying act has been described (Bosma, 1973; and Lind, 1965, pp. 61–92), the tongue remains relatively immobile for several weeks after birth (Lieberman et al., 1971), and the finer coordination required for consonantal production is relatively slow to develop. The reasons for this can be related to the rate at which neural mechanisms become fully functional (Bosma, 1973; Humphrey, 1970; Nash, 1970; Thomas and Lambert, 1958; Schulte, Albert, and Michaelis, 1969; Ulett, Dow, and Larsell, 1944; and Winick and Greenberg, 1965).

In man, as in other species, myelogenesis is a progressive phenomenon. It begins during the second half of gestation, first appearing in the spinal cord and proceeding upward through subcortical structures toward the cerebral hemispheres. Fiber pathways relating to equilibrium and sensation start to myelinate by about the sixth fetal month and, in the term infant, are already heavily medulated. Fiber pathways related to voluntary movement develop at a far slower rate (Dubowitz et al., 1968; Hursh, 1939; and Schulte et al., 1968): myelin first is deposited only a few weeks before term and heavy medulation is not found until well after birth. It should be noted, however, that there is no 1:1 relation between myelinization and reflex activity (Langworthy, 1928 and 1933). In the cortex, neither the corpus callosum, the band of nerve fibers connecting the hemispheres, nor its associated tracts in the fornix have begun to appear.

The articulatory musculature is controlled by fibers passing from the lower portion of the left frontal lobe, via the corpus callosum, to a corresponding area in the right hemisphere. From there, the fibers pass downward via pyramidal tracts, various cranial nerve nuclei, and their corresponding motor neurons, to innervate the larynx, tongue, and associated structures of the speech apparatus. The muscles of the face and lips are innervated by the facial (seventh cranial) nerve, those of the jaw by the trigeminal (fifth) nerve, and those of the tongue by the hypoglossal (twelfth) nerve. The diaphragm and other muscles involved in respiration are innervated by corticospinal fibers and, as in the case of other motor activities (Lawrence and Kuypers, 1965), they are regulated through extrapyramidal centers and pathways, including the cerebellum (Abbs and Eilenberg, 1975; Brain, 1961; Dubner and Kawamura, 1971; Fletcher, 1973; Karlin, Karlin and Gurren, 1965; and Penfield and Roberts, 1959).

In sum, the crying and sucking activities of early infancy reflect the early maturation of brain stem centers that serve vital functions,[9] while

---

[9] Crying, for instance, involves inspiratory and expiratory reactions as well as vibration of the vocal cords, and the first extrauterine cry serves vital functions by oxygenating the blood.

the changing patterns of vocal utterance discussed in the Introduction reflect later maturational processes at higher levels in the nervous system. At any stage of development, however, speaking normally depends upon the integrity of the efferent structures and pathways noted so briefly above.

Language and the Perception of Speech Sounds

Questions relative to the nature of language, the mechanisms that subserve it, and the processes by which it is acquired are far beyond the scope of this book. The purpose of this short section, therefore, is merely to indicate the place of central mechanisms in a hypothetical communicative network and to remark upon current thinking and information that is pertinent to the study of auditory competence in early life.

There is a great deal of evidence to indicate that the primary center for comprehension of spoken language, Wernicke's area, is located in the temporal lobe, immediately adjacent to auditory cortex (Lenneberg, 1974). The primary center for production of spoken language, Broca's area, lies in the frontal lobe, immediately adjacent to that portion of motor cortex controlling the speech musculature (McAdam and Whitaker, 1971). These association centers are connected with each other and also with centers in the occipital lobe that have to do with processing written language. Thus, the telephone conversation considered in the Preface to this volume would involve, among a great many other things, the passage of information from Wernicke's area to Broca's area, via a tract known as the arcuate fasciculus, to relevant efferent pathways. Further, if the telephone exchange had involved spelling out a term, writing down directions, or similar activities, the arcuate fasciculus would serve to route impulses appropriately between either of these centers and the angular gyrus of the parietal lobe, which constitutes the association area for communicative systems (Brodal, 1969; and Geschwind, 1970).

There is today some limited but fairly strong anatomic evidence showing that the left side of the brain is larger than the right during both newborn (Witelson and Paillie, 1973) and adult life (v. Bonin, 1962 and 1963; Geschwind, 1964, 1965, 1970, and 1972; and Geschwind and Levitsky, 1968). These findings in conjunction with a mounting body of data on functional asymmetries in hearing, have aroused enormous interest since they suggest that, in most humans, the left hemisphere somehow is specialized for speech perception (Sutker, Altman, and Satz, 1974). It is hardly surprising, then, that a sizable number of experiments and clinical studies has been undertaken in an effort to tease out underlying factors. Sparked by Kimura's pioneer work (1961*a* and 1961*b*), a host of investigations involving dichotic stimulation (Bever and Chiarello, 1974) almost

[handwritten margin note: ASSOCIATION AREAS]

uniformly has shown that even in childhood (Dorman and Geffner, 1973; Goodglass, 1973; Kimura, 1963; Knox and Kimura, 1970; and Nagafuchi, 1970), right ear (left hemisphere) mechanisms are dominant in the processing of verbal inputs while left ear (right hemisphere) mechanisms are dominant in the processing of nonspeech inputs (Berlin et al., 1973; Chaney and Webster, 1966; Curry, 1967; Dirks, 1964; Kimura, 1964; Kimura and Folb, 1968; King and Kimura, 1972; Shankweiler, 1966; Shankweiler and Studdert-Kennedy, 1967; Spellacy and Blumstein, 1970; Springer, 1971; Springer and Gazzaniga, in press; Studdert-Kennedy and Shankweiler, 1970; and Zurif and Mendelsohn, 1972).

These results tend to be supported by related studies involving other kinds of interventions with normal subjects,[10] by findings on patients with temporal lobe or other CNS pathology,[11] and by the patterns of EEG activity associated with speaking and listening tasks.[12] Although there are some data to suggest that differential processing of short-duration sounds, sequential factors, and possibly repetition rates may underlie the various kinds of functional asymmetries that have been reported,[13] the determining factors remain speculative.

As might be expected, then, a number of models already has been proposed to explain the differential processing of speech and nonspeech sounds (Mattingly, in press). Perhaps the most influential notion has been the so-called motor theory of speech perception (Allport, 1924; Lane, 1965; Lenneberg, 1967; Liberman et al., 1963; Liberman et al., 1967; and Mattingly et al., 1971), which, having stimulated many investigators, now seems disputable on several counts (Bailey and Haggard, 1973; Baumrin, 1974; Fujisaki and Kawashima, 1969 and 1970; Griffiths, 1968; Haggard, Ambler, and Callow, 1970; Lane, 1968; McCaffrey, 1971; Morse, 1973;

---

[10] Cohen, Noblin, and Silverman, 1968; Cooper and O'Malley, 1974; Doehring and Bartholomeus, 1971; Doehring and Ross, 1972; Gerber and Goldman 1971; Haggard, 1971; Herman, 1972; Hicks, in press; Murphy and Venables, 1969 and 1970; Perl, 1968; Sparks and Geschwind, 1968; Spellacy, 1970; Spreen, Spellacy, and Reid, 1970; Tsunoda, 1969; and Warren et al., 1969.

[11] Albert et al., 1972; Annett, 1973; Berlin Porter et al., 1973; Dobie and Simmons, 1971; Faglioni, Spinnler, and Vignolo, 1969; Gazzanaga, 1972; Hutchinson, 1973; Kaas and Diamond, 1969; Lynn and Gilroy, 1972; Milner, Taylor, and Sperry, 1968; Nagafuchi and Suzuki, 1973; Pinheiro, 1973; Sato and Dreifuss, 1973; and Speaks et al., 1974.

[12] Cohn, 1971; Grabow and Elliott, 1974; Greenberg, 1974; Greenberg and Graham, 1970; Matsumiya et al., 1972; McAdam and Whitaker, 1971; Morrell and Huntington, 1971; Morrell and Salamy, 1971; Ratliff and Greenberg, 1972; Tobin and Graham, 1968; Wood, 1973, 1974, and in press; and Wood, Goff, and Day, 1971.

[13] Bartholomeus, in press; Crowder, 1973; Dooling, in press; Godfrey, 1974; Gregory, Harriman, and Roberts, 1972; Halperin, Nachson, and Carmon, 1973; Hannah, 1971; Horenstein, LeZak, and Pitts, 1966; Klatt, 1974; Nachson and Carmon, 1974; Papcun et al., 1974; Peters, 1967; Rosenthal, 1971; Tallal, 1974; and Zaidel, 1974.

Pisoni and Lazarus, 1974; and Tsunoda, 1969 and 1971). Other speculations revolve around the existence of feature detector systems,[14] the possibility of "synthesizer," "integrator," or "extractor" mechanisms of sorts,[15] and the role of attentional and memory processes.[16] Some of these models, together with recent data on the perception of speechlike signals during infancy, will be considered in later sections of this book.

---

[14] Abbs and Sussman, 1971; Ades, 1974; Cooper, 1974; Cutting, 1973; Cutting and Eimas, in press; Eimas, 1975; Eimas, Cooper, and Corbit, 1973; Eimas and Corbit, 1973; Naeser and Lilly, 1970; Peters, 1967; Stevens, 1973; and Stevens and Klatt, 1974.

[15] Cole and Scott, 1974; Cutting, in press; Dowling, 1967; Fujisaki and Kawashima, 1971; House et al., 1962; Robertson and Inglis, 1973; Savin, 1967; Stevens and House, 1972; Warren and Obusek, 1972; Warren, Obusek, and Ackroff, 1972; and Webster, Woodhead, and Carpenter, 1970.

[16] Broadbent, 1971; Deutsch, 1969 and 1970; Dorman, 1974; Haydon and Spellacy, 1973; Inglis, 1965; Klatzky and Atkinson, 1971; Pisoni, 1971, 1973; and Wilson, Dirks, and Careterette, 1968.

CHAPTER 2
Methods for Studying Auditory Behavior in Infants

"Want of Care does us more Damage
than Want of Knowledge."
  Benjamin Franklin, *Poor Richard's*
  Almanack (1758)

Whatever the background in which infant studies are approached, the same
sorts of methodologic rules apply. Procedures must take into account both
environmental factors and the developmental status of subjects. Criteria
for response must be established. Response, if it is to be meaningful, must
be defined operationally, in terms of specific referents.

Operational definitions of stimulus-bound behavior are difficult to
come up with, regardless of the modality under investigation or the
response indices employed. Particularly in situations where the aim is to
obtain valid experimental data under *clinically viable conditions,* problems
implicit in all infant study are compounded many times (Cairns and
Butterfield, in press). It must be assumed, for instance, that no subject
cooperation will be forthcoming and that none but the most indirect
external constraints can be imposed. From a methodologic standpoint,
then, the task reduces to manipulating the study situation in ways that can
yield reasonably foolproof answers to the questions under investigation.
The purpose of this section is to analyze the problems posed by infant
studies in audition to consider how they properly can be approached.

A MODEL OF INPUT-ORGANISM-OUTPUT RELATIONS

The first step in dealing with problems is to define them clearly and Figure 2 represents one way of doing so.

The diagram is merely a device for reducing variables that operate in all perceptual studies to simple input-output dimensions in order to think concretely about them. Thus, the complex infant discussed in the previous chapter becomes no more than a "black box" incorporating feedback mechanisms.

External components of input are schematized as *nonauditory* (all classes of environmental signals other than sound) and *auditory* (all classes of sound stimuli). Internal components of input, considered according to their conditions of operation, are schematized as *intrinsic* (all classes of steady-state signals arising among interrelated physiologic systems) and *output* (all classes of intersystem feedback signals that are consequent upon the combined effects of repeated stimulation and repeated response).

Detectable portions of output are schematized as *nonauditory* (that pattern of activity observed in the absence of acoustic signals) and *auditory* (that pattern associated with acoustic stimulation). Output accordingly can be seen as a subject's aggregate response to all of the variables in his internal and external environment; and any significant change in any of these factors necessarily will be reflected in behavioral and/or instrumentally measurable change. The question for an observer, then, is how to differentiate some change in output that is specifically auditory.

As perhaps is evident, the approach represented by Figure 2 owes a good deal to concepts of automatic process control (Buckley, 1968; Johnson, 1962; and Powers, 1973) that go under the name of living systems theory (Cromwell et al., 1973; Leibovic, 1969; Milhorn, 1968; and Miller, 1965). Its application to auditory study seems almost inevitable because the auditory system has attributes characteristic of all control systems. Once this application is made, it follows that the entire organism

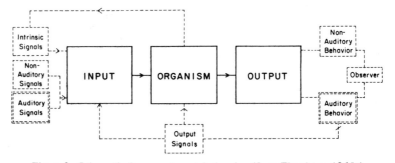

Figure 2. Schematic for experimental planning (from Eisenberg, 1965*a*).

must be examined as if it were, in some respects at least, a control system. Thus, the "state" of the organism, which relates the auditory system to other systems in the CNS and thereby both conditions and reflects its dynamics, becomes a critical variable. The sole object of presenting acoustic signals is to force the auditory system out of equilibrium in order to effect detectable changes in performance. These transient changes, which are labeled "response," become meaningful only when they are evoked by known signals, under specified conditions, and according to specified criteria. By the same token, the absence of detectable change, which is labeled "no response," attains significance only in reference to defined states and conditions under which response normally might be expected.

THE DEVELOPMENT OF STUDY PROCEDURES

The major value of a model like that shown in Figure 2 is that it literally forces one to think operationally. The six general classes of variables schematized represent potential sources of error and, because the study situation is exposed in its entirety, the investigator is led to consider implicit problems as well as explicit ones. It becomes obvious, for instance, that the only way to approach definition of auditory behavior is to reduce the number of operating variables: factors that are manageable have to be controlled and factors that are unmanageable have to be specified. To suppose that stimulus-bound activity can be defined with total precision is unrealistic, however. In the first place, the two internal sources of input are interrelated simply because they have their origin in physiologic systems that are interrelated: this means that the nature and extent of intrinsic signals and feedback stimuli cannot be specified exactly. In the second place, both internal equilibrium and its measurable correlates are dynamic, that is, they change from moment to moment: this means that no matter what variables are controlled or specified, a given signal may exert different effects each time it operates. In the third place, the accuracy with which any change in output activity can be detected depends upon the degree of change as well as the sensitivity of the observer(s) or measure(s) employed. Realistically, then, one purpose of study design must be to reduce the degree of experimental (or clinical) error by treating the sources of error as adequately as possible.

INTERNAL SIGNALS AND THE USE OF STATE INDICES

The treatment of internal stimuli is a difficult matter, although their effects can be minimized somewhat if study periods are fixed with reference to feeding schedules (Berg, Adkinson, and Strock, 1973; Bridger, 1962b; Carlson and Ginsburg, 1915; Hendry and Kessen, 1964; Irwin, 1933; Silverio, 1964; and Turkewitz et al., 1966), sleep patterns (Dittrichova and Lapackova, 1964; and Parmalee, Brück, and Brück, 1962), and other situational variables (Eisenberg, 1965a; and Eisenberg et al., 1964). Unfortunately, given individual differences in temperament as well as a host of indeterminate factors no diagram can specify, there is no way they can be reduced to insignificance (Birns, 1965; Bridger and Birns, 1963; Bridger, Birns, and Blank, 1965; Brown, 1964; Escalona, 1968; Korner, 1964 and 1973; Kron, Ipsen, and Goddard, 1968; Newton and Levine, 1968; Prechtl, 1965; and Steinschneider and Lipton, 1965). The only option remaining, then, is to develop some way of measuring the aggregate effects of internal stimuli; and, since all such signals serve in the maintenance of physiologic equilibrium, it seems logical to treat them with reference to their collective regulatory function.

Procedures used at the Bioacoustic Laboratory stem from an assumption that the state of a subject, as reflected in his degree of behavioral arousal and/or his level of somatic function at any given time, represents a temporary balance between some internal signals that are excitatory in nature and others that are inhibitory. Given this assumption, one can grade the effects of internal stimuli along some defined continuum pertaining to the measures employed. Thus, overt behavior can be rated on an arousal scale ranging from deep sleep to extreme excitation while cardiac and brain wave patterns can be treated with reference to period or rate distributions over time (Anders, Emde, and Parmalee, 1971; Eisenberg, 1974a and 1975b; Eisenberg, Marmarou, and Giovachino, 1973, and 1974a and b; Graham and Jackson, 1970; Jennings, Stringfellow and Graham, 1974; Khachaturian et al., 1972; Lewis, 1974; Procter and Adey, 1965; and Rechtschaffen and Kales, 1968). Although behavioral and electrophysiologic continua clearly are related, the treatments to which individual indices can be subjected are to some extent arbitrary. Where correlative studies are undertaken, therefore, concomitance among indices must be tested rather than assumed (Eichorn, 1951; Hutt, Lenard, and Prechtl, 1969; Johnson, 1970; Monod, Eliet-Flescher and Dreyfus-Brisac, 1967; Podvoll and Goodman, 1967; Prechtl et al., 1969; and Schmidt, Rose, and Bridger, 1974).

Electrophysiologic measures of internal equilibrium are far more difficult to deal with than behavioral ones, partly because such measures present intrinsic problems and partly because methods for data treatment remain a subject for debate (Clifton, 1974a; Donshin and Lindsley, 1969; Graham and Jackson, 1970; Lewis, 1974; McCallum and Knott, 1973; and Prescott, Read, and Coursin, 1975). Since adding another voice to the debate cannot resolve the issues and discussing the issues can add little to an understanding of infant hearing processes, HR and EEG measures are considered in this volume only insofar as they apply to data obtained at the Bioacoustic Laboratory (see Chapter 5).

Behavioral Measures of State

The net effect of intrinsic signals (those that operate whether or not acoustic stimuli are introduced) can be indicated by *basal* measures obtained during specified rest periods prior to and subsequent to presentation of a study schedule. The effects of feedback signals (those that arise as a consequence of acoustic stimulation) can be indicated by sequential measures obtained as the schedule progresses. Putting this another way, defined rating scales can be used for obtaining measures applicable to given conditions under which the two sources of internal input operate: (1) *nonstimulus,* or basal state, values that refer to a subject's resting equilibrium; and (2) a series of *prestimulus,* or activity state, values that refer to his dynamic balance during some specified interval immediately prior to each stimulus presentation. Although the term, prestimulus state, commonly is used to denote baseline values, measures obtained during the course of a stimulus run, in fact, cannot refer to steady-state conditions: each signal presentation in a sequence and each response in that sequence must exert effects upon an organism's subsequent activities, whether or not those effects can be isolated (Eisenberg et al., 1964).

For purposes of behavioral study, each point on a sleep to waking continuum must be defined by a differential pattern of overt activity and, given the fact that indices of infant state have received attention for over 40 years (Kessen, Haith, and Salapatek, 1970; and Pratt, 1960), criteria for judgment are reasonably well specified (see Appendix C, Table I.1). Indeed, by this time, most of the useful points have been validated statistically, either by correlations among independent observers[1] or by correlations with related measures.[2]

In Bioacoustic Laboratory work, the number of states differentiated has increased from four (Eisenberg, 1965a; Eisenberg et al., 1964) to seven (Eisenberg, 1970b; and Eisenberg, Coursin, and Rupp, 1966) as studies

---

[1] References: Bell and Haaf, 1971; Birns, 1965; Brazelton, 1962; Brazelton and Freedman, 1971; Bridger, Birns, and Blank, 1965; Brown, 1964; Dittrichova and Lapackova, 1964; Korner, 1968; Lamper and Eisdorfer, 1971; Rosenblith, 1961; Rosenblith and Lipsitt, 1959; Wagner, 1937; and Wolff, 1959, 1965, 1966, and 1967.

[2] References: Aeserinsky, 1965; Ashton, 1971a; Birns, Blank, and Bridger, 1966; Brackbill, 1970; Campos and Brackbill, 1973; Desmedt and Manil, 1970; Eichorn, 1951; Graham and Jackson, 1970; Hutt et al., 1968a; Hutt, Lenard, and Prechtl, 1969; Parmalee, Stern, and Harris, 1972; Parmalee et al., 1967; Petre-Quadens, 1967; Pomerleau-Malcuit and Clifton, 1973; Prechtl, 1965 and 1974; and Prechtl et al., 1969.

have proceeded (see Appendix C, Table I. 1). No matter what the intervals, however, scales employed to define the arousal continuum uniformly have been based upon correlation coefficients (among observers and/or with related measures) or 0.76 or better at each of the points specified. This is consistent with criteria established by other investigators. Both basal states, or nonstimulus measure of equilibrium, and activity states, or stimulus-bound measures of equilibrium, have been rated numerically on a defined scale covering the intervals from deep sleep (I) to extreme excitation (IV→VII).

The Significance of State Measures

These state indices have been dwelt on at some length because, as noted earlier in this chapter, measures of internal equilibrium are equally measures of nonspecific influences that govern the operating characteristics of eighth nerve channels. By definition, then, relations between state and auditory behavior constitute a functional property of sounds that bears upon neuronal organization. The value of a study framework based upon automatic process control theory is that it permits two critical assumptions about these relations. On the one hand, it can be said that *relations which hold constant for all stimulus conditions* (or for all sensory modalities) *reflect the organization of nonspecific mechanisms in the central nervous system.* On the other hand, it can be said that *relations which vary systematically according to stimulus conditions reflect the organization of specific coding mechanisms in the eighth nerve system.*

THE TREATMENT OF NONAUDITORY EXTERNAL STIMULI

In studying any sort of sensory processing, it is obvious that information yield will increase directly with the number of valid responses obtained. The object of controlling external variables, then, is to create conditions that are weighted toward response and against artifact. This section considers environmental factors that can exert untoward effects during infancy and suggests optimal study conditions for newborn subjects. Optimal conditions for older infants have not been studied systematically at the Bioacoustic Laboratory so that specific recommendations are precluded. Whatever the developmental status of subjects and whatever conditions prevail, however, maintaining a *constant* environment is critical.

Room Temperature

During earliest infancy, when compensatory heating is limited by a feeble skeletal musculature and compensatory cooling is limited by inadequate sweat gland activity (Adams et al., 1964; Athavale, 1963; Cooke, 1952;

Eichorn, 1970; Mestyan and Varga, 1960; Pratt, 1930; Silverman and Agate, 1964; and Stern, Lees, and Leduc, 1965), room temperature becomes an important variable. The 75°F temperature (at 50% humidity) recommended for the newborn nursery by the American Academy of Pediatrics (1974) is not adequate for study of the nude or nearly nude infant (Halverson, 1942). As temperature is varied below 78–79°F, the unclothed neonate tends to become progressively more lethargic and correspondingly less responsive to most kinds of external stimulation. As it is varied above 81–82°F, on the other hand, he tends to become progressively more irritable, to the point where auditory behavior cannot be detected in the background of gross bodily activity, even when the evoking signals are not masked by loud crying.

Bioacoustic Laboratory data suggest optimal study conditions for the exposed neonate to be 50% humidity, with room temperature maintained at some fixed level in the 78–82°F range (Eisenberg, 1965a). All other things being equal, these limits provide reasonable assurance that intermediate states (doze or quiet wakefulness) favoring responsivity will be maintained for periods up to about an hour.

Light

Despite certain accommodative deficiencies and a fovea centralis that is developed only partially, all parts of the eye necessary for sight are formed completely at birth (Pieper, 1963, p. 54). The pupil contracts to light and dilates to other external stimuli, the lids close reflexly in response to signals of many kinds, and fixation is possible under favorable circumstances. Indeed, given favorable circumstances, the neonate is capable of remarkably fine visual discriminations (Cohen and Salapatek, 1975; and Kessen, Haith, and Salapatek, 1970). Thus, light as a medium for the introduction of competing visual signals becomes an important variable in the study of auditory behavior.

Although there are data to the contrary (Anderson and Rosenblith, 1964; and Ashton, 1971a), studies at the Bioacoustic Laboratory and elsewhere (Irwin, 1930 and 1941; and Weiss, 1934) suggest that the *amount* of light present in the environment probably does not exert significant effects. Increasing luminance seems to be associated with increasing infant motility and higher basal levels (Irwin and Weiss, 1934a and 1934b), but irritable states tend to diminish over time when brightness is held constant. Data on the effects of brightness are too limited to permit recommendations respecting optimal intensities, however, Doubtless, it is wise to use the lowest adequate level, allowing for a settling down (adaptation) period in the study setting (Eisenberg, 1965a).

The *source* of illumination, on the other hand, is a significant factor in auditory research. Direct lighting, by dividing the visual field into contrast areas, maximizes an infant tendency to turn in the brightest direction and clearly increases the possibility of artifact: the neonate can focus only on targets in the 19-cm range, but the range of flexible accommodation approximates adult levels by 4 months of age (Haynes, White, and Held, 1965) and infants of 6–20 weeks can fixate for prolonged periods at distances between 30–90 cm (McKenzie and Day, 1972).

All conditions of direct lighting explored at the Bioacoustic Laboratory have been found unsatisfactory in some respect. Overhead illumination, although desirable because it tends to elicit the supine position most favorable for behavioral observation, also tends to reduce responsivity to sound, possibly by inducing fixation on the light source (Richmond, Lipton, and Steinschneider, 1962a). With illumination on either side, the best vantage point for observation becomes that directly in the infant's line of vision. Rear illumination, though a reasonable expedient when direct lighting must be employed, affords the least adequate conditions for any observational technique.

By and large, experience suggests that infants placed in a supine position will maintain that position for considerable periods of time when indirect lighting is used. Thus, conditions can be considered optimal for observational research in audition when the method of illumination assures diffusion of a constant light intensity throughout a distraction-free environment.

THE TREATMENT AND SELECTION OF AUDITORY SIGNALS

Basically, the object of studying auditory behavior is to make connections between physical attributes of sounds and their functional properties, or what subjects do in response to sounds. Thus, if the relationships sought are to have validity, it is axiomatic that the evoking stimuli must be known exactly, and procedures for measuring them (Coombs, 1972) are specified in manuals that are provided with all calibration gear. In addition, if these relationships are to provide insights into the nature of auditory processing operations, the signals employed must be viewed as "probes" which, under properly controlled conditions, can be made to yield information on underlying mechanisms. Accordingly, it becomes important to think about how different kinds of signals relate to auditory coding in the nervous system and to communicative behavior in everyday life.

Classification of Auditory Stimuli

To start with, one can adopt Cherry's view (1961) that the linguistic information in sounds is merely a potential. Then, assuming that this potential resides in particular attributes of sounds, language can be viewed as a physical phenomenon. Specifically, all language sounds can be defined simply as multidimensional patterns that vary in the time domain (Flanagan, 1965) within known parameter limits prescribed by the speech apparatus (Lieberman, 1971; Lieberman and Crelin, 1971; and Lieberman, Klatt, and Wilson, 1969). This general definition is applicable despite such variables as age, culture, or specific language code. Moreover, if the aim is to examine the effects of given parameters such as frequency or intensity, a choice is available: they can be studied either in isolation, using "constant" signals, or in combination, using "patterned" signals. In making the choice, however, it must be recognized that these two general classes of stimuli vary significantly both in their manner of coding within the central nervous system and in their degree of significance for a hearer (Eisenberg, 1966b, 1967, 1970a, 1970b, 1974a, and 1975a).

Constant, or fixed-dimension signals can range in band width from pure tones (sine waves) to white noise. The nervous system can code such stimuli in "bits" *because their physical properties are invariant in time.* They are easy to control and, consequently, very useful for both clinical and laboratory purposes. However, such signals rarely if ever are found in nature and, because they are abstract, their significance for a hearer depends heavily upon such factors as learning or the "set" induced by instructions.

Patterned, or multidimensional, signals, on the other hand, can range in complexity from modulated tones to complex environmental noises and the sounds of spoken language. The nervous system somehow must code these stimuli in "chunks" or "ensembles" *because their component physical parameters are invariant only in relation to each other.* Obviously, since they are less easily controlled than constant signals, patterned stimuli must be used with caution (Bench, 1973; and Hutt, 1973). All the same, such signals variously approximate sounds in the natural environment, and, consequently, they may have varying degrees of built-in significance (Eisenberg, 1965a, 1967, 1970a, 1970b, and 1975a; Worden and Galambos, 1972).

Relations between Physical and Functional Properties of Sounds

At least seven parameters of sound are clearly relevant to some of the fundamental processes discussed in Chapter 1. *Sound pressure level* (SPL) and *duration* apply to the spatiotemporal configuration of activity in neural aggregates. *Repetition rate,* as it refers to the pulses within a stimulus envelope, applies to the integration of acoustic energy. *Intersignal interval* (ISI), as it bears upon following characteristics at varying levels of the auditory system, applies to the relative distribution of excitatory and inhibitory mechanisms. *Frequency* and *band width* apply to the locus of stimulation in the cochlea and to the tonotopographic layout of the transmission pathway. *Dimensionality,* as it refers to the kind and amount of variance within a stimulus envelope, applies to the existence of feature detectors and to the characteristics of the transmission pathway. Only a few of these parameters have clear-cut correlates in perceptual function. Loudness and pitch judgments, for instance, vary systematically with the respective physical dimensions of SPL and frequency, but qualitative judgments of speech, music, or environmental sounds relate to a complex of factors, most of which are ill defined (Bever and Chiarello, 1974; Hochberg, 1965; Kincaid and Cooper, 1972; Kryter, 1966 and 1968; and Perret, Grandjean, and Lauber, 1963).

Effects exerted by representative constant and patterned signals have been studied, to greater or lesser extents, both in neonates and in older infants, and relevant data, including information on optimal values for given parameters, will be considered in subsequent chapters. For present purposes, only a few points need be made. First, no stimulus battery can be weighted in favor of response unless the signals composing it are well above the threshold of hearing. Second, in schedules containing both constant and patterned signals, it is critical that stimuli be equated for intensity.[3] Third, whatever the specific SPL values employed, a stimulus battery must be designed with reference to the effects of interactions among sequential sounds, recovery time in the system(s) being measured (which is partly a function of developmental status), and an organism's responsivity over time.

Interstimulus Interval (ISI) and the Sequential Arrangement of Acoustic Signals

Any attempt to study sensory behavior in infants or to evaluate the validity and significance of data on infant audition is doomed to failure unless the nature of the acoustic battery is taken into account. Thus, though ISI is not so much a parameter of sound as a critical determinant of response to sound, its effects warrant consideration here. The importance of ISI derives from the fact that any sequence of signals involves parameter interactions and, by and large, the shorter the time between successive stimuli, the greater the chance of obtaining ambiguous data (Sutton et al., 1967). Indeed, many of the studies listed in Appendix B are

---

[3] In Bioacoustic Laboratory work, small scale psychoacoustic studies with normal hearing young adults uniformly are undertaken before schedules of this kind are employed with infants.

omitted from discussion in this book precisely because the design of the stimulus battery makes the data suspect.

The easiest way to avoid ending up with ambiguous data is to define ISI operationally, with reference to the total time required both for response and for return to baseline conditions. On this basis, it is doubtful whether ISIs shorter than 10 sec can be used effectively in the study of newborn hearing processes. The incidence of overt response to sound during neonatal life, which remains quite stable when ISI is varied upward from 10 sec, decreases markedly when shorter delay periods are used (Irwin, 1946; and Eisenberg, 1965a). The duration of respiratory non-excitability (Peiper, 1963), which varies with arousal and other factors, lies somewhere between 10 and 15 sec. Recovery time for sound-evoked potentials may be 10 sec or longer (Davis et al., 1966; and Goodman et al., 1964). The amount of time required for the heart to return to baseline following stimulation with constant signals is of like order (Lipton, Steinschneider, and Richmond, 1961a, 1965a, and 1966; Steinschneider and Lipton, 1965; and Steinschneider, Lipton, and Richmond, 1966) and when high-potency patterned signals are used, this time may be increased appreciably (unpublished Bioacoustic Laboratory data). Moreover, the incidence of cardiac response to constant signals tends to fall systematically as ISI is reduced below 40 sec (Bartoshuk, 1962a and 1962b; Brazelton, 1962; Bridger, 1961; and Lipton et al., 1965a).

It further must be borne in mind that repeated bombardment of a single sensory modality results in a more or less systematic decrement in responsivity over the course of a stimulus sequence. The limiting number of trials has been explored variously in neonates and young infants (Graham, 1973; Graham and Jackson, 1970; and Kessen, Haith, and Salapatek, 1970). Bronshtein et al. (1960) reported "adaptation" of the sucking diminution response to sound after 10 trials and Bridger (1961) reported "habituation" of the startle response in 15–18 trials, depending on frequency. Eisenberg et al. (1964) found no significant reduction in responsivity to a randomized 20-signal sequence containing four constant signals, but complete cessation of response activity after 20–37 trials with a tonal pattern (Eisenberg et al., 1966). On the other hand, Wertheimer (1961) reported "reliable" eye movements in response to a series of 52 clicks, presented within a 10-min period shortly after birth.

Differences of the order cited tend to be found only when a measure is dependent upon several interacting variables and, allowing for procedural differences, small-scale studies at the Bioacoustic Laboratory (Eisenberg, 1965a) suggest that some of the significant factors reside within the signal battery. The incidence of detectable responses increases systematically with the number of differing stimulus events and ISIs and also with the degree to which these events and intervals are randomized. Accordingly, it would appear that, for studies designed to disclose the functional properties of sounds, the effective number of trials varies inversely with homogeneity.

THE TREATMENT OF BEHAVIORAL OUTPUT

Dealing with the output side of Figure 2 presents three main problems. First, stimulus-bound activity must be differentiated. Second, specific indices of auditory processing, referable to given measures of response activity, must be defined. Third, general descriptors of auditory function, referable to any or all measurement procedures, must be defined.

In the material that follows, discussion centers on how behavioral responses to sound can be differentiated, analyzed, and related to correlative data. Treatment of cardiac and EEG responses is considered in Chapter 5, with reference to specific research.

The Validity of Observational Data

The validity of observational studies essentially depends upon the degree to which assertions about the existence and nature of response events can be confirmed. When the assertions stem from filmed behavioral sequences and no-stimulus "catch trials" are included, their validity can be tested statistically (Bench, Hoffman, and Wilson, 1974). When the assertions stem solely from on-the-spot judgments in situations where observers are biased by their exposure to stimulus events and other factors (Eisenberg, 1965a; Foss, 1961, p. 150; and Moncur, 1968), high correlations among observers testify to the uniformity of the independent assertions, but not necessarily to the validity of the judgments (Bench et al., 1972).

One way to assure validity under the latter conditions is to use only highly trained observers who are thoroughly familiar with the measures employed (Eisenberg, 1965a, pp. 170–171). Another is to introduce the stimulus sequence only after each observer has had sufficient time to evaluate nonstimulus patterns of activity that characterize individual subjects (Eisenberg et al., 1964). A third and most useful way is to require not merely that response be scored on a yes-or-no basis, but that it be scored according to the nature and sequence of the alleged response events.

Specific Measures of Overt Auditory Behavior

In studying overt activity at the Bioacoustic Laboratory, the object has been to relate that activity to the communicative process. Each of the classes of behavior employed defines a system(s)-specific output that reflects a differential mode of origin in the nervous system. Each applies equally to nonauditory and auditory behavior. Each is scored with reference to clearly defined dimensions of activity.

Response behavior is viewed solely as a "display" (Busnel, 1963; Hinde, 1970; Sebeok, 1968; and Worden and Galambos, 1972) from which information referable to underlying mechanisms can be extracted. Therefore, the indices, which vary in detail according to whether the detector is a human observer or a motion picture camera, relate to system(s)-specific behavior of three kinds. Motor reactions are of interest because vocal utterance in infancy, like speech later in life, can be considered a subset within this category. Visual reactions are of interest because sight and hearing are interrelated distance senses and also because auditory processing abilities are thought to bear upon the acquisition of reading skills (Kavanagh and Mattingly, 1972; Klasen, 1972; Levin and Williams, 1970; and McNeil and Keislar, 1963). State-dependent reactions are of particular interest because they reflect RAS mechanisms and, thereby, bear upon the ontogeny of listening behavior.

Motor Reactions Motor reactions have been employed extensively in observational studies of infant auditory behavior (Downs and Sterritt, 1964; Eisenberg, Coursin, and Rupp, 1966; Eisenberg et al., 1964; Steinschneider, Lipton, and Richmond, 1966; Stubbs, 1934; and Suzuki, Kamijo, and Kiuchi, 1964), probably because they are more amenable to definitive analysis than other classes of behavior. Treatment is based almost uniformly upon the use of an intensity continuum along which response strength can be graded. Dimensions of this scale are dictated by the capacities of the infant; its lower limits may be defined, as a matter of preference, in terms of "no detectable motor response" or the "smallest detectable motor response:" its upper limits must be defined by the maximum motor response that can be elicited, that is, movements of startle- or Moro-like intensity (Berg, 1973). The size of component increments is dictated by the method of observation, and there is no doubt that the use of film techniques (Bench, Hoffman, and Wilson, 1974) permits refinements unthinkable under conditions of direct observation: detail of the continuum can be defined precisely on the basis of limb displacements and so on. Experience at the Bioacoustic Laboratory strongly suggests that on-the-spot observers cannot be expected to discriminate more than six points on a motor scale with reasonable assurance. Moreover, when motor activity constitutes only one of several response classes to be observed, even this degree of refinement may be excessive: a continuum containing only half as many points tends to gain in validity what it lacks in detail. The scale found most generally useful for study purposes is a four-point continuum: (1) a single segment activity; (2) bisegmental movements;

(3) mild whole body movements of the quasi-Moro type; and (4) reflexes that approximate startle or Moro intensity.

Eye Movements   Eye movements differ from larger body movements in that there is no way to grade response strength: it is as impossible to define the dimensions of an eye blink scale, for instance, as it is to assess the intensity of a blink relative to pupillary dilation or some other form of visual response. For this reason, visual reactions frequently are analyzed according to whether they serve to expand or limit the visual field. Unfortunately, except under special conditions that lend themselves poorly or not at all to naturalistic studies in auditory behavior, it is usually difficult and sometimes impossible to specify response mode in terms of discrete activities. When diverse aspects of visual behavior were evaluated at the Bioacoustic Laboratory, correlation scores for examiner judgments on two or more subclasses of activity seldom were found to be above 0.50. This is hardly surprising since eye movements are, of their nature, fleeting in time and difficult to specify. For purposes of "on-the-spot" judgments, then, an investigator can choose between setting up a generic index relative to eye movements or selecting a specific reflex for observation. Over the years, we have found the eyeblink to be the only aspect of visual behavior that yields adequately to independent treatment. This cochleopalpebral reflex, or CPR, is both ubiquitous and quite resistant to extinction, so it proves a useful index, especially over prolonged study periods (Eisenberg, Coursin, and Rupp, 1966).

State-Dependent Reflexes   State-dependent reflexes logically must be treated according to the direction of change from a prestimulus level of activation: those serving to increase that level usually are termed arousal responses; those serving to decrease it most commonly are considered orienting responses (OR). At the Bioacoustic Laboratory and elsewhere (Stechler, Bradford, and Levy, 1966), reflexes of the OR type have been termed "orienting quiet" (OQ) during early infancy, in order to distinguish them from the more mature directional responses of later life. They are defined solely on the basis of signal-induced behavioral changes involving either a significant decrease in activation or the complete cessation of ongoing activity.

The behaviors associated with state-dependent responses, though complex, tend to be prolonged and, hence, readily detectable (Maltzman and Raskin, 1965; and Wolff, 1966). Arousal responses are characterized by functionally "negative" reactions (Peiper, 1963) such as increased body movement, blinking, pupillary contraction, and closing of the eyes or mouth. From a functional standpoint, these kinds of increased activity serve to decrease the potency of external input signals. OQ responses, on the other hand, are manifest in "positive" reactions, such as decreased body movement, cessation of sucking, pupillary dilatation, widening of the eyes, opening of the mouth, and so on. Functionally speaking, these kinds of stimulus-seeking behaviors serve to increase the potency of external inputs.

General Measures of Auditory Behavior

For purposes of auditory study, general measures can be defined as nonspecific descriptors that are equally applicable to any measurement technique. Such descriptors have to do with the potency of signals, the profiles of evoked activity with which they are associated, and the temporal dimensions of response activity. Given such descriptors in addition to indices pertaining specifically to the techniques employed, it becomes possible not only to consider relations among measures, but also to compare the effects of specific inputs as a function of age or other variables of interest.

Potency The potency, or response-eliciting properties of signals, can be quantified very simply by determining the incidence of response in a study population. In Bioacoustic Laboratory practice, we obtain what are called *response ratios* (Eisenberg, 1965*a*; Eisenberg et al., 1964; and Eisenberg, Coursin, and Rupp, 1966) for individual stimulus conditions. That is to say, for each measurement procedure, we divide the number of response events scored by the total number of signals presented in order to come up with a percentage value. Depending upon how finely one cares to treat the response data, this value can be very helpful both for research planning and for clinical purposes. It can provide information on the probability of response to a given signal under varying conditions of arousal. It can indicate the relative effectiveness of different signals under like conditions of arousal, and the relative efficiency of different measurement techniques under like conditions of study. When the number of presentations is varied in a systematic way, it can afford an index of optimal battery dimensions for a given stimulus condition.

Modes of Response In measuring the distribution of stimulus-bound activity among defined categories, one is concerned solely with response events and, in this case, the measure obtained is termed a *response pattern* (Eisenberg, 1965*a*; Eisenberg et al., 1964; and Eisenberg, Coursin, and Rupp, 1966). The method here is equally simple: for each measurement procedure, the number of responses scored for each category is divided by the total number of responses detected. The derived percentage values are useful from a research standpoint because they provide information on the relative frequency with which specific signals are associated with defined effector systems (Field et al., 1967) or wave forms (Eisenberg, 1974 and 1975*b*; Eisenberg, Marmarou, and Giovachino, 1973, 1974*a*, and 1974*b*). Such data ultimately may serve a clinical purpose in that characteristic profiles for given signals provide a standard for evaluating aberrant response activity.

Time Characteristics of Response   In laboratory investigations, quantitative measures of latency and response time are obtainable by suitable treatment of filmed behavioral data and/or by statistical treatment of cardiac and EEG wave forms. On-the-spot observations of overt activity present obvious problems, however, and they are problems we have been forced to address at the Bioacoustic Laboratory because our controlled studies almost invariably are preceded by pilot work on the nursery floor.

The most useful method we have found for evaluating the time characteristics of response on at least a relative basis is to extrapolate indirect measures from the pattern of response events. This can be done because experienced observers, whether they are dealing with individuals or with populations, tend to establish internal criteria about timing (Eisenberg, 1965a). They learn to recognize that some particular range of intervals between stimulus presentation and response onset is characteristic of a given subject or a given population. In the same way, they learn that the amount of response time required for several behaviors seen in sequence is greater than that required when sequence cannot be differentiated. Given several highly trained observers and reasonable safeguards, we have found that such indirect measures correlate surprisingly well with filmed data. Latency is considered only when the interval between stimulus presentation and response onset consistently exceeds some unspecified "average" value for the study population. Response time is considered only comparatively, according to the number of behavioral components observed in consecutive order (see Appendix C) (Eisenberg, 1965a; Eisenberg et al., 1964; and Eisenberg, Coursin, and Rupp, 1966). Gross indices such as these, which obviously have limited research application, are worth mentioning simply because they prove useful clinically.

CHAPTER 3
A Frame of Reference For Studies in The Development of Auditory Competence

"How have all those exquisite adaptations of one part of the organization to
another part, and to the conditions of
life, and of one organic being to another,
been perfected?"
  Charles Darwin, *The Origin of Species* (1859)

Thus far, discussion has been limited to evolutionary and physiologic determinants of infant behavior and the methods whereby audition, as one aspect of that behavior, can be examined. This chapter serves to outline specific ideas that can usefully guide research strategy. It places the developing human organism in biologic perspective and, by stating some testable hypotheses about the organization of auditory behavior, provides a framework within which the factual material to be considered subsequently can be evaluated.

Basic to these hypotheses is a notion that nature is orderly and its various aspects subject to rules. Given this working assumption, it follows that the behavior of infants, however unorganized it may appear at first glance, must reflect self-regulatory mechanisms in the nervous system and similarly follow rules. The theoretical task, then, is to establish these rules a priori by attempting a synthesis of current biologic information.

40   Determinants of Communicative Behavior

ONTOGENETIC DETERMINANTS AND MECHANISMS OF DEVELOPMENTAL CHANGE

For purposes of discussion, it is useful to resort once again to the "black box" approach employed in Chapter 2. One thus can schematize the various kinds of ontogenetic determinants and consider how, and through what sorts of mechanisms, they might operate.

In Figure 3, which can refer to any organism and any form of stimulus-bound behavior, these factors are grouped, perhaps somewhat unconventionally, according to their pre- or postnatal times of operation. The historic vs. developmental dichotomy is helpful because it places the determinants of newborn behavior on a past to future time scale and leads one to think in comparative terms.

In considering these factors, there is no need to dwell on evolutionary theory or other accepted concepts. It can be assumed that all differential patterns of newborn behavior are correlates of neuronal events that, in some environment peculiar to a species, have evolved phylogenetically and proved their adaptive value (Barnett, 1971; Bass, 1959; Campbell, 1966; Cohen, 1968; Evans and Bastian, 1969; Mayr, 1965; and Washburn, 1963). Likewise, it can be assumed that species-specific patterns of adaptive behavior reflect the biologic structure and organization of mature organisms in a society (DeVore, 1965; Fox, 1966; Hinde, 1970 and 1972; Richter, 1966; Schiller, 1964; Simpson, 1966; Tax, 1964; and Teilhard de Chardin, 1965). Implicit in this last assumption is the idea that develop-

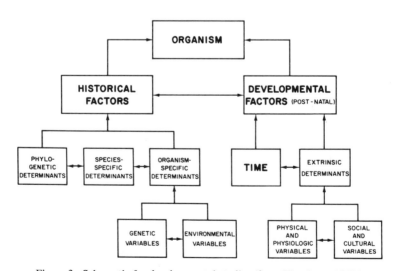

Figure 3. Schematic for developmental studies (from Eisenberg, 1970b).

mental functions must follow patterns directed toward adaptation in that society. The first proposition, therefore, is that the developmental time table for any given function will be a historically determined "best fit" between a given species and a given external milieu.

To account for species-specific patterns of developmental change, two general kinds of mechanisms are postulated: (1) discrete units, or structurally differentiated organs, receptors, and effectors; and (2) feedback systems, or functionally differentiated neural nets.[1]

One can conceive of such mechanisms as unequally susceptible to alteration by environmental forces. Discrete units attaining greater or lesser degrees of significance during development may be seen as relatively unmodifiable. Thus, biochemical or structural change, like functional use or disuse, results merely in some form of "amplification" or "attenuation;" that is, the units may become hypertrophied, or they may become vestigeal or atrophied. Feedback systems, on the other hand, are relatively plastic (Buckley, 1968; Jacobson, 1969; Leibovic, 1969; and Powers, 1973) and subject to subtle forms of qualitiative and quantitative control (Crain, Bornstein, and Raine, 1974; Douglas, 1973; Pfeiffer and Smythies, 1962; and Wiener and Schadé, 1965). Systems that cease to be adaptive during growth can be inhibited or otherwise rendered inoperative, except perhaps under pathologic conditions, by biochemical change at any or all levels of the network. Alternatively, they can be shunted as initial functional purposes become obsolete. Systems that favor viability in a given milieu can be augmented by changes in both channel capacity and efficiency. New channels can be created either by elaboration of new mechanisms adapted to new requirements or by linkage of preexisting mechanisms to newly operative units and/or networks (Crain and Peterson, 1975). Operational improvements can be brought about by facilitative change at cellular and transmission levels or by alterations in the pattern of excitatory and inhibitory influences.

Since we know from embryology that programming for development begins at oogenesis (Carmichael, 1960; Holliday and Pugh, 1975; Munn, 1965; and Peiper, 1963), mechanisms for ontogenetic change presumably are operative during gestation. Under normal conditions, however, the intrauterine environment is relatively undemanding while the extrauterine one requires continuing adaptation at all biologic levels (Eichorn, 1970; and Lorenz, 1965). The second proposition, then, is that most changes occurring during gestation are geared to long-term, species-specific require-

---

[1] The term, neural nets, as used in this volume, serves only to describe some sort of lateral association between functionally related systems. It does not refer to specific synaptic mechanisms, nor does it imply an adherence to formal network theory.

ments (Schiller, 1964). Following this line of reasoning, one can say: (1) that functional similarities among species (Dallos, 1972; Fay, 1974; Finck and Sofouglu, 1966; Hinde, 1970; Krushinskii, 1962; Marler and Hamilton, 1966; Prestrude, 1970; Sebeok, 1965 and 1968; and Schrier, Harlow, and Stollnitz, 1965) reflect common adaptive mechanisms; and (2) that the stage of development at which such mechanisms emerge reflects the relative position of a species on the phylogenetic continuum (Dethier and Stellar, 1961; Gottlieb and Klopfer, 1962; Stein, Rosen, and Butters, 1974; Warren, 1965; and Webster, 1966). By the same token, significant differences among species reflect stabilized mutational changes of proved adaptive value (Marler, 1967; and Marler and Tamura, 1964), while individual differences within a species reflect interactions of genetic and environmental variables (Capranica, Frishkopf, and Nevo, 1973; Singh, 1968; and Thorpe, 1968).

Given these assumptions, individual developmental patterns are contingent upon all of the determinants in Figure 3. The status of discrete units and feedback systems during newborn life reflects both the history of an organism and the history of his species. Consequently, the age at which such units and systems become operational postnatally, like the efficiency with which given mechanisms operate during growth, depends upon pre-uterine and intrauterine factors that condition (1) the physiologic integrity of the organism, (2) the degree of maturity in given units, and (3) the degree to which related systems are organized for effective interaction. In the intact organism, the extent to which individual circumstances can alter a predetermined course depends upon how much and how long these circumstances differ from some biologically expected norm. In the damaged organism, it depends additionally upon interactions within and among organism, environment, and caretakers (Korner, 1973; and Sameroff, 1974).

ADAPTIVE PROCESSES AND
THE ORGANIZATION OF PERCEPTUAL MECHANISMS

Since developmental studies essentially are concerned with adaptation over time, one obviously must consider the organization of newborn behavior according to whether the mechanisms postulated serve immediate or potential demands for survival.

It can be reasonably assumed that the stage of development present at birth, or the maturational status of adaptive mechanisms, depends primarily upon immediate requirements for survival in the external world. On this basis, the degree of maturity in discrete units and feedback systems, like the number of effectively organized networks, would vary according to (1) the kind and amount of caretaking available during early life, and (2) the kind and amount of independent activity required (Hulse, 1963; and Mason, 1968). This implies that species of infants denied protection will retain neonatal reflex patterns only for short periods of time and that they will have certain relatively mature receptor and feedback systems as well as a historically determined repertoire of stimulus-bound motor skills.

The degree of complexity in the CNS, on the other hand, is seen to depend largely upon potential requirements for adaptation in a species-specific environment and society. On this basis, the number of intrinsic networks associated with a given perceptual channel, and the maturational status of its receptors, would vary according to the biologic significance of the channel for the species. The number of plastic networks associated with the channel and the degree to which these might be elaborated during growth would vary, in turn, according to the complexity of the species and the society (Hulse, 1963). This implies that, for any given organism and any given point on the developmental continuum, the organization of perceptual-motor skills normally will reflect both species-specific and society-specific attributes. The final proposition, then, is that perceptual channels are organized in a functional hierarchy such that the degree of built in indeterminancy increases directly with the order of phyletic and neuronal development.

In applying these general constructs specifically to hearing, it is pointless to speculate about the form or function of mechanisms that can be manipulated experimentally. There are adequate comparative data to show that: (1) the auditory system has evolved mainly by addition rather than substitution (Davis, 1961; and Sedlacek, 1971); and (2) phyletic change is accompanied principally by alteration of peripheral structures (Katsuki, 1965; Peterson, Pate, and Wruble, 1966; and Schwartzkopf, 1967). For instance, loss of the pinna, or external ear, has no appreciable effects in man (Flanagan, 1965; and Webster, 1966) while the pinnaless cat sustains a significant loss of acuity, particularly in the high frequency range (Flynn and Elliott, 1965). The cochlea, which in man shows frequency-dependent response modes (Teas, 1966) that possibly serve to improve low frequency resolution (Davis, 1961), is absent in primitive forms of life and fully developed only in mammals.

One is forced to conjecture about neuronal relays associated with the eighth nerve system because feedback mechanisms remain difficult to isolate for investigation (Szentágothai and Arbib, 1974). However, Desmedt's work (1965), showing electrical signs of activity in the efferent auditory pathways of congenitally deaf cats, supports the existence of such mechanisms, while his comparative findings suggest that inhibitory controls may increase in potency with phyletic order. In any case, the notion that feedback mechanisms operate has led to a great many experiments with animals and a few suggestive studies with humans. Since the findings bear directly upon current thinking about the organization of human hearing mechanisms, it may be useful to note briefly two general kinds of data that are available.

First, a host of studies in ethology and related sciences (Busnel, 1963; Hewes, 1973; Hinde, 1970; Lanyon and Tavolga, 1960; and Sebeok, 1968) suggest that certain organizational principles are common to many species. Decoding and encoding mechanisms for sound appear to be matched in species-specific ways (Beer, 1969; Capranica, 1966; Ewing, 1969; Lieberman, in press; Marler, 1969; Nottebohm, 1970; Schusterman, Balliet, and St. John, 1970; and Thorpe and North, 1965). Such mechanisms are related systematically in a manner that assures species survival (Busnel, 1963; Dittus and Lemon, 1969; and Konishi, 1969), and *relevant* sensory stimulation plays an important role in regulating the development of adaptive behavior (Fischer, 1966; Gottlieb, 1965, 1966, and 1968; Snapp, 1969; and Thorpe, 1968). In species of fish (van Bergeijk, 1964), mice (Berlin, Majeau, and Steiner, 1969), and turkeys (Maiorana and Schleidt, 1972), the auditory apparatus is exceptionally well matched to the characteristics of the species calls. Naive chicks and ducklings, shortly after hatching, can discriminate the maternal call of their own species in simultaneous discrimination tests involving the maternal call of other species (Gottlieb, 1968). Rats (Hamm, 1971), chicks (Tolman, 1967), and other species seem to have a natural preference for intermittent sounds. Sparrows, exposed to recorded songs of their own and other species, selectively learn their species-specific vocal patterns, even when raised in isolation (Sebeok, 1968). The bull frog has been shown to have a sensitive auditory system that is specifically adapted for response to the mating call (Frishkopf and Goldstein, 1963). The frequency sensitivity of the auditory system in amphibians (Blair, 1958), cicadas (Simmons, Wever, and Pylka, 1971), and cricket frogs (Capranica, Frishkopf, and Nevo, 1973) is so closely matched to the spectral energy in mating calls that species in different geographic areas respond preferentially to calls in their local dialect. Monkeys, reared in isolation during the first 6 months of life and later exposed to a normal social environment, develop grossly aberrant vocal patterns, characterized by unusual temporal organization and abrupt fluctuations in intensity (Newman and Symmes, 1974a).

Second, not only do a wide variety of acoustic cues serve similar purposes in man and lower animals, but also a number of acoustic parameters have been shown to be processed similarly in man and lower animals (Dewson and Burlingame, 1975). Humans, like other vertebrates, rely on intensity cues for orientation in space. Nonhuman primates process SPL in much the same way as humans (Gates, Romba, and Martin, 1963; Stebbins, 1966 and 1973; and Stebbins, Green, and Miller, 1966), although they seem less sensitive than man in detecting frequency differences and rates of frequency change over time (Sinnott, 1974). Data on time-intensity trading relations in the bottlenosed porpoise show that this species, which integrates acoustic energy similarly to man (Johnson, 1968), may be far more efficient than man in detecting small temporal increments (Thompson and Herman, 1975; and Yunker and Herman, 1974), although evidence on chimpanzees suggests that primates and humans may have more or less equivalent capacities for discriminating among intermittent signals (Prestrude, 1970). Monkeys make use of formant information in communicating with each other (Rowell, 1962) and they can be taught to discriminate among spoken vowels (Dewson, Pribram, and Lynch, 1969). Cats can be conditioned to discriminate among word pairs (Warfield, Ruben, and Glackin, 1966). Chinchillas recently have been shown to distinguish between pairs of phone classes (Burdick and Miller, 1974; and Kuhl and Miller, 1974). Sinnott (1974), in a fascinating comparative study involving humans and old world monkeys, has just shown that the ability to discriminate phonemic contrasts is not exclusively human. Morse and Snowden (1975), in a less definitive study with rhesus monkeys, have obtained suggestive supporting data.

Information on humans, although sparse and perhaps subject to varying interpretations, supports the notion that mechanisms analagous to those disclosed for lower animals may be present in early life. Certainly, data on the precocious development of auditory mechanisms (cited in Chapter 2) suggest that preadapted auditory functions of some kinds may be present in newborn life. A close correspondence between articulatory patterns and the acoustic patterns they generate is well recognized (Lane, 1965; Lane and Tranel, 1971; Lane, Tranel, and Sisson, 1970; Mattingly et al., 1971; and Menyuk, 1971). There are limited data to suggest the existence of intrinsic audiovocal relays (Allen, 1971; Cairns and Karchmer, 1975; Chase et al., 1961; Cullen et al., 1968; Elliott and Niemoller, 1971; Fargo et al., 1973; Irwin and Mills, 1965; Karlovich and Luterman, 1970; Mavilya, 1969; and Naeser, 1970), innate acoustic preferences (Eisenberg, 1965a, 1970a, and 1970b; and Friedlander, 1968 and 1970), and perhaps race-specific differences in speech and hearing mechanisms (Dickson, 1968; Jarvis and Heerden, 1967; Laughlin, 1963; Petrakis, Molohon, and Tepper, 1967; Post, 1964; Shepherd, Goldstein, and Rosenblüt, 1964; Spielman, Migliazza, and Neel, 1974; and Yeni-Komshian, Preston, and Benson, 1968).

A BASIS FOR PREDICTING
DIFFERENTIAL PATTERNS OF INFANT HEARING

It is reasonable, then, to postulate the existence of auditory feedback channels and to consider how hearing organisms might become organized during the course of development. One way to approach this question is to contrast auditory behavior in lower animals and man.

In the animal kingdom, a limited number of highly specified acoustic signals have obvious biologic value (Busnel, 1963; Hinde, 1970; Mattingly, in press; and Sebeok, 1968) and, in most species, deafness in early life precludes survival (Marler and Mundinger, 1971; Nottebohm, 1972; and Nottebohm and Nottebohm, 1971). Signals from the environment or from other group members lead either to motor activity or to motor inhibition, evoking highly specified behavioral patterns that have to do with flight, feeding, reproduction, and the like. Since the behavioral patterns and the functions to which they relate remain relatively constant over the life span, the biologic significance of sounds (Worden and Galambos, 1972) can be considered more or less invariant. One must suppose, therefore, that intrinsic networks associated with the eighth nerve are elaborated only to a minor degree during development.

By the same token, one must suppose that such networks become greatly elaborated in man. Adaptation in most human societies, and economic survival in acquisitive societies, depends more upon effective processing of the communicative code than upon strength or rapid motor reflexes. A vast number of environmental and social sounds attain differing degrees of significance during growth, and deafness becomes maladaptive when it precludes verbal communication (Fry, 1973). In most western cultures, for instance, children with defective hearing remain in what are essentially caretaker situations for long periods of time. Those who fail to acquire the requisite coding skills (in some cases, despite considerable residual hearing) never really become integrated into the body of society, but splinter off into so-called deaf-mute groups. For man, then, the biologic significance of sound can be defined with reference to the physical properties of spoken language, and one can posit a hierarchy of auditory feedback circuits having degrees of relevance to verbal communication.

If the general constructs deriving from Figure 3 are valid, this hierarchy should be operant at birth. Preadapted mechanisms referable to phylogenetic history should be demonstrable as stimulus-bound behavior having correlates in infrahuman performance. Preadapted mechanisms referable to species history should be demonstrable as stimulus-bound behavior having exact correlates in adult life. Plastic mechanisms, referable to future communicative functions, and existing as a potential in the form of morphologic and physiologic specializations, should be demonstrable in discriminative responses to speechlike signals and in "precursor" vocal activities.

In considering material which follows in the next section then, the question at issue is whether the rules governing auditory behavior in early life can be shown to vary according to a stimulus hierarchy. The emphasis is on "pragmatics," in the linguistic sense of trying to understand the significance of signals to communicants (Cherry, 1961; Marler, 1961 and 1967; and Sebeok, 1965). The fact that the communicants considered in this volume mainly are prelinguistic is irrelevant as long as the procedures used and the definition of significance bear upon communicative processes.

Part II FUNCTIONAL PROPERTIES OF SOUNDS AND THEIR ONTOGENETIC IMPLICATIONS

CHAPTER 4
Overt Responses to Sound in Newborn Infants

"The neonate is not deaf, but there is
little evidence that it makes pitch discriminations or differential responses
correlated with the complexity characteristic of auditory stimuli."
   Karl C. Pratt, The Neonate (1960)
   (in Carmichael's *Manual of Child Psychology*)

As noted in Chapter 1, questions about the nature of auditory competence
can be posed either with reference to the auditory system or with reference to central mechanisms. This chapter, which considers two pilot
studies undertaken at the Bioacoustic Laboratory, illustrates these complementary approaches. The first of these "fishing expeditions" defines
certain relations between physical and functional properties of sound and
shows how the measures of auditory behavior discussed in Chapter 2 can
serve in disclosing the differential effects of acoustic parameters. The
second inquiry, which bears upon relations between the auditory system
and the RAS, shows how these same measures can apply to the disclosure
of individual and group differences.

   The two investigations differed markedly from each other in several
important respects. In the first case, the stimulus battery consisted of four
different constant signals presented in randomized order at variable intervals; in the second case, a given patterned signal, presented at fixed
intervals, was used. Taken together, then, these exploratory studies serve
to contrast the functional properties of constant and patterned signals and
the differential effects of varied and monotonous stimulation.

THE EFFECTS OF CALIBRATED NOISEMAKERS

The first study to be considered (Eisenberg et al., 1964) constituted a follow-up of observational work discussed in the Introduction to this volume. A prime aim was to show that methods worked out earlier were applicable to a large population and, since little then was known of newborn hearing abilities, the inquiry was designed to yield maximum information in minimum time. Specific questions had to do with the effects of selected parameter variables upon an unselected population of infants and the effects of procedural and subject variables upon selected measures.

The subjects were 170 clinically normal babies who happened to be available in the newborn and premature nurseries at St. Joseph Hospital during study days. A vast majority of these infants had 1-min Apgar ratings in the 8–10 range, and all but 17 of them were full-term babies.

Four spectrally complex noisemaker stimuli, chosen for their amenability to controlled use as well as for their frequency and time characteristics, were provided by: (1) a drum beat, 300 msec in duration, with a narrow band, low frequency range (approximately 500–900 Hz); (2) the crumpling of a fresh sheet of onionskin paper (put through an autoclave prior to each study period to assure uniform characteristics under varying atmospheric conditions), 1.3 sec in duration, with a broad band, essentially white noise spectrum; (3) the striking together of a pair of pierced wooden sticks, 200 msec in duration, with a spectrum closely approximating that for white noise; and (4) the toot of a small plastic whistle, 250 msec in duration, with a narrow band, high frequency range (4,000–4,500 Hz).

Sequential recordings with a sound level meter, octave band analyzer, and sound spectrograph showed the physical properties of all four signals to remain relatively constant over a series of manual presentations. A uniform signal intensity of 65 dB (re 0.0002 μbar) was assured by sound level meter calibrations that defined precise presentation distances from the midline of a subject's head for each noisemaker.

Except in the case of eight premature infants who could not be removed from incubators, all subjects were studied in an acoustically quiet room (SPL < 35 dB) near the newborn nursery. With all clothing except diapers and hospital shirt removed, the babies were placed supine in a standard hospital bassinet, and the shirt was raised so that respiratory movements could be seen easily.

Observations were made by three highly trained investigators who were variously positioned with respect to the infant's head. Individual study sessions uniformly were preceded by an observation period of 1–5 min that permitted evaluation of nonstimulus activity patterns. During this time, each investigator independently recorded on a standardized score sheet information on his observation site, the infant's basal arousal level, and other factors. Basal state ratings, like activity state measures obtained during the subsequent stimulus period, were defined on a four-point continuum (Rosenblith, 1961; and Wagner, 1937), ranging from (I) deep sleep, through (II) doze or light sleep, and (III) less than full wakefulness, to (IV) full wakefulness.

Stimuli were presented only by the investigator, positioned, at the precalibrated distances, behind the infant's head. Each of the noisemakers was introduced five times, in randomized (latin square) order, and at random intervals in excess of 10 sec. Immediately preceding each signal presentation, observers were advised by a hand signal to note their activity state ratings.

Immediately following any presentation, each of the independent observers coded stimulus-associated behavior according to whether a response event was judged with assurance to have occurred (+), judged doubtfully to have occurred (?), or judged with assurance not to have occurred (−). Whether a response judgment was scored as assured or doubtful, however, an observer was required to note the sequence of reactions upon which that judgment was based.

Number codes (see Appendix C, section I) were used to designate the four behavioral indices discussed in Chapter 2, that is, motor reactions, visual reflexes, arousal, and OQ. These, in conjunction with specified modifiers, provided a basis for obtaining both quantitative and qualitative information on stimulus-bound behavior. For analytic purposes, the only response events considered valid were those scored in like fashion by at least two observers.

Relations between signal variables and auditory behavior were considered quantitatively, in terms of the number of responses meeting these criteria and qualitatively, in terms of the kinds of stimulus-bound activities observed. Response ratios were used to describe the incidence of response to each of the signals. Response patterns were analyzed with reference to the single behavioral class best describing a given response, or its "major component," and the number of components appearing in that response, which provided some index of its complexity. Data on latency and response time were extrapolated by scoring as latent only those responses so noted by all three observers and scoring as sequential those responses characterized by the appearance of several components in consecutive order. In the latter case, it was presumed that response time was prolonged to the extent that different behaviors could be distinguished in like sequence by two or more observers.

The Effects of Signal Variables

As descriptions of the noisemakers suggest, this inquiry was designed to yield preliminary information on the differential effects exerted by frequency, duration, and complexity (defined in terms of band width). Table 1 shows response ratios and modes of response to the individual signals under unspecified state conditions.

Response Ratios   From the response ratios, it was clear that the signals differed in potency. The poor response-eliciting properties of the whistle could be related only to its frequency characteristics. Maximum effectiveness of the onionskin, on the other hand, might have resulted from interaction between band width and duration. However, given the sizable difference in response ratio between this signal and its spectrally matched counterpart (the sticks) as well as the higher ranking of the narrow band low frequency signal (the drum) in the response ratio array, it seemed likely that duration was the critical determinant.

Response Patterns   As the behavioral repertoires associated with each of the four signals were considered, a systematic relation between response ratio and response pattern became evident. The proportion of major component motor responses, like the proportion of sequential responses, varied directly with response ratio. The proportion of major component responses dependent upon activity level, the proportion of latent responses, and the total proportion of eye reflexes all varied inversely with it. Response pattern data, then, yielded much the same trends disclosed by the response ratios. The ineffective high frequency signal was uniquely associated with a preponderance of activation-dependent responses. Band width per se seemed to exert no overriding effects in that the two white nose signals were associated with substantially different response repertoires. Duration again emerged as a critical factor in that response patterns for the two shortest signals were similar in almost all respects and clearly different from those calculated for the two longer signals.

Study of the response ratio and response pattern data, accordingly, suggested that the duration and frequency characteristics of signals were critical determinants of auditory behavior during newborn life. On the other hand, a presumed measure of stimulus complexity exerted no marked effects. This last finding was important since it led to a conclusion that band width was an unsatisfactory index of acoustic complexity. Thus, very early in program development, the question of what constitutes a complex auditory signal assumed significance.

The Effects of Sequence

In examining auditory behavior as a function of sequence, the aims were twofold. From a practical standpoint, information on interactions between

Table 1. Response Ratios and Response Patterns as a Function of Stimulus Variables

Spectrum Duration	Noisemaker Stimuli			
	Onionskin (White Noise) (1.3 Sec)	Drum (5,000–900 Hz) (300 Msec)	Sticks (White Noise) (200 Msec)	Whistle (4,000–4,500 Hz) (250 Msec)
Response Ratios				
No. of presentations	850	850	850	850
No. of responses	602	561	511	399
NR/NP = R-R (%)	70.8	66.0	60.1	36.7
Distribution of Responses by Major Component (%)				
Motor reflexes	58.0	41.9	27.2	12.2
Eye reflexes	11.8	24.1	36.2	26.6
*	(42.9)	(57.4)	(63.2)	(71.3)
Arousal	14.4	21.9	19.4	32.4
Orienting-quiet (OQ)	15.8	12.1	17.2	28.8
**	(30.2)	(34.0)	(36.6)	(61.2)
Distribution of Responses by Number of Behavioral Components (%)				
One component	64.5	64.3	71.3	68.3
More than one component	35.5	35.7	28.7	31.7
(Two)	(32.1)	(32.8)	(25.0)	(28.2)
(Three)	(3.3)	(2.5)	(3.7)	(3.5)
(Four)	(0.1)	(0.4)	(0.0)	(0.0)
Distribution of Responses by Time-Associated Indices (%)				
Latent	2.7	3.2	4.1	5.4
Sequential	13.0	11.8	10.8	8.0

*Total proportion of eye reflexes, including those subsumed within major component.
**Total proportion of responses dependent upon activity level.

ISI and other stimulus-related variables was required for future experimental planning. At a theoretical level, it was hoped that such information might cast light on the nature of the CNS events underlying infant responses to repeated acoustic stimulation. Stimulus-bound behavior was accordingly studied with reference to the distribution of signals over all 20 trials in the acoustic battery and also with reference to the distribution of given signals within their particular sequence of 5 trials.

Response Ratios   Analysis of the response ratio data over the 20-signal sequence showed the percentage of responses to be somewhat lower during the final 10 trials than during the initial 10 trials, but the decline in responsivity was statistically insignificant. It was concluded, therefore, that for randomized schedules employing ISIs of 10 or more sec, overt responsivity would be little affected over a series of 20 trials or fewer.

Response Patterns   Data on modes of stimulus-bound behavior as a function of sequence were interesting in several respects.

The most significant finding, confirming the existence of a systematic relation between physical and functional properties of sound, was that given signals elicited relatively specific response profiles regardless of the order in which they were presented.

So far as could be determined, neither the complexity nor the time characteristics of response behavior were affected significantly by sequence and visual reflexes appeared with approximately equal frequency throughout the test battery. However, in agreement with Pratt's early data (1934), the strength of motor responses was found to decrease more or less systematically as the stimulus schedule progressed. This tendency toward decreased response strength over trials also was disclosed when higher intensity responses (motor and arousal reactions) were compared with lower intensity ones (eye and OQ reactions). Under those conditions, responses were divided about equally between the two categories over the first eight presentations, but a majority of the subsequent behaviors (61.4%) fell into the lower intensity group.

Findings on arousal and OQ responses as a function of sequence were provocative in that they were distinctly at odds with popular Soviet concepts of the OR as a response to "novel" stimuli (Cole and Maltzman, 1969; Elkonin, 1957; O'Connor, 1961; and Sokolov, 1963). When relations between these two classes of RAS-dependent behavior were examined, it was found that the proportion of arousal responses tended to decrease, and the proportion of OQ responses tended correspondingly to increase, as the schedule progressed. It seemed possible, then, that the newborn's "what is it?" reflex represented something rather different from the orienting behavior of later life. If this indeed were the case, the OQ term, originally coined on a purely descriptive basis, had potential significance with respect to the organization of underlying mechanisms.

The Effects of Activity State

Activity state, as used in this study, referred to four defined levels of internal arousal that could be differentiated with reasonable certainty on the basis of overt behavior. To examine its effects upon auditory behavior, the data summarized in Table 1 were segregated according to the pre-stimulus activity state ratings scored by at least two of the observers. Table 2, which shows the distribution of subjects and signal presentations under each state condition, indicates that the four noisemakers were represented with approximately equal frequency at each point on the continuum.

Response Ratios Figure 4 shows the effects of activity state upon the newborn's responsivity, and it contains several important indications. First, the relative potency of the four noisemaker signals was unaffected by state variables. Second, activity state exerted systematic efforts on the response-eliciting properties of all noisemakers. Third, the shape of the response ratio functions not only was in accord with data reported for nonauditory neonatal reflexes (Murray and Campbell, 1970; and Parmalee, 1963*a* and 1963*b*), but also closely resembled functions describing relations between state and performance level in adult subjects (Freeman, 1940; and Stennett, 1957). Fourth, the high frequency whistle was the only signal associated with peak responsivity during wakefulness.

Given these indications, it could be said with some assurance that: (1) signal variables were critical determinants of responsivity under all condi-

Table 2. Distribution of Study Population by Activity State Ratings Immediately Prior to Stimulation[a]

		Activity State			
Stimulus	Index	Deep Sleep (I)	Doze or Light Sleep (II)	Less than Full Wakefulness (III)	Wide Awake(IV)
Onionskin	I	27	57	97	95
	II	86 (10)	131 (15)	295 (35)	338 (40)
Drum	I	29	62	93	91
	II	82 (10)	136 (16)	296 (35)	336 (39)
Sticks	I	27	53	101	91
	II	83 (10)	131 (15)	314 (37)	322 (38)
Whistle	I	27	56	98	87
	II	89 (11)	131 (15)	303 (36)	327 (38)

[a]The number of subjects per signal is greater than 170 since individual infants were represented at more than one point. The two indices indicate, in order, the number of subjects (I) and the number of signal presentations (II) represented at each point on the state continuum. Bracketed figures for index II show, for each signal, the percentage of total presentations ($N = 850$) represented by each state.

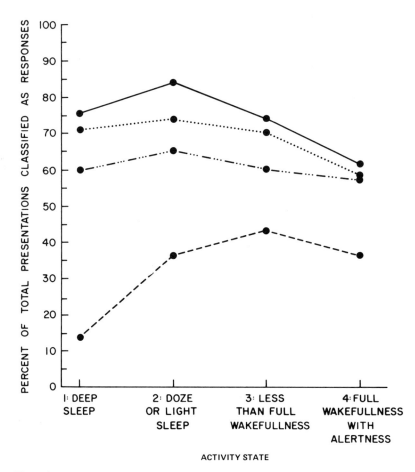

Figure 4. Response ratios as a function of prestimulus activity state. State, graded on a four-point continuum, is shown on the abscissa. The functions graphed refer, in descending order, to the onionskin paper (———), drum (· · · · ·), sticks (—· · ·—), and whistle (- - - - -).

tions of arousal; (2) auditory study procedures could be weighted in favor of response if infants were studied during intermediate states of arousal; (3) relations between activity state and responsivity in newborn life were governed by mechanisms akin to those underlying relations between state and performance in adult life; and (4) the significantly different shape of the response ratio function for the high frequency signal reflected equally significant differences in underlying mechanisms.

Response Patterns   Figure 5, showing the effects of activity state upon response patterns, supported other indications that signal variables were critical determinants of newborn auditory behavior.   As can be seen from

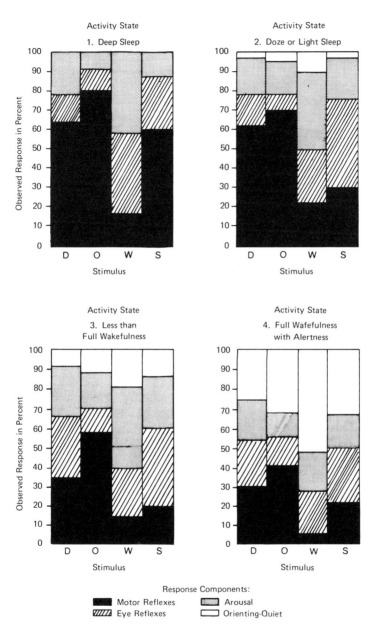

Response Components:
Motor Reflexes   Arousal
Eye Reflexes   Orienting-Quiet

Figure 5. Effects of signal variables upon the distribution of major response components (from Eisenberg et al., 1964). The graphed percentages (based upon the numerical values given in Table 2) indicate, for each of the stimuli presented during a specified activity state, the proportion of major component responses distributed among the four behavioral indices. Signals are indicated on the abscissa as D (drum), O (onionskin), W (whistle), and S (sticks).

the individual histograms, activity state affected all stimuli similarly and given signals elicited differential response patterns at every point on the continuum. The two signals shorter than 300 msec (sticks and whistle) consistently were associated with a higher proportion of visual reflexes than the longer signals. The high frequency whistle consistently elicited the highest proportion of arousal and OQ reactions.

Rank order of the signals for percentage of motor reflexes, which remained constant under all conditions of arousal, followed the same pattern found for response ratios. For all signals, the ratio between higher intensity and lower intensity reactions varied more or less systematically with state. In agreement with other data (Bartoshuk, 1962b; and White, Castle, and Held, 1964), the strength of motor reflexes tended to decrease systematically with arousal much in the manner predicted by the so-called law of initial values, or LIV (Bench, 1970; Lipton, Steinschneider, and Richmond, 1961b; Richmond, Lipton, and Steinschneider, 1962b; and Wolff, 1967). Reactions of Moro-like or startlelike intensity, like tonic neck reflexes (Vassella and Karlsson, 1962), characteristically were observed under conditions of deep sleep, occasionally were observed during doze states, and never were observed under waking conditions.

The relative distribution of arousal and OQ reactions in Figure 5 clearly supported response ratio data suggesting a reciprocal relation between the two reflexes. The changing distribution of OQ responses with increasing arousal was of considerably greater interest, however, in that it could be related directly to an "awake-alert-aware" continuum postulated for the RAS (French, 1960; French, Hernández-Péon, and Livingston, 1955; and Moruzzi and Magoun, 1949). It seemed possible, therefore, that systematic study of relations between state and auditory behavior eventually might apply to the development of diagnostic procedures bearing upon CNS integrity in early life.

Factors Affecting Activity State

It is well recognized that the ability to sustain sleep or arousal, which is dependent upon functional maturation of the RAS and related systems (French, 1960; French, Hernández-Péon, and Livingston, 1955; and Hess, 1957 and 1964), is poorly established before about 8 months of age (Aeserinsky and Kleitman, 1955; Kleitman, 1965; Oswald, 1962; and Parmalee, 1961). It is equally well recognized that the human neonate cannot maintain a constant state over long periods of time (Moore and Ucko, 1957; Parmalee, 1961; and Parmalee, Schultz, and Disbrow, 1961). Thus, in examining activity state as a function of sequence, we mainly sought to determine whether variations in arousal level during the study period were affected in any way by stimulation per se or by other external factors.

Figure 6 shows the distribution of activity state ratings during 19 successive signal presentations as a function of basal state.

The first presentation is omitted since, in this experiment, the activity state associated with the initial stimulus was identical with basal state.

From these distributions, it is evident that states I (deep sleep) and IV (full wakefulness) were associated with a degree of short-term stability that could not be easily altered by repeated auditory stimulation. There was some tendency for sleeping infants to become more wakeful and for aroused infants to become less so as the schedule progressed but, as can be seen, most of the population maintained basal state throughout the stimulus period.

It is not especially surprising that findings for the two intermediate states were less clear-cut, since the points labeled "doze" and "less than

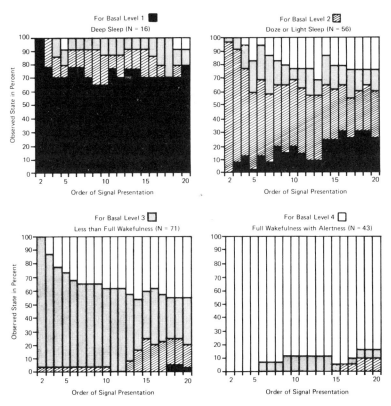

Figure 6. Activity state as a function of sequence and basal state (from Eisenberg et al., 1964). The individual histograms show, for the population at each basal level, the proportional distribution of activity states during each of 19 sequential presentations. The number of subjects at each basal level (*coded block*) is indicated above each graph. The time span covered by these observations ranged from 6–15 min, with a mean of 10 min.

full wakefulness" covered a fairly wide range of arousal levels in this experiment. Moreover, then as now, there were no hard and fast behavioral criteria for judging interim stages between deep sleep and full wakefulness. Respiration pattern is by no means an infallible index of state, and visual behavior sometimes can be flatly misleading: it is not unusual for the neonate to doze with his eyes open or to maintain a variety of wakeful states with his eyes closed. Nonetheless, inasmuch as intermediate states were associated with a relatively low degree of short-term stability and more easily altered by external stimulation, it seemed possible that they differed in fundamental ways from states at the poles of the arousal continuum. It certainly seemed likely, since the direction of state change over time was far from systematic, that factors other than basal level might account for the changes found during intermediate stages of arousal.

The findings might well have been explained by rhythmic variations in state (Dodgson, 1962; Lipsitt, 1963; Moore and Ucko, 1957; and Parmalee et al., 1969). However, given data showing that this cyclic pattern could be modified by external factors (Irwin, 1930; Lipton, Steinschneider, and Richmond, 1960 and 1965b; Marquis, 1931; Parmalee, Brück, and Brück, 1962; and Sherman, Sherman, and Flory, 1936), we chose to examine hunger, which was the only such variable on which adequate information was available. Figure 7 shows the distribution in percent, as a function of time lapse since the last completed feeding, of (I) basal levels and (II) activity states during the study period.

The graphed values in Figure 7 leave little doubt that behavioral arousal was significantly affected by whether infants were hungry or satiated. Over 70% of the babies studied within 1 hr after feeding had basal state ratings of I or II. During the next 1-hr period, the proportion of sleep and doze ratings dropped precipitously to less than 30%. During the third hour (immediately preceding the next scheduled feeding for most of the population), the first-hour distribution of states was almost exactly reversed, with over 70% of the infants scored as wakeful.

Data on babies studied more than 3 hr after feeding suggested that cyclic variations in state might be modifiable only within a limited time period. However, since many of the infants included in the latest postprandial interval were on 4-hr or demand feeding schedules, no conclusions could be drawn. Nor could conclusions be drawn respecting the poor match between data on infants who had never been fed and those who were on regular schedules. The unfed group included only 13 subjects, all of whom were less than 12 hr old, and the differences found could have been related to basic changes attendant merely upon the institution of a feeding schedule or, indeed, to any number of other factors not considered in the experiment. However, a tentative conclusion that repeated auditory stimulation tends to sustain short-term arousal could be drawn from the

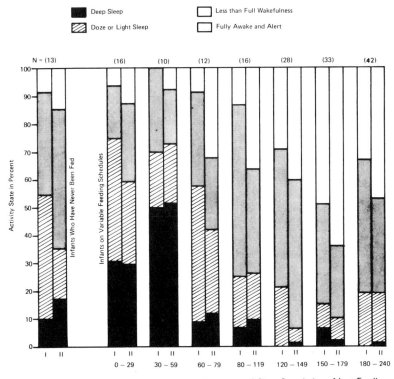

Figure 7. Relations between feeding schedule and activity state (from Eisenberg et al., 1964). The first histogram-set refers to infants who never have been fed. Histogram-sets at half-hour intervals along the time continuum refer to infants who have been fed a variable number of times since birth. (Most of these were on 3-hr feeding schedules.) The number of subjects within each set is indicated by the *figures in parentheses* at the top.

relations between basal and activity state ratings. As can be seen from Figure 7, wide awake states were markedly more prevalent under stimulus conditions than under nonstimulus conditions.

Perhaps the most constructive outcome of this analysis was that it led us to consider whether more selective observations on state as a function of feeding schedule could serve to define specific periods during which most of a newborn population could be found in the intermediate states optimal for auditory study. Such follow-up inquiries, which yielded data slightly different from those shown in Figure 7, suggested that the best time for instituting procedures was between 70 and 90 min postprandially. Whenever possible in recent years, therefore, Bioacoustic Laboratory investigations with infants under 1 month of age have been scheduled on this basis, and the results consistently have been in line with these later data.

Auditory Behavior as a Function of Age

Inasmuch as several investigators had reported the behavior of newborns to vary with age (Bartoshuk, 1962*b*; Engen, Lipsitt, and Kaye, 1963; Fantz, 1963; Foss, 1961, pp. 29–33; Kaye, 1964; Kaye and Lipsitt, 1964; Kessen, Williams, and Williams, 1961; Lipsitt, Engen, and Kaye, 1963; Lipsitt and Levy, 1959; and Sherman, Sherman, and Flory, 1936), data were segregated by 12-hr intervals to determine whether either response ratios or response patterns changed in an orderly way with time elapsed since birth. Analysis of these findings indicated that the only two aspects of auditory behavior to vary systematically were those bearing upon time relations in the CNS.

Latent responses, which were considered valid only when all 3 observers were in agreement and at least 50% of a subject's responses were so scored, were characteristic only of 7 infants, all of whom were under 72 hr of age. Given the strictness of these criteria, it is doubtful whether such responses were artifacts. Given the absence of such responses in 32 additional subjects in the same age range, as well as the lack of any other common denominators among these 7 infants, however, it could not be determined whether the existence of latent responses reflected some sort of underlying dysfunction or transient factors without clinical significance.

Sequential responses were not confined to a particular age range, but their incidence varied systematically with age and with no other factor explored in this investigation. For graphic purposes, therefore, data showing relations between sequential behavior and hours of life were grouped without reference to state or stimulus variables (Figure 8).

The linearly accelerating function in Figure 8 seems to be so clearly a growth curve that even at this writing no alternate explanation presents itself. There is every reason to believe that this evidence for increased behavioral response time over the first 9 days of life is valid, even though the determinants remain speculative.

The composition of sequential responses, unlike the incidence of such responses, showed no systematic relationship with age. In agreement with reports on somewhat older infants (Aeserinsky and Kleitman, 1955), eye reflexes tended to precede other types of behavioral reactions: for all subjects in the study population, they were recorded as initial components over 80% of the time.

Summing up the results of this large-scale exploration, some of the rules governing newborn responses to sound are suggested rather clearly.

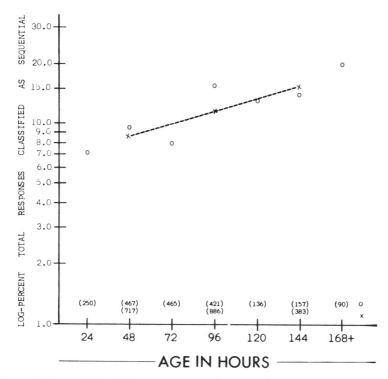

Figure 8. Sequential behavior as a function of age (from Eisenberg et al., 1964). The *circles* indicate, for each 24-hr interval, the percentage of total responses classified as sequential; the *crosses*, connected by the dotted line, indicate the percentage of sequential responses calculated for 48-hr intervals. The total number of responses from which the graphed values derive is shown by the *figures in parentheses* above each interval.

First, parameter variables, such as duration and frequency, exert differential effects upon the incidence of response to auditory stimulation (response ratio), the kinds of behavior elicited during response (response pattern), and the intensity of response.

For constant signals of the kind used in this study, response ratio and response pattern are related systematically. More effective stimuli tend to be associated with a preponderance of higher intensity (motor and arousal) responses and less effective ones with a preponderance of lower intensity (eye and OQ) responses. Regardless of signal potency, however, the proportion of motor reflexes, like the strength of such reflexes, varies directly with response ratio.

Second, differences in infant state exert significant effects upon all aspects of auditory behavior. Response ratio varies systematically with activity state much as performance level varies with it during adult life. Response pattern varies systematically in accordance with an awake-alert-aware continuum that has been posited for the RAS. Response strength varies systematically in accordance with LIV.

Activity state can be modified by hunger and by repeated auditory stimulation. Wakefulness tends to increase systematically with time elapsed since completion of a feeding. Intermittent auditory stimulation tends to sustain short-term arousal, even among infants who have not been placed on a feeding schedule.

Third, sequence effects (that is, those relative to the influence of a given response in a series upon subsequent ones) are reflected primarily in a reduction of response strength over trials and in a reciprocal relation between arousal and OQ reactions. The last finding accords poorly with notions that the OR during infancy represents a response to novel stimuli.

Fourth, a high frequency signal seems to have unique functional properties. Its response-eliciting properties are strikingly limited under all conditions of arousal. It is the only signal to elicit peak responsivity during wakefulness. It is associated with a far higher proportion of RAS-dependent reactions than low frequency noisebands or white noise stimuli.

THE EFFECTS OF MONOTONOUS STIMULATION
WITH AN ACOUSTIC PATTERN

The investigation to be considered now was a landmark of sorts in terms of the direction of further research efforts. It led us, for the first time, to consider whether complexity could be defined with reference to stimulus dimensionality. It provided the first solid indication that predictive auditory test procedures eventually could be devised. It afforded new and valuable insights into central mechanisms underlying the development of listening behavior.

The inquiry grew out of a chance rereading of the classic Sharpless and Jasper paper on "Habituation of the Arousal Reflex" (1956). Noted somewhat casually in this report of an experiment with cats was the provocative, if hitherto overlooked, finding that, given ablation procedures, "Pattern-specific habituation was . . . never observed in animals in which the auditory system had been damaged in any way" (p. 662).

Applying this hint to studies with human infants posed an obvious problem in that eighth nerve integrity hardly could be specified in the absence of direct physiologic measures. This problem was bypassed by adopting the working hypothesis that any form of dysfunction affecting the integrity of relations between auditory channels and other CNS systems, especially those governing activation and attention, would be re-flected in differential rates of habituation and/or in differential modes of stimulus-bound behavior. Then, to test the validity of this notion, the Sharpless and Jasper experiment was replicated with infants drawn from selected risk categories (Eisenberg, Coursin, and Rupp, 1966).

The subjects were 18 newborns,[1] 12 hr to 7 days of age, who became available during a 2-month period set aside for pilot studies. All had passed standard neurologic tests and all but one were full-term babies. Thirteen infants were classed as controls on the basis of Apgar ratings of 9 or 10, completely unremarkable physical histories, and negative familial back-ground (that is, no evidence of genetic or other problems). Three infants with Apgars in the 8–10 range were considered "suspect," two because they were drawn from a biased population (Eisenberg, 1963b; and Eisen-berg et al., 1964) in which nutrition and/or genetic factors conceivably might exert untoward effects, and one because of multiple (though minor) physical anomalies. Two babies were classified as "high risk," in one case because of prematurity and in the other because of a 1-min Apgar rating of 4.

The patterned "habituation" stimulus, repeatable 100 times at 10-sec intervals, was "a modulated tone falling in pitch from 5,000 to 200 cps in a period of four seconds" (Sharpless and Jasper, 1956, p. 662). The "dishabituation" signal, introduced subsequent to habituation, was an exact reversal of this tonal sequence.

Stimuli were generated by an audiooscillator (HP 200 ABR), tape recorded (Ampex SP-300) in the control room of the Bioacoustic Labora-tory, and then dubbed onto a portable tape recorder (Roberts 1600). Speed of modulation was monitored by chronoscope to assure a uniform rate of frequency change over the 4 sec of stimulation; ISIs were timed by stopwatch. SPL varied mostly between 77 and 80 dB re 0.0002 μbar, falling below (68–73 dB) only in the 200- to 400-Hz range, and peaking (83 dB) at 1,000 Hz. Careful calibrations with a Bruel and Kjaer artificial ear revealed no standing waves during the experiment.

All of the infants were subjected to exactly the same procedures under exactly the same conditions. They were brought into the acoustically quiet test room on the nursery floor by our staff nurse about 1 hr after feeding and given whatever time was required for adaptation to their new sur-roundings. As in all Bioacoustic Laboratory experiments, nonstimulus behavior patterns were observed carefully during the adaptation period. Behavioral data were recorded only by the senior investigator, whose

---

[1] This number includes 5 subjects on whom no data were available when prelimi-nary results of this habituation study were reported in the literature (Eisenberg, Coursin, and Rupp, 1966).

detection scores consistently had shown a high correlation with autonomic measures (0.89–0.94) and with other observers (0.92–0.97).

At the end of the adaptation period, and immediately before introducing the taped schedule, two pretest indices were recorded: respiration rate, which was counted by the nurse; and basal state, which was scored by the observer. In contrast to the noisemaker study discussed earlier, the behavioral state scale employed in this inquiry covered a seven-point continuum, as follows: (I) deep sleep; (II) lighter or irregular sleep; (III) doze; (IV) minimal wakefulness; (V) alert inactivity; (VI) active arousal; and (VII) extreme excitation (see Table I.1, Appendix C).

Once a tape was started, the nurse became responsible for controlling it according to a specified protocol; and the observer became responsible for scoring stimulus-bound behavior. Each stimulus presentation was associated with two kinds of coded information: activity state, recorded during the second immediately prior to stimulus-onset and mode of response behavior, which included "no response" and was recorded somewhere between 5 and 8 sec following stimulus onset. Fluctuations within a given state were indicated by directional arrows. Response events detected over the course of the schedule were coded, within newly enlarged behavioral categories, as motor, visual, or vocal. RAS-dependent behavior, although still classified according to the direction and degree of change from prestimulus activity level, included a new *irritation* category as well as the previously used arousal and OQ designations. Time characteristics of response events were extrapolated from the recorded behavioral data in the manner already described for the noisemaker study.

Subjects were considered habituated whenever 10 consecutive misses (no responses) for the descending tonal sequence were followed by a clear-cut hit (response) for the reverse (ascending) pattern. If habituation could not be achieved, stimulation was terminated when all 100 signals were used up or, as sometimes happened before then, when the observer became too tired to record information properly. In any case, both respiration rate and basal states were recorded once more, 5–8 sec after the final descending trial was presented.

Before considering the results of this pilot study, it must be noted that the criteria used for habituation seemed to be entirely adequate. Infants who missed 10 consecutive trials with the descending pattern continued to miss even after the ascending (dishabituation) pattern was interposed. In a few cases, where test signals in addition to the reverse pattern were employed, a sequence of responses to novel stimuli could be obtained without reinstating response to the descending pattern: a 20-dB reduction in SPL values, like reversal of the tonal elements, evoked immediate behavioral arousal; a sharp click of the reverse switch on the tape recorder elicited generalized startle activity.

In planning this study, we were interested both in the nature of the habituation process and in the effects of the patterned stimulus. Thus, in analyzing the data, we were concerned with four things: (1) speed of habituation, or T_{hab}, as defined by the last presentation of the descending pattern to evoke a response; (2) changes in state over time, as a reflection of RAS mechanisms; (3) response ratio, as an index of stimulus potency; and (4) response pattern, as a clue to the functional properties of a hitherto unexplored class of stimuli.

The Habituation Process as an
Index of Individual Differences Among Infants

To consider the habituation process, each subject's prestimulus activity state ratings were plotted over all trials to T_{hab}. These plots, grouped in ascending order according to basal (nonstimulus) state, are shown in Figure 9.

As is clear from Figure 9, speed of habituation, which tended to decrease somewhat with higher basal states, varied systematically with risk category. Control infants, despite wide differences in basal state, ceased to respond to the descending pattern after 20–37 trials, or approximately within 4 min of each other. The two suspects who habituated took almost twice as long as controls to do so; and three infants, including one of the suspects, did not habituate at all. (The second graph is deceptive since, in the case of S5, examiner fatigue forced termination of the schedule after 73 trials.)

Controls, although hardly identical in their reaction to repeated stimulation, showed certain typical patterns of behavior. All gave immediate and clear-cut responses to the first 3 stimuli, and all reached peak arousal within 7 to 8 trials. Responsivity over 5-trial blocks remained at 90–100% through the period of maximal activation, and prestimulus state was regained within 16–20 trials. During declining activation, responsivity tended to vary with individual rates of habituation. When the process was rapid, it decreased almost linearly. When the process was slower, fluctuations in responsivity more or less paralleled changes in activation. In no case was the activity state rating at the final trial higher than basal state. Infants who were wakeful during the nonstimulus period either were sleeping or approaching that state when stimulation was terminated. Infants who had been dozing went to sleep. Infants who initially were sleeping returned to sleep.[2]

---

[2] Hutt, Lenard, and Prechtl (1969), using a somewhat different analysis technique, since have reported very similar results.

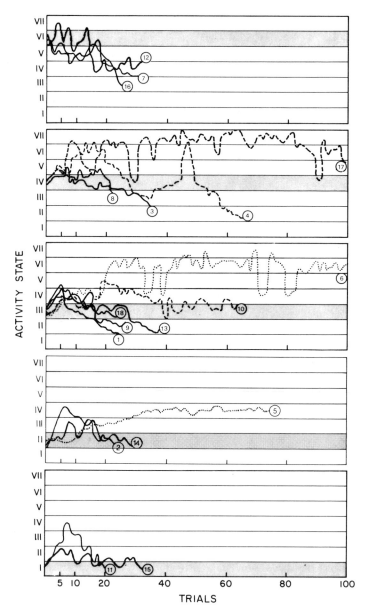

Figure 9. Changes in state as a function of monotonous stimulation with a tonal pattern. Subjects, indicated by number, are plotted as ——— (controls); - - - - - (suspects); •••••• (high risk). *Curves*, based upon sequential prestimulus ratings by a single observer, should be interpreted cautiously: respiration rates, measured immediately prior to introduction of the dishabituation signal, almost uniformly were lower than those noted under basal conditions; and the judgmental values shown here probably are a specious index of depth of sleep. (Infants were exposed to stimulation about 70–90 min following completion of feeding, at which time a majority of subjects were in optimal basal states for study.)

The two groups of risk infants showed category-specific patterns of state change. Suspects tended toward more labile activation patterns than controls and, just as they required double the number of trials for habituation, they took twice as long to attain peak arousal. Responsivity fluctuated between 80 and 100% over the first 45 trials, declining erratically thereafter, and activity state ratings at the final trial were either within or below the basal state range. The three subjects who failed to habituate were slower to arouse than other infants. Once they did arouse, however, they remained in a state of more or less tonic activation. Indeed, they seemed, quite literally, to be stimulus-bound: they responded without a miss to all of the initial 40 trials and, even during later trials, continued to respond at least 95% of the time.

Functional Properties of a Tonal Pattern

The differential activation patterns in Figure 9 had their correlates in differential modes of response behavior that will be considered further when clinical implications of these data are discussed. The question at issue for the moment is whether, for patterned signals of the kind employed in this experiment, relations between state and auditory behavior are governed by the same rules that apply to constant signals such as noisebands.

Relations between State and Auditory Behavior   Since changing levels of activation during the habituation process tend to mask relations between state and overt responsivity that are obvious when a stimulus battery is more variable, data on control subjects first were analyzed without reference to sequence, that is, they were segregated solely on the basis of prestimulus activity state ratings. From the results, it seemed likely that certain relations between state and auditory behavior were unaffected by stimulus variables: the response ratio function for the tonal pattern showed the same inverted U shape found for constant signals (Figure 4); the proportion of major component responses distributed among the four behavioral categories varied systematically in much the manner illustrated by Figure 5. It seemed equally likely, as relations between response ratios and response patterns were examined, that the functional properties of patterned signals differed substantially in several ways from those already disclosed for constant signals.

Modes and Incidence of Responsive Behavior   To consider functional properties of the tonal pattern in experimental context, control subjects were separated into two categories according to whether their basal state ratings fell into the sleeping or the waking range, that is, states I through III as opposed to states IV through VII. Then, for the pooled data within each category: (1) response patterns were calculated, in separate 5-trial blocks, over all responses to T_{hab} , and (2) response ratios were calculated for the 4 initial 5-trial blocks common to all control infants. Values resulting from this analysis are shown in Table 3.

From the response ratios at the bottom of Table 3, it can be seen that the tonal pattern proved far more potent than any of the noisemakers considered earlier. Over the 20 consecutive trials common to all infants, including the 16–20 block during which some subjects were approaching habituation, subjects responded to the signal almost 85% of the time. This contrasts sharply with findings in Table 1, showing that 5 widely separated presentations of the maximally effective onionskin stimulus evoked response only about 71% of the time.

The differential functional properties of the tonal pattern were qualitative as well as quantitative and they are reflected only partially in the behavioral displays listed in Table 3.

Motor Responses   As can be determined from Table 3, the incidence of motor responses, including body stirrings during arousal, was markedly low under sleeping and waking conditions alike. Some equivocal support can be found for LIV in that the incidence of such responses tended to be higher when infants were in lower basal states, but response strength showed no systematic relation with level of arousal. The Moro-like or startlelike reflexes characteristically evoked by constant signals under sleep and doze conditions (Eisenberg, 1970a and 1970b) were conspicuously absent: in somnolent babies as in wakeful ones, motor reactions consisted solely of grimaces and small movements of the limbs or even the digits.

Cochleopalpebral Reflexes and the Temporal Characteristics of Response Behavior   Percentage values in Table 3 hardly reflect the ubiquity and persistence of the CPR in normal newborns: 80–90% of the responses observed immediately prior to habituation consisted solely of eyeblinks. This consistent trend toward simple responses during declining activation, together with a differential distribution of latent and sequential responses, shows that the temporal characteristics of response behavior probably were affected by the monotonous stimulus schedule. Latent responses, which easily can be confused with "no response," especially when they occur atypically, were almost invariably recorded just before complete habituation. Sequential (longer) responses, on the other hand, characteristically were scored during the first 10 trials and never were scored during the final 10 trials. Considering the sources of error implicit in this pilot study, these trends were highly consistent. They suggest rather strongly that behavioral response time decreases and stimulus-response interval correspondingly increases during the habituation process.

RAS-Dependent Reflexes   The two indices relating to vocal behavior fall into the new irritation category mentioned in the discussion of study procedures, and the fact that such indices were set up only after this pilot

Table 3. Effects of Basal State and Repeated Stimulation on Response Activity in Clinically Normal Newborns

Basal State	Sleep or Doze (I–III: $N_s = 8$)					Wakeful (IV–VII: $N_s = 5$)				
Trial Intervals	1–5	6–10	11–15	16–20	21+	1–5	6–10	11–15	16–20	21+
	Response Patterns (Percent of all Detected Responses)									
DISPLAY										
Grimacing	6	10	9	8	2	6	1	—	1	—
Body movement	18	5	3	7	6	3	4	—	4	—
MOTOR$_T$	24	15	12	15	8	9	5	0	5	0
CPR in isolation	26	34	47	51	65	5	16	34	14	46
Body stirs	18	15	2	—	—	17	9	—	—	—
Opening eyes	27	30	24	26	27	4	0	0	0	3
Crying or whimpering	5	—	8	7	—	—	—	—	8	21
AROUSAL$_T$	50	45	34	33	27	21	9	0	8	24
Cessation of movement	—	—	—	—	—	10	15	11	13	15
Visual attention	—	6	7	1	—	55	55	55	50	7
Cessation of crying or whimpering	—	—	—	—	—	—	—	—	10	8
OQ$_T$	0	6	7	1	0	65	70	66	73	30
RAS-dependent$_T$	(50)	(51)	(41)	(34)	(27)	(86)	(79)	(66)	(81)	(54)
No. of response events	39	38	37	26	31	23	22	21	18	29
Response ratio (%)	98	95	93	65	*	92	89	84	72	*

*No response ratios calculated.

study was initiated reflects the far more important fact that responsive vocal behavior is almost never evoked by constant signals. It is, in Bio-acoustic Laboratory experience, one differential functional property of patterned stimuli (Eisenberg, 1967 and 1970*b*). As Table 3 indicates, however, such behavior represented only a fraction of the RAS-dependent activity scored for the tonal sequence. The overall incidence of arousal and OQ behaviors among the normal newborns in this study was comparable only with that evoked by certain ineffective constant signals in the high frequency range (Eisenberg, 1965*a*; Table 1). Relations between arousal and OQ reactions, as Table 3 suggests, once again were found to vary reciprocally in accord with activation theory and an awake-alert-aware continuum.

A crucial outcome of this pilot study, then, was the demonstration that patterned signals had functional properties that could prove singularly useful for further studies bearing upon the nature of auditory competence in early life. The tonal sequence was remarkably potent under sleeping and waking conditions alike. It was associated with a preponderance of RAS-dependent reactions that could be related to listening behavior later in life. It evoked selective motor responses, including vocalizations, rather than generalized startle reactions.

Differences Associated with Risk Category   While no conclusions can be drawn from the behavior of individual newborns, differences associated with risk category warrant comment because they correlated, in nature and degree, with the divergent activation patterns seen in Figure 9.

The only index to differentiate clearly among the three infant groups was the lapse of time between stimulus and response. Both suspect and high-risk babies tended to respond more slowly than controls during both early trials and late ones: responses scored as latent were twice as frequent in suspect infants and 5 to 6 times as frequent in high-risk infants. The data, although judgmental, seem to have been valid because very similar findings later were obtained by Schulman (1970*a* and 1970*b*), who used autonomic measures.

Suspect infants, who tended to be less responsive than control subjects and more labile in their activation patterns, did not show grossly aberrant reactions of any sort. High-risk babies, on the other hand, differed vastly and in clinically significant ways both from controls and from suspects. The incidence of motor responses was extremely high, comprising 50–70% of the behavior displayed in any 5-trial interval. Some 10–30% of this behavior after the 15th trial was characterized by tremor, asymmetrical movement, or other aberrant signs. Eye movements, including those asso-ciated with arousal and OQ, were present no more than 25% of the time. RAS-dependent responses, seen only in the full-term subject (S6 in Figure 9), consisted mostly of crying (40–60%) or cessation of body movement. It is possible, since the additional high-risk infant (S5) weighed less than 3 lb, that the total absence of OQ behaviors was related to her prematurity.

There is every reason to suppose that these differences among infant groups were real and, in some cases at least, predictive of CNS dysfunction. The one suspect infant who failed to habituate (S17 in Figure 9) and who also had a mild hearing loss (disclosed during evoked potential studies undertaken a few days after participation in this pilot study), died at 6 weeks, although his Apgar rating was 8. Moreover, despite an apparently negative maternal history, he was found at autopsy to have the classic rubella triad.

Predictive Potential of Habituation Measures

It was, of course, very encouraging to find a procedure that seemed to discriminate so neatly among groups of newborns. The major question at issue for clinical purposes, however, was whether the results of that procedure proved to be a reliable indicator of future developmental differences.

To address this question and to confirm pilot indications on the number of trials required for habituation during the newborn period, a follow-up inquiry was instituted. This study involved an additional 31 neonates, 5 of whom were controls and 26 of whom were divided equally between suspect and high-risk categories. Among the population were a number of control and high-risk subjects who could be studied longitudinally.[3] In contrast to the pilot investigation, this inquiry was undertaken in the test chamber of the Bioacoustic Laboratory under well-controlled conditions. Behavioral data, retrieved from filmed sequences which included no-stimulus "catch trials" as well as bona fide stimulus trials, were analyzed exhaustively.

Further Findings on Newborns Additional data, for the most part, were compatible with those already discussed. The 5 control subjects habituated within 25–28 trials, returning either to basal level or to some lower state of activation when stimulation was terminated. Eight of the 13 suspect babies continued to respond after 50 or more trials, showing state patterns of the kind graphed in Figure 9 while 5 of them proved, in all respects, indistinguishable from control subjects. One of the high risk

---

[3] Although every effort was made to have parents from the clinic bring their infants back to the laboratory for follow-up studies, not one of them in this group was willing to cooperate. In Bioacoustic Laboratory experience, cooperation from clinic parents seldom is forthcoming in the absence of incentives (free formula, medical care, or the like); even then, the attrition rate in longitudinal studies runs as high as 60%.

infants was unresponsive; one habituated by the 57th trial; and all of the remaining 11 infants continued to respond until the 100-stimulus schedule was terminated.

Thus, the follow-up study confirmed preliminary indications that habituation measures could discriminate among infant groups. Further, since about 60% of the suspect infants differed significantly from control babies, these further findings substantiated a long held conviction that normative values derived from clinic groups are subject to considerable error.

Longitudinal Findings   The results of longitudinal follow-up suggested that habituation measures might be reliable predictors of normal developmental patterns, but they were unreliable predictors of deviant ones. Specifically, although none of the 5 control subjects was found to have problems of any kind when seen again at 1 year, a substantial proportion of the high risk population seemed problem-free when seen again during later infancy. By and large, measures of the habituation process tended to be diagnostic of future dysfunction only in those cases where problems easily might have been predicted on other grounds. Perhaps the best way to illustrate this last point is to consider four representative high risk subjects who were followed longitudinally.

The group to be reported consists of one infant with Down's syndrome, one dysmature subject, one baby with Rh incompatibility, and one severely distressed infant.

The infant with Down's syndrome, who could be followed only until 5 months of age, remained grossly retarded in all areas of development when last seen. She demonstrated consistent and singular patterns of auditory behavior over 6 separate study sessions conducted at 1-month intervals. Specifically, failure to habituate over 100 trials was associated with remarkably little variation in state (rather than increasing excitation)[4] and, in waking states, fewer than 20% of the responses observed were scored as OQs.[5]

The dysmature infant, who was tested at daily intervals during his first week of life, gave no reliable responses to either patterned or constant

---

[4] Correlative HR measures, obtained at 1 month and again at 2 months, showed a similar trend. The range of HR values was very limited in comparison with normal infants of the same age, that is, the difference between the highest and the lowest HRs over the entire study period was no greater than 30 beats, whereas in clinically normal subjects such differences range upward of 60 beats. In general, the data suggested that for this Down's infant, the dynamic range of the cardiac system was significantly restricted. It might be speculated that this kind of "damping" reflects underlying biochemical abnormality (Coleman, 1973).

[5] Moskowitz and Lohmann (1970), who have reported closely related findings for adult subjects with Down's syndrome, concluded that deficits in attention may be critical determinants of the learning problems associated with this entity.

signals as intense as 110 dB. (Given reported threshold values for neonates, this means an effective SPL of 70–75 dB.) At 5 weeks, response to constant signals still was entirely absent, although a patterned stimulus of 60 dB or greater was thought to elicit equivocal responses. Evoked potential studies, undertaken at 3 months in order to define threshold values for the speech-hearing frequencies, ruled out hearing loss, however. Later habituation studies, attempted at 4 months and again at 5 months, were unsuccessful due to artifact. At 6 months, the subject was clinically unremarkable except for mild motor retardation, and his prelinguistic utterance was appropriate for his age.

The Rh incompatible baby, who was last in a long line of offspring having such problems (gravida x), had a bilirubin of 17.1 prior to exchange transfusion shortly after birth. During none of 4 tests undertaken between 1 and 3 months of age did he show any signs of habituation. On all occasions, repeated stimulation evoked aberrant motor activity and tonic activation. Serial evoked potential studies showed increasing seizure activity, and this youngster, who was demonstrably retarded in all areas of development when last seen at 8 months, is currently on an anticonvulsant drug regimen.

The distressed infant, product of a precipitate delivery, had a 5-min Apgar of 4. During each of 4 follow-up sessions prior to her fourth month, she consistently failed to habituate and, just as consistently, showed tonic activation. Nonetheless, when last seen at 6 months, she was clinically unremarkable, habituated within 30 trials, and showed temporal conditioning to a tonal pattern after only 6 trials.

Summing up the results of these habituation studies, it can be said that they were important in a number of ways. First and foremost, they showed that patterned signals had differential and singularly useful functional properties. Second, since the nature of the habituation process in normal infants was almost identical with that described by Sharpless and Jasper (1956) for cats, they showed that relations between state and auditory behavior could be related to brain stem mechanisms and ultimately to listening behavior. Third, they showed that differences among risk categories of newborns were significant, systematically related, and in accord with the hypothesis that the integrity of CNS organization could be measured in early life. Finally, if disappointingly, they showed that differential responses to a habituation schedule were constant with age only about 60% of the time in the case of high-risk subjects. As a consequence, studies designed to explore the clinical applicability of habituation measures were shelved in favor of work with patterned signals that were speechlike in nature.

CHAPTER 5
Electrophysiologic Measures of Auditory Behavior During Early Life

"Our increase of knowledge . . . is like
that of a traveler approaching a moun-
tain through a haze; at first only certain
large features are discernible and even
they have indistinct boundaries."
　Bertrand Russell, *Human Knowledge, Its Scope and Limitations* (1948)

Discussion of infant hearing patterns so far has centered on the measurement of overt responses by newborns to constant and patterned signals
that bear directly upon auditory processing operations but only indirectly
upon the coding of language sounds. This chapter, which considers the
functional properties of patterned signals that are speechlike in nature, is
mainly concerned with the HR and EEG changes associated with acoustic
stimulation during selected developmental stages. Because the modes of
overt activity elicited by synthetic speech sounds seem indistinguishable
from those elicited by the tonal pattern considered in the previous chapter
(Table 3), behavioral data will be cited only to the extent they relate to
the electrophysiologic findings.

　The chapter deals specifically with correlative information stemming
from an ongoing inquiry into the effects of conversationally loud synthetic
vowel sounds. Thus, the findings to be reported here refer to work in progress
and, unlike the behavioral material, they must be regarded as exploratory.

Portions of this chapter were originally published in *Physiological Measures of the
Audio-Vestibular System* (L. J. Bradford, editor; Academic Press, New York, 1975)
and are reprinted here by permission of Academic Press, Inc.

BACKGROUND INFORMATION ON HEART RATE

The use of cranial blood pressure and related cardiac measures dates back some 60 years (Kessen, Haith, and Salapatek, 1970), and cardiac measures in particular have acquired wide currency within the past decade. Indeed, HR now is employed quite regularly to disclose the effects of stimulus parameters, to monitor fetal status, and to study the organization of behavior (Graham and Jackson, 1970; Lewis, 1974; and Steinschneider, 1971). There has been little interest in using cardiac measures to study infant audition, however. Beadle, who first reported work in this area (Beadle and Crowell, 1962), did not persist beyond a preliminary inquiry. Bench, who used the electrocardiogram (EKG) to study intensity and frequency discrimination by neonates (1969*a* and *b*) as well as relations between HR and arousal (1970), has not pursued the clinical implications of his data. Barrager (1974), who compared the efficacy of behavioral and cardiac indicators, concluded that the former provided considerably more information about hearing than the latter, and at considerably less expense. Lassman (personal communication), at the University of Minnesota, has attempted to measure auditory thresholds by HR and found the experience frustrating. Jerger (personal communication), at Baylor University, explored the possibility of transmitting cardiac data by telemetry with some success, but shelved this effort in favor of more rewarding activities. Schulman, who has done a great deal of work on cardiac measures of auditory sensitivity during early life (Schulman, 1970*a* and 1970*b*; Schulman and Kreiter, 1970; Schulman et al., 1970; and Schulman and Wade, 1970) and has developed an automatic device for computing threshold responses to pure tones, recently qualified earlier statements on the validity of HR measures during the neonatal period (Schulman, 1973).

Our group at the Bioacoustic Laboratory first became interested in cardiac measures of auditory behavior around 1962, during a period when a number of electrophysiologic indicators were under investigation (Eisenberg, 1965*a*). We got interested in cardiotachometry somewhat later, when reports from the Department of Pediatrics at the New York Upstate Medical Center in Syracuse came to our attention (Lipton and Steinschneider, 1964; Lipton, Steinschneider, and Richmond, 1960, 1961*a*, 1961*b*, 1964, 1965*a*, 1965*b*, and 1966; Richmond, Lipton, and Steinschneider, 1962*a* and 1962*b*; Steinschneider and Lipton, 1965; and Steinschneider, Lipton, and Richmond, 1964 and 1966).[1]

---

[1] We learned the tools of the HR trade by visiting at Syracuse, and some of the technical procedures, for instance, electrode placements, are based upon Steinschneider's recommendations.

Physiologic and Technical Considerations

Limited progress in developing HR measures of infant hearing relates partly to a traditional audiologic focus upon threshold definition (Bradford, 1975; Eisenberg, 1970a, 1971, and 1974) and partly to difficulties inherent in working with immature subjects. Although the cardiovascular system is the first organ system to attain functional capacity (Eichorn, 1970; and Phillips et al., 1964), mechanisms regulating HR remain immature for some months after birth (Eisenberg, 1974b and 1975b; Eisenberg, Marmarou, and Giovachino, 1973, 1974a, and 1974b; Emmanouilides et al., 1964; Lipton and Steinschneider, 1964; Lipton, Steinschneider, and Richmond, 1966; and Vallbona et al., 1963; and Vallbona, Rudolph, and Desmond, 1965). Accordingly, cardiac patterns differ markedly as a function of developmental status (Namin and Miller, 1974; Sroufe, 1971; and Sroufe and Morris, 1973). The cardiac pattern of the young infant normally is characterized by a marked sinus arrhythmia (Lipton, Steinschneider, and Richmond, 1964; and unpublished Bioacoustic Laboratory data)[2] that poses sizable problems in data analysis. Particularly during the first 2 months or so of life, heart rates tend to be grossly unstable, sometimes showing instantaneous changes on the order of 20–30 beats in the absence of any external stimulation. The range of HR values encountered in early infancy is roughly twice as high as that found during adult life (Eichorn, 1970; and Eisenberg, 1974b and 1975b) and genetic factors possibly may contribute to differences among infants from different racial groups (Schachter et al., in press). Therefore, if maturational factors are to be considered or cardiac data are to be treated correlatively, the descriptors employed must deal with these age- and group-related factors and, in addition, must be comparable with ancillary measures.

Derivation of HR Data   The electrocardiogram, which reflects action potentials in cardiac muscle cells, yields a pattern of strip chart deflections referable to intervals of the cardiac cycle. These deflections, which conventionally are characterized as P, Q, R, S, and T waves, yield a great deal of important diagnostic information respecting mechanisms of heart action. However, numerous investigations have shown little of this information to be pertinent when the purpose of cardiac measures is to study perception or some other selected aspect of human behavior. Under these conditions, HR has emerged as the least troublesome and, consequently, the most widely applied indicator of function (Eichorn, 1970).

The salient deflection in the EKG record is the R wave, which appears as a prominent spike (see Figure 11 and Appendix C, Figure II.1), and the

---

[2] A pattern which, in mature life, characteristically is found for subjects who smoke (unpublished laboratory data).

HR measure accordingly can be extrapolated from the full EKG complex by counting the number of R waves per unit of time. However, this is a tedious, time-consuming exercise that tends to be short on accuracy, hard on the eyes, and seemingly endless in arithmetic computations. Fortunately, cardiotachometers are available now and experimental chores have been reduced appreciably.

The cardiotachometer is essentially a beat-to-beat metering device that is triggered by the R wave of a subject under test. Electronic circuits built into the instrument continuously measure the time intervals (tau, or τ) between successive R waves, convert them to instantaneous rates, determine the reciprocals of those rates ($1/\tau$), and display and/or record the resulting values on a calibrated scale, as "Nixie" read-outs of instantaneous heart rates and/or as strip chart deflections convertible to such rates. Reciprocals must be determined because the period between successive R waves, measured in milliseconds, is not identical with HR in beats per minute (bpm) (Khachaturian et al., 1972). This means, then, that the formula:

$$HR = 60/\tau$$

must be applied for conversion. For instance, a tau, or R-R interval, of 0.3 sec (300 msec) would yield an instantaneous HR of 200 bpm.

The example cited above is a clue to the massive amounts of data generated by HR studies. A half-hour recording on an average adult, whose HR usually varies between 60 and 70 bpm, would generate approximately 2,000 data bits; a similar recording on an average 1-month old infant, whose HR may span a 100-beat range, would generate about 6,000 data bits. Thus, cardiac measurement presents serious problems with respect to data reduction and retrieval. Resolution of these problems depends partly upon the questions under investigation and partly upon the resources available, but, under most conditions, computer treatment of the data is mandatory.

BACKGROUND INFORMATION ON ELECTROENCEPHALOGRAPHY

Although the discovery of electrical potentials in the brain dates back to the nineteenth century (Regan, 1972; Reneau and Hnatiow, 1975; Skinner, 1972; and Thompson and Patterson, 1974), recordings of such potentials first were made only 50 years later (Berger, 1929). EEG work began to accelerate only after World War II and, sparked by the advent of computer technology in the 1950's, numerous studies related to the effects of age, physiologic status, and other factors now have been undertaken. Studies of sensory evoked activity have proliferated only within the past 15 years however, and many of the problems they present remain to be resolved (McCallum and Knott, 1973; and Prescott, Read, and Coursin, 1975).

Essentially, the EEG is a measure of relatively slow electrical processes occurring in the nervous system. Obtained conventionally with scalp electrodes, it reflects variations in brain potentials that relate not only to activity in areas immediately beneath the electrodes, but also to activity in specific and nonspecific channels lying well below the surface of the brain. Such variations produce wave forms that can be analyzed with reference to their frequency, amplitude, and time characteristics, their spatial distribution among cerebral regions, and so on. Unfortunately, the wave forms also reflect artifacts (Low, 1973; and Milnarich, 1958) and other phenomena that make the interpretation of data very difficult, particularly for the unsophisticated investigator.

EEG data are usually evaluated with reference to the arousal conditions under which they are obtained and the kinds of experimental manipulations to which subjects are exposed. Recordings derived in the absence of experimental manipulations (resting records) serve as the standard by which the effects of sensory stimulation can be measured. The sensory evoked potential refers to changes in wave form associated with particular kinds of sensory stimulation. Thus, the wave form associated with auditory stimulation is termed the auditory (or acoustic) evoked response (AER), that associated with visual stimulation is termed the visual evoked response (VER), and so on.[3]

The first reports of EEG responses to auditory stimulation date back to the late 1930's (H. Davis et al., 1939; P. Davis, 1939; Loomis, Harvery, and Hobart, 1938) and, indeed, such terminology as K complex (Loomis, Harvery, and Hobart, 1938) and V potential (H. Davis et al., 1939) stem from this early work. Since the advent of the average response computer, studies have proceeded apace (Regan, 1972, pp. 162–166; and Skinner, 1972).

Most work with infants and young children has involved the use of clicks, pure tones, or other constant signals (see Appendix B), and the vast majority of studies has centered about threshold definition.

Bioacoustic Laboratory work in the EEG area has proceeded sporadically since about 1963 (Eisenberg, 1966a and 1975a; Eisenberg et al., 1974c), but studies undertaken prior to those discussed here contributed relatively little to our current thinking.[4]

---

[3] In clinical audiology, standardized procedures for measuring the AER now are referred to as electroencephalic response audiometry (ERA). Also, it should be noted that the terminology, auditory evoked potential (AEP), is preferred by some.

[4] Early work, involving the use of pure tone stimuli and signal detection techniques for analysis, was based upon suggestions by A. J. Derbyshire, to whom I am greatly indebted for my introduction into the mysteries of EEG.

Physiologic and Technical Considerations

A major factor contributing to slow progress in the measurement of sensory evoked potentials is the gap in our understanding of scalp potentials (Donshin and Lindsley, 1969; Prescott, Read, and Coursin, 1975; Regan, 1972; Reneau and Hnatiow, 1975; and Thompson and Patterson, 1974). However, problems of working with developing subjects are in themselves substantial. The resting EEG of the young infant, for instance, is extremely diffuse, so that state definition presents challenges that vary in magnitude according to age and the availability of ancillary measures such as EMG (electromyography) and ERG (electroretinography) (Barnet, Bazelon, and Zapella, 1966; Barnet and Lodge, 1967a and b; Groth et al., 1967; Hutt et al., 1968a; Hutt and Hutt, 1970; Hutt et al., 1968b; and Monod and Garma, 1971). Although activity in the alpha band of frequencies may be discerned during neonatal life in central leads (Churchill, Grisell, and Darnley, 1966), the occipital alpha rhythm becomes prominent only within 3 or 4 months after birth. The tracé alternant pattern (Dreyfus-Brisac, 1964 and 1966), differentiating quiet sleep from active sleep (Ellingson, Deutch, and McInteir, 1974; and Parmalee et al., 1968), is present in the full-term infant, but parietal humps characteristic of doze states later in development are difficult to discern even at 6 weeks of age and reasonably synchronous sleep spindles appear only at about 3 months. The inability to specify state with great precision is critical because this source of variability, which affects both the magnitude and latency of AER components (Himwich and Himwich, 1964, p. 16) becomes difficult to tease out. There are additional sources of variability, however. For instance, movement artifacts of one sort or another (Low, 1973) are commonplace; and although sedation may serve to reduce them (Suzuki, 1973), it contributes still another source of variability (Skinner, 1972).

Derivation of EEG Data   The electroencephalogram, or EEG, which reflects electrical potentials recorded between linked electrode sites, yields patterns of strip chart deflections that represent differences in potential between those sites. Each set of two electrodes, one of which is considered "active" and the other of which serves as a reference, composes one channel of information.

The electrical activity being monitored is a minute voltage of continuously changing amplitude, phase, and frequency and an amplifier, built into the EEG instrument, serves to increase its magnitude up to a million or more times. Since phase shifts occur during each stage of electronic amplification, it is critical that all channels be adjusted within given precise limits. High- and low-pass filters, also built into the EEG, selectively amplify those portions of the EEG signals arising within the brain and selectively attenuate those portions arising from environmental interference (for instance, 60 Hz) or from unwanted biologic potentials (for instance, muscle) that are within the EEG frequency range.

Conventionally, electrode placements are specified according to the 10–20 international system (Low, 1973). Active brain areas are indicated alphabetically as F (frontal), C (central), T (temporal), P (parietal), and O (occipital), and numerically, according to whether derivations are on the left side of the scalp (odd numbers) or the right (even numbers); midline placements are indicated by the modifier, "z." Inactive reference sites are indicated similarly by number, the ears being specified as A_1 (left) and A_2 (right).

Monopolar placements are usually preferred for evoked potential studies, and, in auditory work, the most frequently selected site for the active electrode is C_z. This derivation yields large amplitude potentials that have been related to activation of frontal cortex (Picton and Hillyard, 1974; and Picton et al., 1974). A relatively inactive area, such as the earlobe or the mastoid, provides a convenient reference site under these conditions.

Davis (1973) has related time characteristics of the vertex AER (V potential) to neural structures as follows: (1) 0 msec latency = organ of Corti; (2) 1–4 msec = auditory nerve; (3) 3–20 msec = cochlear nucleus through inferior colliculus; (4) 25–50 msec = medial geniculate and primary cortical projection area; (5) 50–280 msec = cortical projection areas (secondary response); (6) >180 msec in sleep and >300 msec in waking = diffuse late cortical responses relating to "certain psychological functions." It is these late responses and the psychologic functions they reflect that are of major concern in Bioacoustic Laboratory work. Accordingly, discussion of EEG work in this chapter relates to the potentials beyond 50 msec.

CORRELATIVE STUDIES OF RESPONSE
TO A CONVERSATIONALLY LOUD SYNTHETIC VOWEL

The study to be considered here is the first of several directed toward long-term clinical objectives. However, it also encompasses basic research questions, and, because the experimental situation is so complex, it may be helpful to spell out the rationale for our procedures.

Briefly, the long-term objective of this and other studies is to develop a groundwork for the design of predictive auditory tests for infants. Such tests must be based upon the facts of performance at various stages of development between birth and adult life. They must yield operational measures of auditory processing that bear not only upon normal coding functions in the eighth nerve system but also upon normal "integrating" functions in the central nervous system. They must be clinically viable.

These requirements impose specific constraints upon the research approach. Study methods must be applicable to control subjects at any stage of development. They must be valid under a wide range of stimulus conditions. They must apply under all conditions of arousal. They must neither require nor assume subject cooperation. They ultimately must prove reliable in average clinical situations as well as in research-oriented facilities.

This particular inquiry best can be viewed as a pilot experiment, designed to disclose whether and to what extent the procedures devised meet these requirements. It is presently an incomplete experiment because few of the data have been subjected to more than preliminary analyses. Nonetheless, even such limited findings suggest that the procedures considered below have substantial clinical potential and that the methods of approach can cast light upon mechanisms underlying auditory competence. Such methods involve complementary procedures whereby the analysis of stimulus-bound behavior per se yields information on perceptual specializations and the analysis of dynamic changes over time yields information on central specializations.

Subjects and Stimulus Conditions

Some 60 subjects were involved in this initial correlative study of responses to speechlike sounds. The population spanned an age range between 13 hr and 27 years, and included a few high-risk newborns as well as male adults with known or suspected CNS dysfunction. However, the bulk of the data was collected on infants under the age of 45 days.

The acoustic stimulus used in the experiment was the synthetic vowel "ah", which is a prominent constituent of the young infant's vocal repertoire. This 1.16-sec signal,[5] with a fixed rise and decay of 25 msec, was recorded on magnetic tape at 90-sec intervals (onset to onset)[6] for sound-field presentation at the conversationally loud level of 60 dB (re 0.0002 μbar). The experimental schedule consisted of 30 trials.

System for Data Acquisition and Storage

A condensed diagram of Bioacoustic Laboratory circuitry can be found in Figure 10. The recorded vowel sounds, controlled by digital logic modules,

---

[5] Generated at Haskins Laboratories, New Haven, Connecticut.

[6] An unconventionally long ISI was employed because we were concerned mainly with statistical means of characterizing the cardiac response, and earlier studies with patterned signals of several kinds had shown delays of this order to be required for attainment of stable poststimulus patterns.

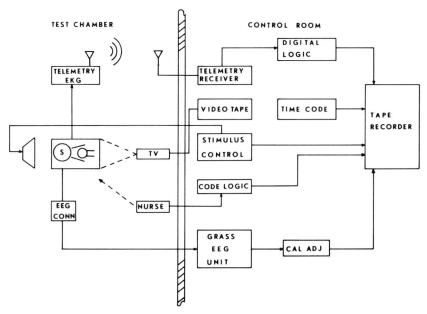

Figure 10. Condensed diagram of Bioacoustic Laboratory circuitry. (A more complete schematic can be found in Appendix C, Figure II.1.)

were fed to amplifier and attenuator networks by way of an electronic switch that gated speakers only when a signal was presented. This precluded the possibility of electrical noise during ISIs. Behavioral, cardiac, and EEG outputs from a subject in the test chamber were routed to appropriate display and monitor units in the control room and also to specified channels of an Ampex FR-1800-L tape recorder. An eight-track recording format on the latter permitted storage of (1) all acoustic events occurring in the test chamber; (2) two channels of HR information (the EKG complex and the heart beat); (3) coded stimulus and artifact markers; (4) three channels of EEG information; and (5) real time, in the form of the IRIG B standardized electrical time code.

Heart Rate Circuitry A block diagram of Bioacoustic Laboratory circuitry for obtaining HR data can be found in Figure 11. Telemetry is employed in our correlative studies for two reasons. From a practical standpoint, it precludes the possibility of electrical hazards arising from simultaneous use of EEG and cardiac indicators. From a long-range planning standpoint, it affords hope for development of auditory test procedures permitting pediatric-aged subjects reasonable freedom of movement in a study environment.

In this investigation, the EKG from a subject in the test chamber was routed to a Lexington neurologic amplifier (model A-103-B) and the

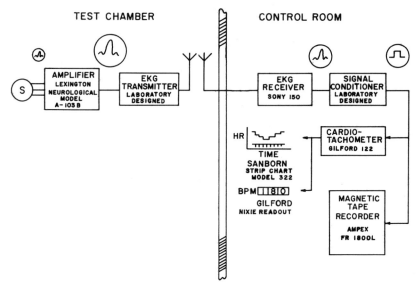

Figure 11. Block diagram of Bioacoustic Laboratory circuitry for obtaining HR data. (More complete schematics can be found in Appendix C, Figures II.1 and II.5.)

amplified cardiac complex thus obtained sent to a special FM transmitter.[7] The transmitted signal was received in the control room by a commercial FM tuner (Sony, model 150) and the output of the tuner, amplified in its turn and conditioned by digital logic circuitry,[8] provided a uniform square pulse for each heart beat. The uniform pulses, representing the successive R waves, were fed into a standard cardiotachometer (Gilford, model 122) for conversion to instantaneous rates. The output of the cardiotachometer, in the form of a DC level proportional to HR, finally was routed to a number of on-line devices: an indicator button on the Gilford, together with its Nixie read-out, permitted visual monitoring of each heart beat; a speaker permitted auditory monitoring; the Ampex FR-1800-L permitted storage of the continuously recorded data; and a two-channel strip chart recorder (Sanborn, model 322) permitted visual inspection of the cardio-tachometer output.

EEG Circuitry Brain wave data were obtained with a Grass (model 78) instrument. These were routed, via a special extension cable, from an

---

[7] This device, like the signal conditioner elsewhere in the circuit, was designed by Dr. Anthony Marmarou of the Bioacoustic Laboratory staff. The transmitter operated at 108 MHZ, a frequency that was relatively free both of commercial transmission in the Lancaster area and hospital equipment interference.

[8] Amplitude thresholds are incorporated into the logic to exclude extraneous noise sources.

electrode board in the test chamber to the unit in the control room. The output of the Grass instrument was adjusted and calibrated before data were stored on specified channels of the Ampex and, at the beginning of each data tape, calibration signals were recorded on each of these channels. This permitted later retrieval of computer data in the form of $\mu v/cm$ for comparison with strip chart deflections.

Electrode Placements   To guard against technical problems, procedures for placement of EKG and EEG electrodes followed strict pretest and test protocols (Eisenberg, 1975b; and Eisenberg, Marmarou, and Giovachino, 1973, 1974a, and 1974c).

The same EKG electrodes (Beckman no. 650944, .062 inch) were employed with subjects in all age groups. These were applied by the attending nurse, and only three were used. Two electrodes were placed on the anterior chest wall, one in the third interspace just to the left of the sternum, and the second (ground) adjacent to the left nipple; the third was attached at the midline over the vertebral column at the same level.[9] Burton Parsons EKG Sol was used as the conductor.

Standard gold disc electrodes, applied by the EEG technician,[10] were used for pick up of the brain wave data. Since we were concerned with the question of whether temporal lead measures were feasible during early life, the experimental montage for study of the AER varied somewhat from that employed by other investigators working with infants (Dreyfus-Brisac, 1964; Ohlrich and Barnet, 1972; and Rapin and Graziani, 1967). The forehead served as a ground and the placements used were the following: C_z-A_2, F_z-A_1, and T_3-A_2. Areas of scalp to be covered were cleaned meticulously before electrode attachment and bentonite paste was used as the conductor. Under these conditions, interelectrode resistances averaged about 5,000 ohms.

General Procedures for Data Collection and Storage

Each experimental session was routinely preceded by a strict "monitor" protocol assuring optimal physical conditions for auditory study, electrical

---

[9] Careful placement of electrodes is crucial to obtaining artifact-free HR data, and an investigator is well advised to work out his own reasonably foolproof physical procedures before any large scale studies are attempted. For instance, the laboratory placements outlined, which have proved highly satisfactory with very young babies and adult males, are not necessarily useful with other kinds of subjects: infants older than about 5–6 months tend to be frightened of the study situation and, unlike younger, relatively passive babies, many of them will struggle actively during the placement process; female subjects, however liberated and cooperative, take a dim view of having their chests exposed for prolonged periods of time.

[10] Mrs. Jane Baker, whose assistance in many aspects of EEG investigation has proved invaluable.

safety, and efficient communication between the test chamber and the control room.

After a subject arrived in the test chamber, the chest was bared so that skin areas to which EKG electrodes, subsequently attached, could be prepared (Eisenberg, 1975b). Infants were fed immediately thereafter by the parent or usual caretaker, and associated care required for their comfort and well being (burping, diaper changes, etc.) was provided. Some 15–30 min later[11] (or, for infants, when feeding and other tasks were completed), all electrodes were attached. Once these physical manipulations and all required subject-in-circuit calibrations were attended to, all personnel other than the subject and the attending nurse-observer left the test chamber.

The subjects, lying supine, remained uncovered above the waist once the experiment actually began, thus permitting a count of respiration rates[12] and easy replacement of cardiac electrodes at need. Depending upon the age of the subjects, the bed in which they rested was an infant crib, an infant recliner, or a standard hospital mattress. The nurse was responsible for seeing to it that all subjects were settled comfortably in a supine position such that an overhead speaker, which constituted the source of study signals, was at the midline between both ears.

The departure of other personnel from the test chamber marked the start of an adaptation period, the duration of which was varied according to subject age, activity level, and pertinent individual factors (Eisenberg, 1965a). At the end of this time, when it was apparent that data acquisition could proceed satisfactorily, a 3-min basal run, providing information on behavioral, cardiac, and EEG patterns under "no sound" conditions was begun.[13] No restraints of any kind (including swaddling) were employed. No subjects were sedated.

Derivation and Storage of Experimental Data   On-the-spot behavioral data were recorded on standardized forms by the nurse-observer in the test chamber and were later coded onto IBM cards (see Appendix C, section I, for comparison with similarly treated filmed data.

---

[11] In the case of adults, this time was utilized for obtaining identifying data, briefing subjects, and so forth. Briefing statements routinely were variations on the following themes: (1) we are interested in how HR and brain wave patterns change over time; (2) you will be hearing some sounds once in a while, but they are not important and you do not have to listen for them or do anything when you happen to hear them; (3) if you feel like it, you can take a nap but, in any case, try not to move about while the experiment is going on.

[12] Respiration rates were counted by the attending nurse-observer at such selected times as experimental conditions permitted obtaining this measurement.

[13] EEG resting records were obtained with the conventional 10–20 International electrode array.

Heart rate and brain wave data alike were derived both from individual strip chart recordings and from the observations stored on magnetic tape. Strip chart recordings served as a basis for obtaining state and response event information on a single trial basis. In the case of EEG, these recordings contained channels in addition to those stored on tape (Eisenberg, Marmarou, and Giovachino, 1974c) as well as on-line indicators of stimulus events. An Astrodata unit (model 5224) provided time code information and, in its search and control mode, was used both to monitor artifacts[14] and to group trials according to prestimulus state or other variables of interest.

HEART RATE RESPONSES

As was noted in Chapter 2, the analysis of electrophysiologic data presents many problems and, not surprisingly, the literature abounds with alternative suggestions for statistical treatment of HR data. These alternatives are discussed in detail in recent review papers (Clifton, 1974a; Graham and Jackson, 1970; Khachaturian et al., 1972; Lewis, 1974; Obrist, Webb, and Sutterer, 1969; Obrist et al., 1970; and Steinschneider, 1971), and there is no need to consider their specific merits and demerits here. However, it is worth remarking that exploratory use of numerous parametric procedures at the Bioacoustic Laboratory has resulted in ambiguous or even conflicting findings. Treatments based upon assumptions that system or response characteristics can be predicted reliably (Jones, Crowell, and Kapaniai, 1969) have not proved out. Specific efforts at analysis in the time domain, testing the use of such diverse techniques as ensemble averaging, time-shifted correlation matrices, analysis of variance, and polynomial regression have been largely unproductive. Not one of these commonly recommended parametric procedures has permitted the extraction of adequate response criteria. Not one of them has proved potent statistically on a single trial basis. Moreover, at a descriptive level, none has yielded more than confirmation of trends that were apparent during preliminary eyeballing.

Although most of the statistical alternatives suggested in the literature have been found wanting, the method of treating cardiac data discussed in this section represents only one of many possible approaches. However, it is useful for Bioacoustic Laboratory purposes because it has already yielded preliminary answers to fundamental questions.

---

[14] For purposes of off-line computer analysis, regions of artifact, determined on a real time basis, can be logged and transferred to punch cards in the form of digital information referable to time of onset, duration, and specific channel location(s).

These questions, briefly, are the following. Can the existence of a cardiac response to sound be proved unequivocally? Can it be demonstrated that cardiac measures are valid under differing conditions of arousal? Can general descriptors be derived that, regardless of stimulus or subject variables, refer to operations in eighth nerve channels? Can dynamic measures be developed that refer to central mechanisms affecting operating efficiency in those channels?

Each of these questions carries with it a set of subquestions, some of which are bound to vary with experimental design. In the present experiment, for instance, the use of a fixed ISI created a whole series of statistical problems related to time-dependent phenomena such as anticipation of and habituation to the stimulus. Although these subsidiary problems remain unresolved at this writing, we have bypassed them in order to attack the more immediate questions noted above. This was managed by adopting a series of simple nonparametric treatments, that, in addition to yielding some of the answers desired, have suggested approaches to the subsidiary problems (Eisenberg, 1975*b*). Such treatments, which uniformly involve the use of interval histograms, are considered below with reference to their applications; and, inasmuch as the statistical manipulations to be covered in this section may be new to some readers, they are discussed with reference to sample data on individual subjects.

When is a Change in Heart Rate a Response?

To answer the question of whether response exists, let us consider data on a typical 13-day-old control subject. A baby of this age is a particularly telling examplar because, as noted earlier, the cardiac system is very labile in early life. To prove the existence of response, then, two things must be shown: (1) that the distribution of heart rates during some sample of time subsequent to stimulus onset (T_0) differs significantly from the distribution found during some like period of time immediately preceding stimulus onset; and (2) that the differences between these two samples differ significantly in degree and/or in kind from differences that characterize contiguous nonstimulus samples. The first set of time intervals obviously must derive from either side of T_0; the second set can be selected from any portion of the data sufficiently remote from T_0 to be assumed independent of stimulus effects.

The samples, or epochs, used in this experiment were selected only after careful visual inspection of many HR records. They covered 40 sec of real time in each trial and permitted comparison of matched samples as follows:

1. A 10-sec stimulus-bound epoch (T_0 to $T_0 + 10$ sec) with the like nonstimulus epoch immediately preceding it in time (T_0 to $T_0 - 10$ sec).

2. An alternate nonstimulus epoch of 10 sec (T_0 + 75–85 sec) with the 10-sec epoch immediately prior to it (T_0 + 65–75 sec).[15]

As a first step toward proving response, interval histograms were extracted from each of these four selected epochs in each trial so that the distribution of taus, or interbeat intervals in seconds, could be obtained. These distributions then were converted to equivalent heart rates according to formula (HR = 60/tau) in order to make the findings comparable with other data in the literature.

As a next step, the matched data sets, that is, those describing the two 10-sec epochs around stimulus onset and those describing the two 10-sec epochs remote from stimulus onset, were accumulated sequentially, in 3-trial blocks, over the entire 30-trial schedule.

Finally, in order to quantify the significance of differences between sample sets, the accumulative distributions (trials 1–3, 1–6, 1–9, and so on) were subjected individually to the Kolmogorov-Smirnov (K-S) two-sample two tail test (Siegel, 1956, pp. 156–158).

The general approach is illustrated in Figures 12 and 13, which refer respectively to HR distributions in the vicinity of stimulus onset (Figure 12) and HR distributions remote from stimulus onset (Figure 13). Statistical (K-S) values for the accumulative groupings are shown in the pertinent graphs, a through j, in each figure and, to point up the effects of increasing sample size, graphs are arranged in descending order. For purposes of graphic treatment, the approximately equal numbers of observations in each of the sample sets[16] were converted to percentage values.

From these figures, there seems to be little doubt that response occurred. Statistically significant differences between HR distributions for the 10-sec period preceding stimulus onset and the like period beginning with stimulus onset are found consistently. Statistically significant differences between the contiguous epochs remote from stimulus onset are found only inconsistently. In the first set of comparisons (Figure 12) it is true that differences between distributions decline from 0.001 to 0.05 as more and more trials are accumulated, but the decline clearly is systematic and the statistical values never reach a point of no significance. In the second set of comparisons (Figure 13), however, differences between distributions, when they occur, are less significant and the statistical values show no systematic relation with sample size.

---

[15] The 5-sec interval immediately prior to T_0 was excluded from consideration when visual inspection of strip chart data showed anticipatory HR changes to occur during this period of time.

[16] Ranging between 82 and 84 for trials 1 through 3 and between 796 and 801 for trials 1 through 30.

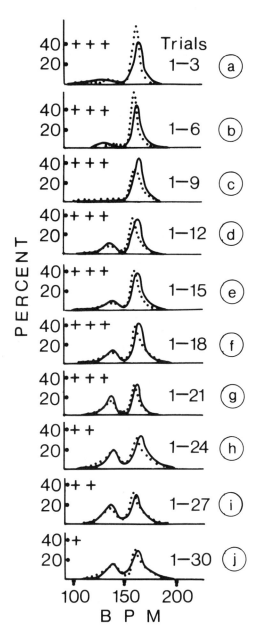

Figure 12. Distribution, by accumulative three-trial blocks, of infant heart rates before and after stimulus onset. Before (———) = T_0 to $T_0 - 10$ sec; after (- - - - -) = T_0 to $T_0 + 10$ sec. The significance of differences between each sample pair, according to the K-S two-sample two-tail test, is shown as + + + (0.001), ++ (0.01), and + (0.05).

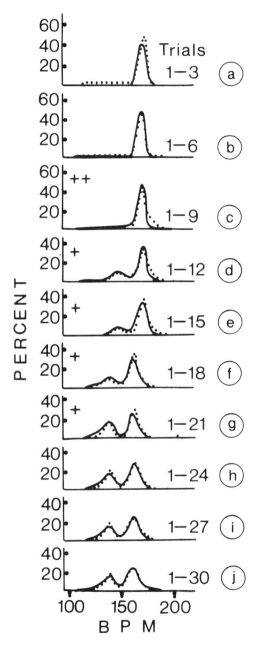

Figure 13. Distribution, by accumulative three-trial blocks, of infant heart rates during contiguous nonstimulus epochs. ——— = $T_0 + 65 - 75$ sec; - - - - - = $T_0 + 75 -$ 85 sec. Where differences between samples are significant by the K-S test, p values are shown in the pertinent graphs as + + (0.01) and + (0.05).

These illustrative findings, which are supported by very similar data on additional control subjects in selected age groups, have obvious implications for further study. First of all, it seems likely that, as more data are accumulated, the approach outlined here can yield strict objective (statistical) criteria for response. Second, since the significance of differences between pre- and poststimulus distributions decreases systematically with sample size, it should prove possible to determine, on an operational basis, the optimal (that is, minimal) number of trials required for standardized clinical procedures. By the same token, the relative potency of sounds having differing physical properties should prove measurable with reference to the number of trials required before statistical significance is lost or appreciably reduced. Third, since the existence of a response event is indicated by the difference between pre- and poststimulus samples, it should prove possible to develop simpler methods of statistical treatment that eventually may apply to the design of automated test instruments.

Arousal Level as a Determinant of Cardiac Activity

As the accumulative histograms in Figures 12 and 13 are studied, it becomes clear that the HR distributions for this subject shifted considerably over the 30-trial (45-min) schedule, whether or not they were associated with stimulus onset. Since the experiment yielded correlative indices of state (that is, behavioral and EEG ratings in addition to the HR values), it can be assumed that these changes reflected alterations in physiologic equilibrium.[17] The question at issue for the moment is not what such changes may mean, but whether cardiac dynamics per se affect the validity of response measures. The answer is that they do not seem to. Although infant heart rates tend to be similarly labile in the presence or absence of stimulation, evidence for the existence of response remains unaffected even when modes of response activity are altered. In the case of this subject, for instance, it is clear that the nature of differences between pre- and poststimulus distributions varied according to the dispersion of HR values along some dynamic continuum. Thus, when the prestimulus distribution was concentrated near the middle of this continuum in Figure 12 (graphs a through c), the sole descriptor was deceleration. On the other hand, when the prestimulus heart rates were distributed more or less in bimodal fashion (graphs g through j), there seem to have been rela-

---

[17] Correlations among the various indices are far from perfect, but for the experimental population as a whole, there is excellent general correspondence among behavioral, EEG, and cardiac measures of arousal: for any given subject, lower HRs are associated with sleep or doze states and slow brain wave frequencies, while higher cardiac rates are associated with wakeful states and relatively faster brain wave frequencies.

tively fewer low heart rates during the stimulus period, suggesting the existence of accelerative changes during at least some trials.

The value of an interval histogram approach is that it provides a reliable and flexible method of treating cardiac data either on a single-trial or an accumulative-trial basis. On a single-trial basis, it holds great promise as an index of prestimulus state because the dispersion of HR values over relatively long epochs is more representative of internal equilibrium than is some arbitrarily selected reference point shortly before stimulus onset. On an accumulative-trial basis, the approach has a number of uses. It permits dealing objectively with response activity that is complex, atypical, or "fragile." It provides information on the inherent variability of the data. It suggests whether a typical response in fact exists.

Heart Rate as a Clue to Auditory Processes

Figure 12 suggests rather strongly that, if there is not a typical response to the synthetic vowel used in this experiment, there certainly is a predominant response. In all of the graphs shown in Figure 12, the heart rates most frequently represented during poststimulus epochs are shifted by an interval (5–8 beats) below those most frequently represented during prestimulus epochs. The same trend has been found for all subjects analyzed thus far, regardless of age or state variables. This trend has not turned up in association with pure tones, noisebands, or any *unmodulated* signals of the kinds explored so far (Eisenberg, 1965a, 1970b, 1974a, 1974b, 1975a, and 1975b; Graham and Jackson, 1970; Segall, 1972; and unpublished Bioacoustic Laboratory data). It seems possible, then, that cardiac deceleration may be one special functional property of complex sound patterns and speechlike stimuli. If indeed this is the case, as we believe it to be, the data reported here have important implications for current thinking about infant perception in general and auditory perception in particular. It has been argued, for instance, that the direction of HR responses reflects the nature of an organism's transactions with his external environment (Lacey et al., 1963; Lacey and Lacey, 1970; and Lynn, 1966): decelerative changes, which presumably are associated with an orienting system (Graham and Clifton, 1966; and Sokolov, 1963), relate to acceptance of stimuli; accelerative changes, which presumably are associated with defense reflexes, relate to their rejection. This hypothesis, which has been extremely influential, gains scant support from Bioacoustic Laboratory data: correlative findings on a number of individual subjects in this experiment show that decelerative responses to the synthetic vowel cannot be associated easily with given patterns of overt or cortical activity.

Figure 14, which refers to the same subject considered in Figures 12 and 13, is a case in point. Here, where six trials were selected which, by

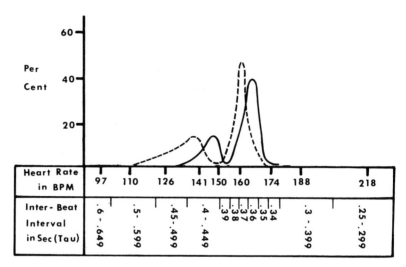

Figure 14. Distribution, for selected decelerative trials, of infant heart rates during 10 sec before (——) and 10 sec after (- - - -) stimulus onset. $N = 6$; p (by K-S two-sample two-tail test) = > 0.0001. Correlative data on behavioral and EEG state ratings are shown in Table 4.

visual inspection, were associated with marked and prolonged cardiac deceleration, and HR distributions for the two epochs encompassing stimulus onset were graphed, an attempt was made to relate the mode of HR response to behavioral and EEG state ratings (Table 4) as well as to the

Table 4. Prestimulus State Ratings Associated with Selected Decelerative Responses (Figure 14)

Trial No.	Behavior		EEG	
	Prestimulus State Ratings			
1	Awake-quiet	(IV)[a]	Awake-quiet	(IV)
2	Sleep	(II)	Doze	(III)
3	Doze	(III)	Doze	(III)
5	Doze	(III)	Doze	(III)
13	Awake-quiet	(IV)	Awake-quiet	(IV)
20	Sleep	(I)	Sleep	(II)

[a]Roman numerals in parentheses with each descriptor refer to Bioacoustic Laboratory codes; they are shown here merely to indicate that correspondence among behavioral and EEG state ratings is not as exact as verbal labels might suggest. State classifications, whether verbal or numerical, are based upon commonly accepted criteria.

kinds of behavioral and brain wave changes observed. From this analysis and from similar efforts with additional subjects, it can be said with some certainty that, whatever the prestimulus HR, purely decelerative cardiac responses are as likely to be found during sleep states as they are during wakeful ones. Although they tend most frequently to be associated with cortical arousal (K-complex-like activity), either localized or diffuse, they appear also in relation to EEG flattening, responsive motor activity, and even (although rarely) no response. There are suggestions, however, that decelerative HR changes bear upon attentive mechanisms, even in earliest life. In the infant considered here, 8 out of 13 trials associated with clearly detectible HR decrement, whether of shorter or longer duration, were classified as OQ behavior of one kind or another, while the remaining 5 were scored under various categories of arousal.

The cardiac properties of synthetic speech sounds obviously cannot be defined operationally with any real precision on the basis of the limited data thus far derived from a preliminary experiment. However, study of responses to the "probe" stimulus used in this study does permit certain general statements bearing upon the organization of auditory mechanisms.

First, for all age groups, including newborns, reliable HR responses to a schedule of 30 trials with a prolonged, steady-state synthetic vowel of 60 dB can be found at least 70% of the time.

Second, the predominant change in the HR pattern is a prolonged deceleration of considerable magnitude (Table 5 and Figure 15). In infants, single-trial changes may be well in excess of 20 beats and persist for periods in excess of 6 sec; in adults, single-trial changes may be in excess of 10 beats.

Table 5. Correlative Data Showing Behavioral and EEG Scores Associated with the Cardiac Response Patterns Shown in Figure 15 (A, B, and C)

| Trial No. | Index | Indicator | |
		Overt Behavior	EEG
1 (A)	State	III (Doze)	III (Doze)
	Response	Finger movement	K-complex (1 lead)
15 (B)	State	III (doze)	III (Doze)
	Response	Visual and Motor arousal	K-complex (all leads)
30 (C)	State	II (Irregular sleep)	III (Doze)
	Response	Undifferentiated attentive behavior	K-complex (2 leads)

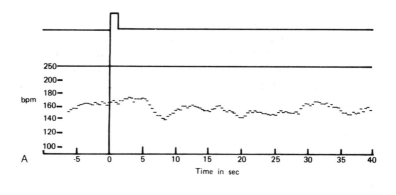

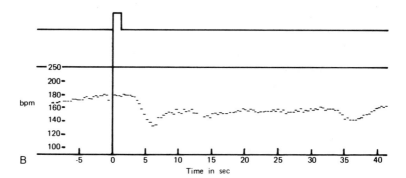

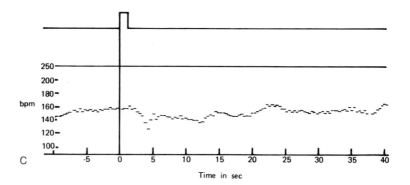

Figure 15. Cardiotachometer strip chart tracings of three selected trials with a 60-dB synthetic vowel ("ah") in one 13-day-old control infant. HR levels in bpm are shown on the *ordinate* while the *abscissa* represents time in seconds over a 40-msec epoch commencing at stimulus onset minus 5 sec. The grpahs show, in descending order, trials 1(*a*), 15(*b*), and 30(*c*); behavioral and EEG scores associated with each are shown in Table 5.

Third, since neither age nor state of arousal seemed to exert significant effects upon mode of response to the "probe" stimulus used in this experiment, the critical determinant of the responsive bradycardia observed here probably relates to the physical properties of the signal. This finding assumes considerable theoretical importance in view of recent data (Newman and Symmes, 1974b) showing the existence, in monkey auditory cortex, of selective "vocalization detector cells" that are independent of arousal level.

Fourth, although latency to peak magnitude of response varies greatly both within and among subjects, such latencies tend to substantially exceed values reported in the literature for other kinds of signals. In infants under the age of about 2 months, peak magnitude most often is found 6 or more sec after stimulus onset.

Heart Rate as a Clue to Central Processes

Discussion of HR work at the Bioacoustic Laboratory thus far has centered on what might be considered "static" measures of hearing, that is, measures relating to the existence of response events during selected periods of time associated with signal presentation. Now, however, a complementary approach will be considered whereby the existence of discrete response events becomes irrelevant and changes in cardiac dynamics over time become both an implicit measure of hearing and an index of individual differences among subjects (Eisenberg, 1974b and 1975b; and Eisenberg, Marmarou, and Giovachino, 1974b). In this frame of reference, the questions at issue are similar to those posed in habituation studies. First, does monotonous stimulation exert systematic effects upon state, as measured by HR? Second, does the nature of these effects differentiate among subjects according to age, neurologic status, or other factors? The major difference between this study and that described in Chapter 4 (under the heading, "The Effects of Monotonous Stimulation with an Acoustic Pattern") is that the conditions of the experiment (a prolonged ISI and a restricted number of trials) are designed to maintain response rather than to abolish it.

The approach toward defining a dynamic curve represents an adaptation of Bioacoustic Laboratory procedures discussed in Chapter 2. Briefly, just as "state" is assumed to constitute a measure of equilibrium in interconnected systems governing overt behavior, the distribution of heart rates over time can be assumed to constitute a measure of equilibrium in systems governing cardiac behavior. Under these conditions, the lowest and highest rates found for any individual subject define the boundary limits within which internal equilibrium can be graded, and all that is required is some set of descriptors equivalent to the "basal" and "activity state" measures used in behavioral study. Such descriptors can be derived by histogram analyses of HR distributions during "sound" and "no sound" periods.

In the procedures to be considered here, the distribution of heart rates over the course of the experimental run was obtained by eliminating 300 msec of information at the beginning and end of each subject tape and segmenting the remaining continuous data into 90-sec epochs that could be treated efficiently by computer. Under these conditions, each experiment yielded 36 histograms covering a period commencing 2.7 min before the first acoustic stimulus and ending 2.7 min after the final trial.

Steady-state, or basal, equilibrium was defined by HR distributions during the rest periods preceding and following presentation of the acoustic schedule (three 90-sec histograms each).

Stimulus-bound, or dynamic, equilibrium was defined on a trial by trial basis, according to 30 individual histograms for 90 sec of real time encompassing stimulus onset, or T_0 (T_0 - 30 sec through T_0 + 60 sec).

At this writing, computer analysis of these data is still in its early stages and it is impossible to report fully on the findings. However, the experimental questions posed at the beginning of this section have been approached on a preliminary basis by selecting two infants and two adults as "prototypes" and subjecting their individual histogram printouts to manual treatments. The nature of such treatments and the results gleaned from them are discussed below with reference to Figure 16.

In order to compress the mass of 120 stimulus-bound histograms for report purposes, each of the thirty 90-sec printouts for each of the 4 subjects was reduced to a set of 5 percentile points, referable to individual HR ranges. It was assumed, since the 90-sec histograms contain values that refer in unequal part to intervals associated with and remote from stimulus presentation, and since responses to a synthetic speech sound tend to be mainly decelerative, that the most representative region for examining cardiac dynamics was that lying between the 25th and 87th percentiles. Thus, the lower boundary of the cardiac range was defined as that heart rate below which 25% of the HR values fell; the higher boundary as that above which 12.5% of the HR values fell; and the intervening points (50, 62.5, and 75% respectively) were included to provide some slight degree of refinement. Then, to compress the data still further, the 30 trials per subject were segmented into 6 consecutive 5-trial blocks and the mean HR value for each block was plotted. Figure 16, then, is designed to yield data on whether and how sequential stimulation affects cardiac dynamics, and it affords a number of provocative trends.

First of all, it is immediately apparent that cardiac boundaries change over trials and, for three out of four subjects, in much the same way—that

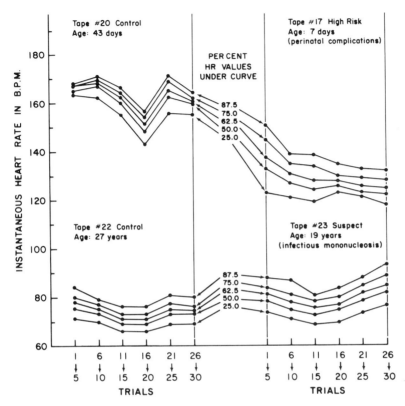

Figure 16. Heart rate change as a function of regular stimulation with the conversationally-loud synthetic vowel "ah" (from Eisenberg, Marmarou, and Giovachino, 1974*b*).

is, HR levels tend to fall during middle trials (11–20) and then to return toward the initial range. It is difficult to evaluate the significance of this trend in terms of such time-dependent phenomena as anticipation[18] or habituation until computer procedures for dealing separately with response and no response epochs (Eisenberg, 1975*b*) have been implemented, but the trend unquestionably is real: analysis of the correlative behavioral and EEG state ratings yields essentially the same results.

Second, the normal infant, despite differences in cardiac function that are reflected in higher HR levels and greater lability over time, behaves

---

[18] Even the most cursory visual inspection of data from this experiment makes it clear that for all age groups, including newborns, temporal conditioning takes place within as few as five trials. This finding, evident by all measures, was totally unexpected: it was assumed, on the basis of considerable pilot work with tonal sequences and other kinds of patterned signals (Eisenberg, 1970*a* and 1970*b*), that time-dependent phenomena of this sort would be precluded by the use of a 90-sec ISI.

very similarly to the normal adult. It seems likely, therefore, that similar control mechanisms in the nervous system, which presumably relate to attentive behavior, are operating in both age groups.

Third, since the high-risk infant is the only subject to show a systematic decline in HR over trials, it seems possible that measures of cardiac dynamics under defined stimulus conditions ultimately may afford important diagnostic information. There is no reason to suppose that the trend seen in Figure 16 relates to age since eyeballed data on control infants in the age range between 28 hr and 11 days shows them to behave much like the 43-day-old infant illustrated here.

The significance of differences between the control and suspect adults cannot be evaluated adequately at this time.[19] However, the tendency toward a wider dynamic range and increased HR lability is of some interest because similar trends have been noted for the few suspect infants on whom 90-sec interval histogram printouts are currently available.

Although basal data could not be analyzed in depth for purposes of considering them in this volume, they were examined on a preliminary basis and there is no evidence for systematic changes in HR during either pre- or poststimulation runs. For both infants and adults, cardiac patterns appear fairly stable during these "no sound" periods. Therefore, whether or not the notion is accepted that dynamic measures bear upon attentive mechanisms and/or the neurologic integrity of subjects, the fact that heart rates and correlative indicators seem to change systematically under conditions of regular stimulation has important implications for the design of study procedures that might prove useful with uncooperative subjects of any age. Unless we are unreasonably willing to assume that systematic changes over time can occur in the absence of sensation, we must reasonably assume that the dynamic curve associated with a train of signals constitutes an implicit measure of hearing. Such a measure conceivably could tell us as much about auditory function as threshold determinations, and it certainly could tell us something different.

Given these preliminary findings and related data on habituation (Eisenberg, Coursin, and Rupp, 1966; Graham, 1973; Graham and Jackson, 1970; and Kessen, Haith, and Salapatek, 1970), it seems evident that sensory evoked changes in physiologic equilibrium over time, however measured, can provide useful information on individual differences. However, since the functional curves obtained under conditions where response is   maintained   seem   relatively   independent   of   developmental

---

[19] This particular suspect adult was included for study because of temporary nervous system dysfunction associated with severe infectious mononucleosis and, unfortunately, data derived from a postrecovery follow-up run have not been treated at this writing.

status, it seems possible that the predictive potential of procedures similar to those considered here may be greater than that for habituation measures.

ELECTROENCEPHALOGRAPHIC RESPONSES

In including EEG measures in this experiment, the purposes were frankly exploratory—that is, we were concerned mainly with assuring that procedures contemplated for a more definitive future study would be productive. It was recognized at the outset that data on the form of the AER to a synthetic speech sound could be regarded only as preliminary and they are presented here in that light.

In studying the EEG data, we relied both on visual inspection of individual strip chart recordings and on electronic averaging (Eisenberg, Marmarou, and Giovachino, 1974c). Visual inspection provided indices of state (Anders, Emde, and Parmalee, 1971; and Rechtschaffen and Kales, 1968) and signal potency as well as the relative distribution of wave form events commonly classified as K-complexes and flattening (desynchronization). Averaging, using a Mnemotron Computer of Average Transients (CAT, model 400B) in conjunction with an X-Y plotter (Houston, model 2000), provided information on variability across trials as well as the basic data from which time and magnitude characteristics of the AER could be extracted. As noted earlier, data from frontal, central, and temporal derivations were stored on tape for off-line analysis.

Information on variability over time was derived by averaging data in cumulative blocks and also in independent blocks of varying size. Thus, trials first were accumulated in groups of 5 (1–5, 1–10 . . . 1–30) and then considered further in subgroups: trials 1–5 were compared with 6–10, 11–15, and so on; trials 1–10 were compared with 11–20 and 21–30; and trials 1–15 with 16–30. Similarly, information relative to the effects of arousal level was derived by averaging subgroups of trials according to prestimulus ratings.

In order to consider both *on* and *off* effects in analysis, CAT data were collected during 2-sec epochs. For stimulus-bound activity, the onset of averaging was triggered by the leading edge of the signal so that each plot covered 840 msec of *off* time in addition to the 1.16 sec of *on* time. Nonstimulus data were collected during 2 sec of "catch trial" time beginning approximately 30 sec prior to stimulus onset.[20]

---

[20] Obviously, it would have been preferable to collect nonstimulus data from the 2 sec immediately prior to stimulus onset, but we were not technically equipped to do so at the time this study was undertaken.

Because of the masses of data generated, statistical analysis was under-taken only on 30-trial data blocks. For each subject and each lead, amplitude values were obtained by sampling the pertinent graphs every 25 msec. Zero amplitude was set arbitrarily at the lowest point in each plot and then, as in HR work, the K-S test was used to examine differences between stimulus-bound and catch-trial data during selected 500-msec epochs. Furthermore, to evaluate the stability of brain wave activity during ISIs, contiguous 500-msec epochs of the catch trial data were compared with each other.

The AER as an Index of Auditory Processes

At this writing, data on 29 control subjects have been treated in the manner outlined above and they strongly suggest that patterned sounds are extremely potent at all stages of development. Individual responses to the probe stimulus used in this experiment were so easily detectible by visual inspection of strip chart recordings that response ratios almost uniformly exceeded 70%. Based solely on amplitude distributions during the initial 500-msec epochs of stimulus-bound and catch-trial data, statistically significant values were obtained in all cases. The statistical evidence is revealing not only because the K-S two tail test is a stiff one, but also because significant results easily might have been vitiated by untoward experimental factors. For instance, subjects were studied under any and all conditions of sleep or wakefulness; movements were not restricted in any way; and artifact trials were not excluded.

Certain general characteristics of the AER to a synthetic vowel can be gleaned from Figure 17. This shows temporal, central, and frontal lead data on four control subjects, two 13-day-old infants (the left-hand graphs) and two young adults (on the right). Each graph represents 2 sec of average brain wave activity beginning with stimulus onset, or T_0.

The probability (by K-S testing) that these wave forms reflect reponse is 0.01 or better, but even cursory inspection of these 30-trial averages suggests the existence of response activity. For a given subject, the form of the AER during the first 500 msec of on time seems to be reasonably specific. For subject pairs, the individual differences, which partly reflect differences in state, fail to mask commonalities among leads and within age groups.

Examining these graphs in detail, certain interesting trends emerge. First, despite individual differences, the infants look remarkably like each other in the first half second or so following stimulus onset, while the adults showed fewer similarities. This suggests, at least as a tentative hypothesis, that, for experiments involving neither tasks nor contingencies, the experienced and well-organized adult may be a less productive source

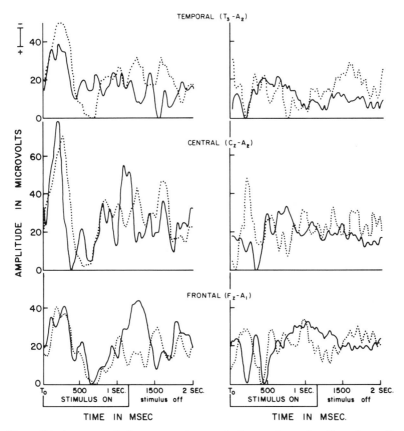

Figure 17. Average evoked responses to a synthetic vowel as a function of age. $N =$ 30 trials. The *solid* and *dotted lines* in each plot differentiate individual subjects, with two 13-day-old infants shown on the *left* and two 21-year-old adults shown on the *right*. Amplitude values for each subject were obtained by sampling 2-sec epochs for each of the three leads at 25-msec intervals. Zero amplitude was set arbitrarily at the lowest point in each CAT plot (from Eisenberg, Marmarou, and Giovachino, 1974c).

of information on auditory processing mechanisms than the infant. Second, differences among leads are smaller than might be expected, particularly in the case of infants. This suggests that speechlike signals may be processed in some relatively specific fashion. Third, two components of the infant AER, although very late in comparison with adult patterns, are readily discernible from 30-trial averages. This supports other evidence that speechlike signals are prepotent in early life. Fourth, amplitude of the major component, usually labeled N_1-P_2, does not seem to increase with age. Indeed, it seems larger during infancy than during later life, an indication that contrasts sharply with data on the effects of clicks, tone pips, and other constant signals. Aside from any implications for the organization of auditory mechanisms, this suggests that amplitude may not be an especially good index of maturational changes in the AER.

In terms of the organization of auditory mechanisms, magnitude and latency of the N_1-P_2 component, as indicated by this experiment, are important insofar as they support a notion that speechlike signals may be processed at relatively high levels of the eighth nerve system (Eisenberg, 1970*b*, 1974, and 1975*a*; Eisenberg et al., 1974*c*). Certainly, the values derived thus far seem substantially in excess of any reported in the literature for constant signals (Regan, 1972; Reneau and Hnatiow, 1975). Tables 6 and 7 summarize what data we are able to group at this writing.

Table 6. Estimated Time and Magnitude of Components of Evoked Potentials for a 60-dB Synthetic Vowel ("ah")

	Age Groups		
Components by Lead	Infants under 1 mo. (*N* = 6)	11 yr. (*N* = 2)	Adults (*N* = 6)
Temporal $(T_3-A_2)^a$			
N_1	125–225	150–175	125
P_2	500–650	475–500	375
N_2	625–825	650–725	500
P_3	675–875	775–800	575
Mean[b]	41	53	32
Range	29–59	31–76	22–43
Central $(C_z-A_2)^a$			
N_1	100–275	150	100–125
P_2	375–550	450–500	325–425
N_2	625–800	675–700	475–525
P_3	750–800	775–800	550–625
Mean[b]	51	67	38
Range	21–82	40–94	32–49
Frontal $(F_z-A_1)^a$			
N_1	175–300	175	100–125
P_2	550–675	500–550	375–450
N_2	650–775	700–750	550–625
P_3	775–825	725–775	600–700
Mean[b]	38	53	39
Range	29–48	26–81	32–51

[a]Latency range in milliseconds.
[b]Amplitude mean and range in μvolts for major AER components (N_1–P_2).

Table 7. Comparative Data on Latency and Magnitude of AER Components during Early Infancy

Constant Signals	Suzuki and Taguchi (1968)	Weitzman and Graziani (1968)	Akiyama et al. (1969)	Engel and Young (1969)	Taguchi et al. (1969)	Lentz and McCandless (1971)	Ohlrich and Barnet (1972)	Bioacoustic Laboratory Data[a] (1969 to Date)
Latency (msec)								
P_1	$60-80^b$	$68-80^b$	64 ± 37^c	182 ± 57^c			63 ± 10^c	$100-275^b$
N_1	$110-210^b$	$70-177^b$	124 ± 42^c	226 ± 26^c		$70-150^b$	92 ± 17^c	$375-550^b$
P_2	$190-340^b$	$163-328^b$	221 ± 79^c			$175-500^b$	220 ± 35^c	$625-800^b$
N_2	$300-690^b$	$349-550^b$	500 ± 110^c		$250-305^b$		470 ± 68^c	$750-800^b$
P_3	$730-860^b$		$>880^b$		$450-650^b$		678 ± 128^c	
Amplitude of Components (μv)								
$P_1 N_1$	36 ± 8^c	$2-11^b$					2 ± 1^c	$\overline{X}(N_1 \rightarrow P_2) = 51$ (Range = 21–82)
$N_1 P_2$		$5-28^b$		18 ± 8^c			13 ± 2^c	
$P_2 N_2$		$6-29^b$			$6-39^b$		23 ± 8^c	
$N_2 P_3$							9 ± 6^c	

[a]Synthetic vowel.
[b]Data presented as range.
[c]Data presented as mean and standard deviation.

Table 6, which considers all three of the electrode placements employed, shows trends for magnitude and latency of various AER components in a small number of subjects at different stages of development. Table 7, which considers only the vertex derivation used by most investigators, compares Bioacoustic Laboratory data on 17 infants under 1 month of age with findings reported by others. To permit such comparison, tradition was followed and the first large positive deflection was labeled P_2.

Whether the apparently increased magnitude of response to this particular synthetic vowel reflects nothing more than the generally enhancing methods employed in this experiment—that is, the use of (1) a sound field rather than earphones (Butler, Keidel, and Spreng, 1969); (2) a fixed schedule conducive to expectancy (Sutton et al., 1967); and (3) a long ISI (Davis et al., 1966; and Roth and Kopell, 1969)—seems doubtful since, much of the time, subjects were in what usually are considered poor states for study. Certainly, these limited data do not permit conclusions, but given a trend that is consistent across the study population and no evidence to the contrary, it may well be that increased magnitude of response relates to the functional properties of speechlike signals.

We are still very far from defining these properties adequately or determining exactly how they vary during the course of development. However, by exploring them in young adults, we are trying to establish a kind of "template" that may tell us what to look for at various stages of maturation. Figure 18, then, is presented in that light. It derives from one 21-year-old control subject and shows three sets of CAT averaged 5-trial blocks for each of the three leads employed.

As can be seen, the wave form here, unlike the right-hand graphs in Figure 17, is quite consistent across trials and among leads. It would appear to meet Vaughn's criteria for a class III evoked potential, that is, one "elicited only when the stimulus carries information of significance for the organism" (Donshin and Lindsley, 1969; p. 47). Moreover, in sleeping and waking trials alike, peak latencies, except for the somewhat inconsistent early components, are in line with those reported by Celesia and his co-workers (Celesia et al., 1968; and Celesia and Puletti, 1969) for click-evoked cortical responses in the region of the superior temporal gyrus.

The data shown in Figure 18 provide some index of the discriminative information lost when a relatively small number of trials is averaged without reference to state variables. In waking trials (1–5 and 26–30), for instance, only those components commonly termed "early" and "late" are clearly discernible. In sleeping trials (16–20), however, the so-called "secondary potentials" beyond 300 msec are outstanding in all leads. Furthermore, these state-related effects, which are much the same for all young adults studied in this experiment ($N = 8$) are at variance with

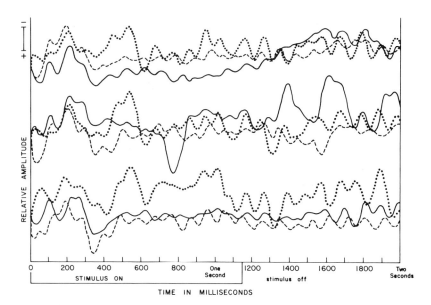

Figure 18. Average evoked responses to a synthetic "ah" sound as a function of state. Plots represent, in descending order, temporal (T$_3$-A$_2$), central (Cz-A$_2$), and frontal (Fz-A$_1$) leads. Average values derived from waking state data are shown as ———— (trials 1–5) and - - - - - (trials 26–30); sleeping trials (16–20) are indicated by the *dotted lines* (••••••) in each data set (from Eisenberg, Marmarou, and Giovachino, 1974c).

reports on responses to pure tones (Cody, Klass, and Bickford, 1967): they are manifest, even in the central lead, not as a change in latency, but rather as a change in wave form. Thus, as in the case of the correlative HR data discussed earlier, it would seem that differential state effects may be one special property of speechlike signals.

The limited EEG data considered here clearly raise more questions than they answer. Nonetheless, it is useful to summarize some of the salient indications that have relevance for new approaches to EEG studies in hearing.

First, statistically significant AERs to a 30-trial schedule of conversationally-loud synthetic vowel signals were obtained in all normal subjects studied, regardless of age, state of arousal, or movement artifacts.

Second, given a potent signal such as a synthetic vowel, it seems evident that the vertex placement commonly employed is not the only useful electrode derivation. The T$_3$-A$_2$ placement used in this investigation, which has the virtue of greater specificity, yielded good-sized evoked responses at all stages of development and, in adult life, the wave form showed some superficial differences, at least in the after discharge area, from patterns seen in other leads.

Third, latency and magnitude characteristics of major response components that could be discerned in all age groups seem to be substantially in excess of most values reported for constant signals.

Fourth, and not surprisingly (Nash, 1970), responses from the frontal lead were least well defined in infant subjects. Perhaps for this very reason, frontal derivations eventually may provide useful clues to maturational processes in hearing. In any event, since frontal lobe lesions have been implicated in "auditory inattention" (Heilman et al., 1971; and Heilman and Valenstein, 1972a and b), information on responses from this region may attain diagnostic significance.

Fifth, a systematic decrease in latency with increasing maturity was clearly evident, a finding which is in accord with other indications in the literature. However, when selected infant responses were segregated by state, the N_1 peak far more closely approximated adult values than did later components.

Sixth, insofar as these preliminary data constitute a valid index, the AER to a synthetic vowel seems to differ from the wave form associated with clicks, tone pips, and other constant signals in respects other than those already discussed: amplitude of the major component seems to show no systematic decrease with age; P_3, which rarely characterizes the evoked response to constant signals during early infancy (Ohlrich and Barnet, 1972), was discerned readily in three out of four 25-day-old subjects.

Finally, there are suggestions that the processing of relatively long signal durations may differ with age: infants tended to show *off* effects during any or all trials throughout a schedule whereas adult subjects tended to show such effects only during initial trials. In line with this, there are indications that the demonstration of *off* effects may vary according to electrode placements. It is tempting, then, to speculate that these differences may relate in part to developmental changes in the capacity to code duration as an independent dimension. That is, the adult, having once ascertained internally that the stimulus is contained within some fixed interval, no longer responds to its disappearance, while the infant, who seemingly cannot make this determination, continues to process the change from sound to no sound.

All things considered, there is every reason to suppose that wider exploration of the AER to synthetic speech sounds should yield a great deal of useful information for application to both clinical and research problems.

Part III RECENT ADVANCES AND FUTURE DIRECTIONS IN DEVELOPMENTAL STUDIES OF AUDITION

CHAPTER 6
Recent Advances in The Study of Auditory Competence During Early Life

"The raw material of every science must always be an accumulation of facts. . . ."
  Sir James Jeans, *Physics and Philosophy* (1943)

The inquiries considered in the previous section constitute only a portion of the work undertaken at the Bioacoustic Laboratory over the years, and the purpose of detailing them has been to provide a context in which the problems and promise of auditory work with infants could be evaluated. From a practical standpoint, they illustrate how logical methods of procedure can apply to diverse study objectives. From a theoretical standpoint, they afford a perspective on the directions infant studies in audition have taken within the past decade or so.

Both at this laboratory and elsewhere, research has increased markedly in sophistication. Investigators have progressed from the use of abstract signals such as pure tones to the use of multidimensional signals and speechlike sounds. If too few audiologists have progressed from asking *whether* infants hear to asking *how* they hear (Eisenberg, 1971, 1972, 1975a, and 1975b; and Stark, 1974), a good many psychologists and linguists have begun to question long accepted ideas about the determinants of verbal communication (Kavanagh and Cutting, in press; Morse and Snowdon, 1975). These changing patterns of research, which are reflected in the contents of Appendix B, have yielded a body of new information bearing upon the organization of auditory mechanisms.

It now seems fairly well established that most newborns, including premature infants and those with known abnormalities of the CNS (Barnet, Bazelon, and Zappella, 1966; Brackbill, 1971a; Eisenberg, 1970a and 1970b; Eisenberg et al., 1964; and Eisenberg, Coursin, and Rupp, 1966; Field et al., 1967; and Schulman, 1973), can discriminate sound on the basis of numerous acoustic variables. Seven parameters, having varying degrees of importance for the decoding of language signals, have been explored as follows: (1) band width, or the frequency content of a stimulus envelope; (2) duration, or the total amount of time consumed by a stimulus; (3) frequency, in Hertz, or the number of sine wave repetitions per second in a pure tone signal; (4) repetition rate, or the number of *on* events per second in a given intermittent signal; (5) rise and decay time, or the interval required for any given acoustic signal to reach or decline from its steady-state intensity; (6) sound pressure level, or physical intensity in decibels with reference to acoustic zero (0.0002 μbar); and (7) dimensionality, or the kind and amount of variance within a complex stimulus envelope.

Dimensionality is an umbrella term covering parameter interactions that can vary according to the kinds of patterned stimuli employed, and it becomes a parameter in itself simply because patterned stimuli, as a class, have functional properties different from those associated with constant signals. Some of these properties already have been discussed in Part II, and they will be considered further in relation to data on the effects of speechlike sounds and other complex stimuli. The other six parameters listed above exert differential effects on the incidence, mode, and intensity of stimulus-bound behavior whether an infant is awake or asleep. Moreover, some aspects of that behavior have correlates in hearing functions of later life (Eisenberg, 1966b, 1967, 1970b, 1974a, and 1975a).

This chapter attempts to synthesize current information. Reasonably definitive data on the hearing of newborns and infants are reviewed. The findings are related to additional Bioacoustic Laboratory data and to correlative information on the hearing of adult humans and lower animals. The implications of the data are related to the organizational principles discussed in Chapter 3.

THE EFFECTS OF DISCRETE PARAMETER VARIABLES

As can be determined from Appendix B, few of the parameters listed have been studied extensively and some of them barely have been approached (Kavanagh, 1971). Furthermore, since only a handful of the inquiries undertaken were designed to yield information on operations in the eighth nerve system, many of the data are difficult to interpret. Therefore, the only experimental results to be discussed in this section are those that cast some amount of light either on the nature of developmental auditory processes or on the ways in which they can be measured.

Band Width

As long ago as 1946, Froeschels and Beebe remarked that pure tones were less effective than noisebands in evoking infant responses to sound, and recent inquiries (Eisenberg, 1965a and 1970b; Hutt et al., 1968a; Lenard, v. Bernuth, and Hutt, 1969; Lenard, v. Bernuth, and Prechtl, 1968; Ling, Ling, and Doehring, 1970; Mendel, 1968; Miller, 1971; and Turkewitz, Birch, and Cooper, 1972a and 1972b) have served only to confirm this early observation. Hutt et al. (1968b) found that square wave stimuli were far more effective in eliciting neonatal electromyographic responses to sound than were pure tones. Lenard, v. Bernuth, and Hutt (1969), who obtained clear-cut evoked potentials to white noise and square wave stimuli, but no reliable AERs to pure tones, found amplitude of the N_2 component to increase more or less systematically with band width. Turkewitz, Birch, and Cooper (1972a), who studied the effects of wide-band noise (50–10,000 Hz) and pure tones at the octave intervals between 250 and 8,000 Hz, found that newborns showed reliable behavioral and cardiac responses to the noise, but not to the sine wave signals. Hoversten and Moncur (1969), who used voice and musical sounds in addition to noisebands, found white noise to be a far more effective stimulus for 3- to 8-month-old-infants than interrupted pure tones. Mendel (1968), who studied the effects of band-limited noises and warbled tones on infants of 4–11 months, found a fairly systematic relation between signal band width and overt responsivity.

Bioacoustic Laboratory studies employing matched conditions (Eisenberg, 1965a) have shown pure tones in the speech-frequency range (500–2,000 Hz) to be comparatively less effective than 200-cycle-or-wider bands centered about the discrete frequencies. However, as noted in Chapter 4, other variables seem to assume major importance as frequency content of a stimulus envelope is increased beyond 200 Hz. Therefore, it is doubtful whether band width per se can be considered a *critical* determinant of auditory function during early life (Eisenberg, 1965a).

Duration

Everything now known about the physical structure of spoken language and acoustic coding in the nervous system indicates that duration, particularly in the short-time range, is a critical determinant of auditory function (Andreeva, Kratin, and Kurbanov, 1972; Gersuni, 1971; Jeffress, 1964; Nabelik and Hirsh, 1969; and Tallal, 1974). Differentiation of speech cues depends upon the perception of acoustic variations that occur within very short intervals, and the duration of these intervals determines the manner of processing in underlying systems (Hirsh, 1974). Acoustic variations occurring within intervals of 20–25 msec are processed as single events (Stevens and Klatt, 1974; and Wood, 1973, 1974, and in press), while sounds separated from each other by longer intervals than this are processed as successive events (Hirsh, 1959; and Hirsh and Sherrick, 1961). The preservation of temporal patterning seems to be crucial for the recognition of both melodic sequences (Dowling, 1967 and 1972) and verbal ones (Pinheiro, 1973). There is mounting evidence that problems in the processing of transients may underlie some developmental disorders of communication (Tallal, 1974; Tallal and Piercy, 1973a, 1973b, and 1974). Unfortunately, duration in the short-time range has been grossly neglected in developmental studies, probably because it poses so many problems: there are no physiologic data on conduction rates, refractory times, or energy integration in the auditory system during human infancy. Duration in the long-time range has received somewhat more attention, mainly with reference to clinical objectives.

Between the 1930's, when there was a brief flurry of work at the Iowa Child Welfare Station (Haller, 1932; and Stubbs, 1934), and the mid-1960's, the literature is almost completely devoid of reports on the effects of duration during early life. Indeed, the only suggestive information available when the Bioacoustic Laboratory program was initiated was Stubb's report (1934) that the incidence of neonatal response to pure tones increased quite systematically as duration was increased between 1 and 5 sec and less systematically as it was increased further. Although a few studies have been undertaken in the years since then, the results contribute very little to an understanding of auditory processing during infancy.

Keen and her co-workers (Keen, 1964; and Keen, Chase, and Graham, 1965) noted that 10-sec signals were more effective than 2-sec ones in eliciting changed patterns of neonatal sucking. Clifton, Graham, and Hatton (1968) found the newborn's acceleratory HR response to square wave stimuli in a range of durations between 2 and 30 sec to be an inverted U function of duration, with a 10-sec signal evoking maximum responsivity. Ling (1972a), who found 50-msec bursts of 90-dB tones to be associated with very low response ratios and few neonatal behaviors other than eye blinks, concluded that such short signals were "less than optimal" for application to infant screening procedures. In a follow-up inquiry (Ling, 1972b), employing 1/3-octave band noises centering on selected frequencies and four conditions of duration between 50 msec and 1 sec, Ling found that the number of whole-body responses increased dramatically at longer durations. However, the incidence of these responses was markedly less than that associated with 3-sec stimuli (Ling, Ling, and Doehring, 1970). Collyer, Bench, and Wilson (1974), who examined the effects of even longer noisebands (5–60 sec), found no significant effects related to duration, while Turkewitz, Birch, and Cooper (1972b), who used correlative HR and behavioral indices to measure neonatal responsivity to a 2,000-Hz pure tone at 4 durations (1, 2, 4, and 8 sec), found the signal to elicit no statistically reliable responses at any duration.

Studies at the Bioacoustic Laboratory (Eisenberg, 1965a) have shown that the incidence of response to pure tones and noisebands increases more or less directly with duration in the range between 300 msec and 5 sec. Contrary to Ling (1972b), it is our feeling that durations of 1 sec or more probably are clinically adequate for most kinds of infant studies employing wide-band signals. Given some of the data cited above, it seems likely that the practical range for pure tone stimuli considerably exceeds this and, provided the use of sine wave signals is considered desirable, further investigation seems indicated.

The time below which trading relations between duration and SPL become demonstrable has not been defined for infants, but given the data reviewed in Chapter 4, it would seem to lie somewhere in the 200-msec range already defined for adult hearers (Eisenberg, 1965a). This is a provocative indication which warrants follow-up under varied stimulus conditions: in adult subjects, 200 msec is the approximate value above which noisiness increases (Kryter, 1966).

Frequency

Frequency is one of the few parameters that has been studied fairly well (Trehub, 1973a), and, consequently, it will be considered in some detail. Findings on neonates derive from a wide variety of independent sources and, with some exceptions that can be related either to the use of unproductive stimulus conditions (Keen, 1964; Keen, Chase, and Graham, 1965; and Ling, Heaney, and Doehring, 1971) or to other factors (Ashton, 1971b; Goodman et al., 1964; Schulman, 1973; and Wormith, Pankhurst, and Moffitt, 1975), the evidence for frequency discrimination during early life is unequivocal. A few useful observations on infants and children are available. There is much psychoacoustic data to which infant findings can be related (Jerger, 1963; and Katz, 1972). The ethologic and physiologic literature is bursting with comparative information on frequency-bound behavior in lower organisms (Busnel, 1963; Hinde, 1970 and 1972; and Sebeok, 1968).

What is important about the data on frequency effects is not so much the quantity of information as the consistency of the experimental results. Despite procedural and other differences of every imaginable kind, reports in the literature uniformly suggest the existence of range-dependent mechanisms for the processing of acoustic information. Indeed, after surveying the literature, one is inclined to believe there is no stage of human development during which low and high frequencies exert similar effects (Pollack, 1968; Rothman, 1970; and Tyberghein and Forrez, 1969). This is not entirely surprising when one considers the material discussed in Chapter 1.

Studies of auditory behavior at various times during the first year of life (Eisenberg, 1970a and 1970b) uniformly suggest: first, that low and high frequencies have differential functional properties; second, that signals in the range of above 4,000 Hz have certain unique properties (see Chapter 4, "The Effects of Calibrated Noisemakers"); and third, that signals in the carrier range for speech are differentially effective. There are even some data on school-age children suggesting that aspects of frequency-detection performance can be improved by training (Soderquist and Moore, 1970).

Findings on infants go back almost to the beginning of the 20th century. Dearborn (1910), who recorded the behavioral responses of a single infant from the 6th through the 67th day of life, concluded that notes in the upper register of the piano keyboard were "disturbing." Haller (1932) found that high-frequency pure tones, which elicited relatively few overt responses, were "more disturbing" for young infants than low-frequency tones. Kasatkin and Levikova (1935), who employed both pure tone and noisemaker signals, showed that infants of 3 months could be conditioned to discriminate frequency differences of one octave. Mukhina-Korotova (1964) found that 6- to 8-month-old children could differentiate between 400 and 900 Hz. Bronshtein et al. (1960), using a conditioned sucking response as their indicator, reported that newborns could discriminate rather finely among sounds of different frequency. Leventhal and Lipsitt (1964), using 10-sec square waves, found that subjects as young as 21 hr could differentiate between signals of 200 and 1,000 Hz. Birns and her colleagues, who studied the relative soothing effects of stimuli, found that 150-Hz tones could be differentiated from 500 Hz tones (Birns et al., 1965) and that low-frequency signals (150 Hz) tended to inhibit infant distress (Birns, 1965). Hutt and co-workers (Hutt and Hutt, 1970; and Hutt et al., 1968a), reporting on the EMG activity associated with sine and square wave stimuli in the frequency range between 70 and 2,000 Hz, noted that signals in the carrier range for speech evoked differential patterns of response. Further, in a related study of EEG responses to these same stimuli (Lenard, v. Bernuth, and Hutt,

1969), amplitude of the N_2 component of the AER (300–500 msec) was found to be larger for a square wave of 125 Hz than for one of 1,000 Hz. Hoversten and Moncur (1969) showed that the 4,000-Hz stimulus used in their study was markedly less potent than other signals at both 3 and 8 months. Bench (1969b; p. 128), discussing relations between frequency and soothing effects during neonatal life, suggested that his experimental evidence best could be explained on the basis of "an innate pitch discrimination or preference." Webster, Steinhardt, and Senter (1972) showed that 7-month-old infants varied in both their responsivity and their patterns of vocal utterance according to the fundamental frequency of selected vowel sounds, higher frequencies being associated with a lower incidence of response.

Briefly, these data support the behavioral findings detailed in Chapter 4, and it can be said with some assurance that almost any index of newborn auditory behavior shows range-dependent frequency effects. Sleeping or waking, signals in the range below 4,000 Hz evoke response two or three times more often than those in the range above 4,000 Hz (see Table 1 and Figure 4). Responses to low frequency signals best can be elicited during doze or light sleep. Responses to high frequency signals best can be elicited during wakeful states. Low frequencies, which are effective inhibitors of infant distress (Birns, 1965; and O'Doherty, 1968), generally evoke gross motor activity. High frequencies, which are associated with relatively shorter cardiac latencies and tend to occasion distress more than to inhibit it (unpublished Bioacoustic Laboratory data), elicit a high proportion of "fixation" responses (Chapter 4; Figures 5 and 6). The behavioral pattern most frequently seen during the first days of life strikingly resembles the "freezing" reactions evoked in lower animals by alarm signals (Busnel, 1963; Harlow and Woolsey, 1965; Hinde, 1970; and Sebeok, 1968). For example, if a high frequency signal happens to be presented when an infant is midway through a spontaneous Moro, one observes a total arrest of movement momentarily, after which the reflex pattern is completed. It is almost as if the stop button of a motion picture projector had been pressed at some particular frame (unpublished Bioacoustic Laboratory data).

These range-dependent frequency differences found in infants have correlates that, later in life, relate to what commonly is termed *affect*. They are reflected in the electrophysiologic responses of adult subjects (Sokolov, 1960), in the acoustical properties of our musical instruments (Roederer, 1973) and alarm signals, in the kinds of sounds we find annoying (Kryter, 1966 and 1968), in the words we use to describe our reactions (Hochberg, 1965), and perhaps even in the ways we store acoustic information (Kincaid and Cooper, 1972; and Wickens, 1970). In summary, whatever the context in which psychologic responses to sound are studied, low frequencies invariably seem to have "good" or pleasurable connotations, and high frequencies seem to have the reverse.

These findings on frequency effects have three very important implications for our thinking about developmental auditory processes. First, they suggest that differential "tuning" to the carrier frequencies of language may be built in during intrauterine life. Second, they suggest that the neonate's unique response to high frequencies may be as much a phylogenetic relic as the Moro reflex (Freedman, 1961; Harlow and Woolsey, 1965; and Prechtl, 1953). Third, they suggest that *qualitative* judgments of sound in adult life, those relating to noisiness, pleasantness, and the like, may have their roots in preadapted mechanisms referable to phylogenetic history.

Repetition Rate and the Effects of Intermittent Signals

Although modulated sounds of one kind or another have been used as stimuli in infant studies (see Appendix B), the effects of differing repetition rates, which might afford information on energy integration and the perception of temporal patterns during early life, have not been studied systematically. The only hint to be found is Eichorn's note (1951) that neonates exposed to "rhythmic" click activity, particularly at "high" repetition rates, show flatter, faster EEG activity in certain leads.

The effects of heartbeat rhythms have been examined by several investigators (Brackbill et al., 1966; Palmqvist, 1975; Roberts and Campbell, 1967; and Tulloch et al., 1964), but Salk's reports (1960, 1961, and 1962) that the overall well-being of neonates can be increased by exposure to the sounds of the human heart have yet to be unequivocally confirmed. This is hardly surprising since the stimuli used in the Salk study were not equated for intensity or other physical variables.

To summarize, there are no really useful data on the effects of repetition rate and most of the findings on modulated tones and noises accord poorly with clinical observations that intermittent sounds tend to be more effective than continuous ones for audiometric testing of the pediatric aged. Berg (1972), seeking to disclose frequency discrimination (1,100 vs. 1,900 Hz) is 15- to 17-week old infants, compared the effects of continuous and pulsed signals at selected frequencies and found pulsed signals to be associated with bradycardia and more resistent to habituation than continuous tones. Birns et al. (1965) found that their low frequency tone exerted soothing effects on neonates when it was continuous but not when it was modulated. Ling (1972b), who used continuous noise as well as 50-msec noise bursts separated by 50-msec intervals, found that the interrupted signals evoked significantly fewer behavioral responses. Sameroff (1970), comparing the effects of continuous and interrupted pure tones on the sucking behavior and respiratory patterns of newborns, came up with very similar results.

Rise and Decay Time

Although it is well recognized that rise and decay times can affect the validity of psychoacoustic data because of the transients generated when signals are switched on and off, systematic studies of these effects during early life have not been undertaken. Goodman et al. (1964), studying the neonatal AER, noted that responsivity to tone pips decreased more or less systematically as rise time was increased. Kearsley (1973), using visual behavior and HR as his indicators, found that the rise time of both noisebands and pure tones was a critical determinant of response patterns. Rapid rise times were associated with what he characterized as defense reflexes (startle, closing of the eyes, and HR acceleration) and slower rise times were associated with what he characterized as orienting responses (opening of the eyes, visual search, and HR deceleration). Berg and his colleagues, using pure tones of 50–90 dB for comparative studies of stimulus-bound cardiac behavior in adults (Hatton, Berg, and Graham, 1970) and 4-month-old infants (Berg, Berg, and Graham, 1971), found rise time to exert differential effects only when the sounds were most intense and subjects were awake. Under these conditions, rapid rise times (3 msec) were associated with acceleration and slow rise times (300 msec) were associated with deceleration. The implications of these data for studies of developmental auditory behavior are obscure since Porges and his colleagues (Arnold and Porges, 1972; and Porges et al., 1971) have reported similar directional HR responses in newborns under conditions where rise and decay time were held constant while very different parameters (duration and ISI) assumed significance.

Sound Pressure Level

Studies of intensity effects in early life, while fewer in number than investigations of frequency, have yielded equally consistent findings. From these findings, it seems possible that *quantititative* responses to sound reflect another historical determinant of human auditory behavior. The data on hearing in early life, like the growing body of information on visual function in infancy (Cohen and Salapatek, 1975), strongly suggest that parameters having to do with our orientation in space are processed in much the same way throughout life.

Before the data on SPL effects are discussed, it must be pointed out that all neonates have what appears to be a conductive "hearing loss" on the order of 35–40 dB. This evidently is not a pathologic condition, but some natural consequence of developmental status, and it disappears within a week or so after birth. Whether it relates to the presence of unresolved mesenchymal tissue in the middle ear (Igarashi, personal communication), to incomplete aeration of the middle ear cavity (Northern and Downs, 1974), or to incomplete development of the tympanic membrane and/or its supporting structures (Keith, personal communication) is not clear at present. In any event, this "loss" factor of 35–40 dB is important because at both the Bioacoustic Laboratory and elsewhere (Engel and Young, 1969; Rapin and Graziani, 1967; Steinschneider et al., 1966; and Taguchi et al., 1969), 35–40 dB is the lowest level at which 2- to 4-day-old infants have been found to show reliable cardiac and EEG responses to sound. By 2 weeks of age, however, these values fall to 10 or 15 dB (unpublished Bioacoustic Laboratory data) and, therefore, it seems likely that auditory sensitivity at birth approximates normal air conduction threshold values for adults (Flanagan, 1965; Katz, 1972; and Licklider, 1951). Changes in the form of sound-evoked potentials during early life (Ohlrich and Barnet, 1972) presumably reflect central changes during maturation (Conel, 1963; and Nash, 1970) rather than significant alterations in eighth nerve mechanisms.

Studies with suprathreshold signals show that SPL exerts a variety of other interesting effects on newborn auditory behavior. The incidence of response to many acoustic stimuli increases directly with intensity (Barrager, 1974; Froeschels and Beebe, 1946; and Kessen et al., 1970), and intense auditory stimuli tend to increase body tension in crying babies (Brazelton, 1962). As indicated in Chapter 4, there is a direct relation between behavioral response ratios and the proportion of motor reactions elicited by constant signals (Eisenberg, 1965a; Eisenberg et al., 1964; Haller, 1932; and Stubbs, 1934). The amplitude of certain components of the sound-evoked potential varies more or less linearly with intensity (Barnet and Goodwin, 1965; Goodman et al., 1964; Rapin and Graziani, 1967; Regan, 1972; Reneau and Hnatiow, 1975; Skinner, 1972; and Thompson and Patterson, 1974).

Studies of the cardiac response to sound almost invariably have shown increasing SPL to be associated with increasing response magnitude and decreasing response latency (Bartoshuk, 1962a; Berg, Berg, and Graham, 1971; Jackson, Kantowitz and Graham, 1971; Lipton, Steinschneider, and Richmond, 1963; and Turkewitz, Birch, and Cooper, 1972a). The magnitude of behavioral, cardiac, and respiratory (Steinschneider, 1968) responses to white noise increases systematically with SPL, and the latency decreases just as systematically with it (Eisenberg, 1965a; and Steinschneider, Lipton, and Richmond, 1966). Bartoshuk (1964) has reported the cardiac intensity function for pure tones above 40 dB to follow the same power low relations that apply to children (Dorfman and Megling, 1966) and adults (Flanagan, 1965; Schneider, Neuringer, and Ramsey, 1972; and Stevens, 1961), although it must be noted that recent attempts to replicate these findings (Morse, 1973) have been unsuccessful.

Taken as a whole, however, these findings on intensity effects have further implications for our thinking on developmental auditory processes. First, neuronal mechanisms for processing intensity may be fully operational at birth. Second, it seems possible that loudness and other so-called "natural dimensions of sound" (Flanagan, 1965) have their roots in preadapted mechanisms referable to species history.

Operationally speaking, optimal intensity for observational studies of newborn auditory behavior lies somewhere in the neighborhood of the 65-dB level Kasatkin (1957) long ago suggested, while reliable electrophysiologic findings usually can be obtained at lower levels (Eisenberg, 1965a). It seems unlikely that these values should be reduced appreciably for studies with older infants (Hoversten and Moncur, 1969), but no systematic inquiries have been undertaken. In any event, given current gaps in our understanding of hearing processes during early life, the use of conversationally-loud levels seems indicated on both theoretical and practical grounds. Aside from adaptive connotations, there are data to suggest that sound localization is most precise within a range of conversationally loud intensities (v. Békésy, 1971).

DIMENSIONALITY AS A
DETERMINANT OF PERCEPTUAL PROCESSES

Whether a signal containing acoustic energy at more than one frequency is perceived as constant or patterned essentially depends upon how that energy is dispersed among the frequencies contained in the stimulus envelope. When the energy is dispersed more or less equally among frequencies, as in the case of pure tones and noisebands (filtered white noise), the signal is perceived as constant. When modulation is introduced so that the dispersion of energy varies over time, the signal is perceived as patterned. However, the kind of pattern perceived depends upon the *structure* of the modulated signal, and alteration along a single dimension cannot change a simple stimulus into one that is highly complex. A pure tone or a noiseband may be transformed into a simple temporal pattern by periodic alterations of intensity, for instance, but it ordinarily cannot be transformed into a musical sound or a phoneme (Kubovy, Cutting, and McGuire, 1974).

Speech Sounds as Multidimensional Signals

In order to interpret current data on infant responses to highly complex, multidimensional signals such as speech sounds, it is important to understand just what synthetic speech sounds simulate and how changes in their physical structure over time serve to convey communicative information. Although some of these matters have been touched upon elsewhere, they are sufficiently complex to warrant repetition.

Distinctive Features of Speech and Speechlike Sounds   Under natural conditions, the production of a CV (consonant-vowel) syllable such as /bæ/ is associated with a series of time-locked acoustic variations (Denes and Pinson, 1963; and Flanagan, 1965). First, there is a very brief burst of high frequency noise (frication) that relates to constriction of the vocal tract at the lips. This is followed by a slightly longer period of silence (aspiration) relating to the build up of air behind this closure. Finally, as the constriction is released and the articulators move toward the configuration required for the steady-state /æ/ portion of the utterance, the acoustic pattern characteristic of /bæ/ is perceived. The consonantal portion of the utterance is an extremely rapid event and, were it prolonged beyond 50 msec or so, the syllable would be perceived as /wæ/ rather than /bæ/. In other words, the nature of the acoustic variations which occur during a transitional period of 50 msec or less, and which determine the nature of the perceived utterance, carry information about both portions of the utterance. This is the phenomenon that has been termed "parallel transmission" (Liberman, 1970).

The variations in time described above, which involve changes among several interacting parameters of sound, best can be understood with reference to representative signals that have been employed in recent experiments with infants. Figure 19 schematizes the salient characteristics of three synthetic speech sounds, /bæ/, /dæ/, and /gæ/; and, for the sake of simplicity, only the second and third formants, which convey information about place of articulation, are shown to be variable.

From the diagram, it can be seen that the formant structure of the three signals differs significantly during the 50-msec transitional period with respect to: (1) the starting frequencies for f2 and f3; (2) the amount of *difference* in frequency between f2 and f3 at onset; (3) the constancy of that difference over time; (4) the direction of frequency change over time; and (5) the rate of frequency change over time. Thus, the ability of a hearer to differentiate among the three syllables can be a function of any or all of five variables, and none of the differences among the syllables will be perceived adequately unless the hearer can code information that is available only within the initial 50-msec period.

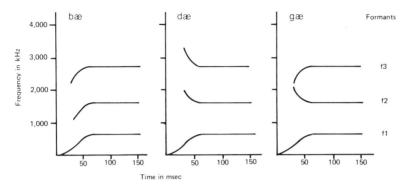

Figure 19. Schematic representation of salient differences among three CV syllables, [bæ], [dæ], and [gæ]. Variations in the second and third formants (f2 and f3, the *upper two bars* in each diagram) during the first 50 msec or so are sufficient for differentiation of the consonants.

Relevance to Current Thinking on Infant Speech Perception It is obvious that most hearers in fact can code short-time acoustic variations of the kind schematized above and, given the physiologic evidence discussed in Chapter 1 as well as recent data showing that fish at least have midbrain "decoders" geared to the recognition of frequency differences (Scheich, 1974), it is entirely reasonable to assume that perception of the speech code depends upon the existence of specialized feature detector neurons or systems (Abbs and Sussman, 1971; Cole and Scott, 1974; Eimas, 1975; Kavanagh and Cutting, in press; Liberman, 1970; Sinnot, 1974; and Stevens, 1973). However, assumptions that such neurons or systems operate in man *only* in the case of speech perception or that they can fully explain speech perception are difficult to justify. Current data on infant performance hardly support such assumptions since few of the experiments undertaken thus far have dealt with isolated stimulus features and none of them has dealt with matched conditions of speech and nonspeech. Moreover, current physiologic evidence supports an alternate assumption (Møller, 1974) that the perception of phonemic distinctions relates to more generally useful mechanisms by which rapid changes in frequency or spectrum are enhanced and slow changes are suppressed. It has been shown, for instance, that for single units in the cochlear nucleus, the *distribution of nerve impulses* changes in characteristic ways as a function of change of rate in frequency (Erulkar, Butler, and Gerstein, 1968; and Møller, 1969 and 1971).

In summary, it seems indisputable that the nervous system must somehow operate to extract critical information from speech signals. However, it seems equally indisputable that what is extracted must somehow be reorganized to arrive at the cortex as a unitary chunk of information which, as some derivative of the peripheral input, can be subjected to linguistic (cognitive) processing.

THE EFFECTS OF MULTIDIMENSIONAL SIGNALS

Studies concerned with the effects of multidimensional signals during early life have taken a variety of forms. Some, directed toward disclosing whether speech, music, or other complex sounds have differential functional properties, have been essentially fishing expeditions in which the stimulus conditions were so complex, so poorly specified, or so poorly matched that the operating variables cannot be isolated. All that can be said with any assurance is that, for normal infants, multidimensional signals, as a class, have different properties from constant signals as a class: when sucking behavior is the indicator, a musical selection can be differentiated from a noise band (Butterfield and Siperstein, 1972) and a vowel sound (Λ) can be differentiated from a pure tone (Shriner, Condron, and Berry, 1973); when vocal activity is the indicator, spoken voice elicits more utterances than music or tonal signals (Lewis et al., 1964); when overt behavior is the indicator, spoken voice elicits more responses at any given intensity level than either music or tonal signals (Hoversten and Moncur, 1969).

Comparative Studies Involving Multidimensional Signals

Few investigators have examined the functional properties of sounds along what might be considered a continuum of dimensionality.

Turkewitz, Birch, and Cooper (1972b), who showed that "independently ineffective" pure tones combined into pairs or triads elicited reliable responses, concluded that their results could be explained on the basis of tonal summation, which they defined as activation of more than one cochlear region. Whether this is a sufficient explanation is at least debatable.

Hutt and co-workers (Hutt et al., 1968a; and Lenard, v. Bernuth, and Hutt, 1969), reporting on the electrophysiologic activity evoked by fixed intensity (70 dB) sine waves, square waves, and word tokens ("baby"), noted that the form of the word-evoked response was differential only when the comparison signals lay in the frequency range above 250 Hz. These findings were taken to support a conclusion that the structure of the stimulating signal was a more important determinant of response activity than was the amount of energy contained in the signal.

Trehub (1973a and 1973b), using dishabituation of the sucking response to study the effects of seven variously complex stimulus conditions, found that infants between 1 and 4 months of age seemingly could not differentiate among pure tones and square waves on the basis of frequency, although they did differentiate among isolated vowels and CV syllables involving frequency contrasts. Commenting upon these discrepant findings and some of the equivocal data on frequency effects in early life (Kessen, Haith, and Salapatek, 1970), she makes the very important point (Trehub, 1973b; p. 94) that "recovery of sucking to a novel stimulus" (may be) "a relatively gross measure which is not" (equally) "sensitive to stimuli of greater or lesser discriminability."

Anderson (1973), in an imaginative doctoral dissertation, used a habituation paradigm to determine the effects of dimensionality upon amplitude of the AER in wakeful infants of 14–18 weeks. With the active electrode placed at a point between C_z and C_3, the babies were subjected to three sounds of graded complexity: (1) a shaped noiseband encompassing the frequencies between 125 and 3,500 Hz; (2) a steady-state synthetic speech signal containing a 150 Hz fundamental and formant frequencies of 489 Hz (f1) and 1,849 Hz (f2); and (3) a synthetic /da/ containing a 114 Hz fundamental and 3 transient-containing formants (f1 = 154 → 669 Hz; f2 = 1,620 → 1,232 Hz; and f3 = 3,500 → 2,525 Hz). Rise and decay times were held constant among signals; duration was held constant at 250 msec; and all sounds were presented at 70 dB. Individual stimuli were combined in trains of eight repetitions separated by intervals of 3.7 sec, and each train, presented 8 times in randomized order, was separated from the next by a 10-sec interval. For purposes of analysis, the first 4 trains (32 trials) were averaged separately from the last 4 trains and the amplitude of a primary AER component occurring in the neighborhood of 200–300 msec was determined from the resultant X-Y tracings.

For purposes of statistical treatment, the only parameter considered was change in amplitude between the initial and final stimulus trains, as measured by difference values. From such values, it was found that amplitude of the primary component was reduced significantly for later trials only in the case of the shaped noise. However, it seems likely that more sophisticated statistical treatment might have yielded other interesting information. When the graphic data presented are examined with respect to the direction of difference between early and late trials, a trend emerges suggesting that habituation rate might have varied systematically with stimulus conditions: for shaped noise, the average amplitude of the primary AER component decreased by about 4 μv; for the steady-state synthetic speech sound, it decreased by about 1.6 μv; and for the transient-containing synthetic sound, it *increased* by about 4 μv. Moreover, if one studies some of the wave forms for individual subjects, it seems possible that statistical treatment of data in the first 100 msec or so following stimulus onset might have yielded evidence of other stimulus-related AER differences. In general, Anderson's suggestion that his data best can be explained in terms of learning phenomena is difficult to accept.

Infant Responses to Speech and Speechlike Sounds[1]

Trehub's caution (1973b; p. 95) that "nonrecovery of" (an) "operant . . . response does not necessarily indicate nondiscrimination" warrants careful attention because most of the information currently available on perception of speech and speechlike stimuli during early life derives from operant procedures designed to disclose whether infants can differentiate among sounds in "phonemically relevant" ways (Eimas, 1975; Kavanagh and Cutting, in press; and Morse, 1973).

Moffitt, who pointed the way to current research in a prescient doctoral dissertation (1968), was the first investigator to report a controlled study of infant responses to speech sounds (1971). Working with subjects of 5–6 months, and using HR as his indicator, he presented babies with a series of 8 stimulus trains, each of which contained 10 repetitions of a 250-msec CV syllable. Intensity, interstimulus interval, and other signal-related variables were fixed so that the ability of subjects to differentiate between "bah" and "gah" could be tested. The population was divided into three groups: the first was exposed to 6 stimulus trains of "bah" followed by 2 trains of "gah;" the second (counterbalanced) group was exposed to 7 trains of "gah" followed by 1 train of "bah;" and the third, a control group, was exposed only to "bah."

All subjects responded initially with HR deceleration and, as was found at the Bioacoustic Laboratory for even younger infants, HR changes to the synthetic speech sounds sometimes were on the order of 20 or more beats (Chapter 5; Figure 15). The magnitude of the decelerative responses decreased systematically over the course of the stimulus schedule; that is, the responses habituated. The evidence for dishabituation (recovery of response magnitude upon introduction of a novel stimulus) varied according to the stimulus schedule: the control group of infants, as expected, showed no signs of dishabituation during the final stimulus trials; the group exposed to 6 trains of "bah" showed only minimal signs of it when "gah" was introduced during the last 2 stimulus trains; the group exposed to 7 trains of "gah" showed reliable evidence of dishabituation when "bah" was introduced.

---

[1] References: Butterfield and Cairns, 1974a and 1974b.

These data occasioned considerable excitement among investigators concerned with communicative behavior since they supported the notion that infants of 5–6 months were able to perceive the primary acoustic cue for place of articulation, that is, the f2 transition which distinguishes "bah" from "gah." Whether the mechanisms underlying their differentiations were specifically "phonemic" or "linguistic" is highly debatable, however, since a number of the purely acoustic variables discussed earlier (see Figure 19) were operating in this study.

However many of these variables may have colored the experimental results, the data are consonant with the possibility that the difference in frequency between f2 and f3. over time may have been a critical determinant. If one assumes the existence in man of neurons analagous to midbrain "decoders" (Scheich, 1974) that are more sensitive to fixed short-time differences than to variable short-time differences, the dishabituation findings fall into place very nicely: the change from "bah" to "gah," which was signified only equivocally by dishabituation, could represent a switch from a very discriminable parameter to a minimally discriminable one, whereas the change from "gah" to "bah," which resulted in reliable dishabituation, could represent a switch from a minimally discriminable parameter to a highly discriminable one. One obvious direction for future research, then, would be to test this possibility by systematically studying the effects of signals encompassing several of the f1-f2 derivatives associated with natural speech.

Results stemming from additional inquiries (Bergman and Shultz, 1972; Eilers and Minifie, 1975; Eimas, 1975; Eimas et al., 1971; Kavanagh and Cutting, in press; McCaffrey, 1971; Morse, 1972 and 1973; Trehub, 1973a and 1973b; and Trehub and Rabinovitch, 1972), like Moffitt's findings, effectively rule out any unmodified "motor theory of speech perception" (Liberman et al., 1967) as well as Lenneberg's thesis (1967) that the infant's ability to employ phonetic categories is determined by his ability to produce these categories in his vocal repertoire.

Eimas and his co-workers (1971) approached the problem of studying speech sound discrimination in early life by using a modified version of the Siqueland and De Lucia (1969) sucking procedures. The technique was an ingenious one whereby, once a baseline rate of high amplitude sucking was obtained under "no sound" conditions, the presentation and intensity of test stimuli were made contingent upon the infant's sucking behavior: the nipple on which the babies sucked was connected (via digital logic modules) in such a way that increased sucking rates activated a power supply to maintain sound intensity at some maximum level and decreased sucking rates (habituation) resulted in presentation of a contrast signal. Given these arrangements, the magnitude of recovery of the sucking response (dishabituation) could be quantified easily and used as a measure of differentiation.

The experiment was as ingenious as the approach in that the synthetic consonants used (/b/ and /p/) involved 6 different manipulations of formant structure encompassing voice onset times (VOTs) between −20 and +80 msec and, additionally, permitted comparison with data already available for adult hearers. The results showed not only that infants as young as 1 month were able to make fine distinctions along the VOT continuum, but also that they were able to do so "in a manner approximating categorical perception, the manner in which adults perceive these same sounds" (p. 306). Stevens and Klatt (1974) have criticized this interpretation on the grounds that 1- to 4-month-old infants cannot discriminate 20-msec differences in VOT and that what subjects may have been differentiating was nothing more than the presence or absence of an fl transient. Furthermore, it is worth bearing in mind Trehub's caution (1973b) that mere difference detection, which is inherent in habituation-dishabituation procedures, may not involve the same processes required for attachment of differential responses to discrete perceptual events. Whatever interpretation one chooses to put upon the Eimas et al. (1971) findings, however, they suggest very strongly that eighth nerve specializations, prerequisite to language acquisition and learning may be present at birth and possibly built in during intrauterine life.

The notion that the human organism, in some ways at least, is perceptually mature at birth gains support from related experimental results. A variety of follow-up studies by Eimas and his co-workers (Cutting and Eimas, in press; Eimas, 1975) has shown that infants as young as 2 months differentiate acoustic cues relating to place of articulation (/bae/ vs. /dae/) and to VOTs for phone pairs such as /t/ and /d/. Whether VOT per se can account for discrimination among phone pairs is open to question, because, as Eilers and Minifie (1975) have suggested, differentiation instead may depend upon presence of absence of a first formant transition. In any case, Morse (1972), also using the sucking procedure, has shown that infants between 40 and 54 days of age can differentiate the acoustic cues for place of articulation and for intonation. The findings on intonation contours are especially interesting since, as discussed in Chapter 4, newborns are seemingly able to differentiate between descending and ascending tonal sequences (Eisenberg, Coursin, and Rupp, 1966). Therefore, it seems probable that had Morse extended his inquiry to neonates, he might have confirmed hitherto unreported Bioacoustic Laboratory observations suggesting that the capacity to code direction of frequency change is present at birth. Trehub (1973a) found that infants of 6–17 weeks not only could differentiate pairs of foreign language contrasts (Czech and Polish) to which they never had been exposed, but also that they could discriminate consonant contrasts in the second syllable of a speech stimulus. Trehub and Rabinovitch (1972) found that infants between 4 and 17 weeks of age could detect differences between synthetically and naturally generated versions of voiced and voiceless sound pairs. McCaffrey (1971), using HR as a measure, found that a number of consonantal contrasts could be detected by infants between 4 and 28 weeks of age. Dorman and Hoffman (1973), who found habituation of the vertex AER to a synthetic syllable in 10- to 14-week-old infants, interpreted their results as suggesting the existence of "at least rudimentary short-term memory."

Perhaps the most exciting clues to developmental auditory processes derive from two recent EEG inquiries that touch upon the question of hemispheric asymmetry as a function of stimulus variables.

The first of these is Molfese's doctoral study (1972) of 31 subjects at various developmental stages. In the experiment, which included 1 newborn and 2 infants under 3 months of age, AERs were recorded from T_3 and T_4 sites during wakeful exposure to 100 replications of nonverbal sounds (a C-major chord and a band-limited noise, nonsense syllables (/ba/ and /da/), and words (boy and dog). Determinations of AER amplitude were based upon magnitude of a primary component labeled N_2-P_3 (occurring roughly between 100 and 160 msec on adult records) and differences between the right and the left hemisphere were calculated according to the Matsumiya et al. (1972) formula. Although some of the study results are suspect either on procedural or on technical grounds, and the stimulus conditions were so ill defined that the effective acoustic variables cannot be specified, the evidence showing the verbal stimuli to have elicited greatest activity in the left hemisphere at all ages seems undeniable.

The second inquiry, and one of great significance, is that of Barnet and her colleagues (1974) on AER differences between normal and malnourished infants under the age of 1 year. In this study, the stimuli, presented under conditions of natural sleep, included 50 replications each of clicks and the child's name. Electrodes were positioned at left and right anterior parietal sites (C_3 vs. C_4), and amplitude ratios for a P_2-N_2 component (occurring roughly between 250 and 450 msec on normal infant records) were examined as a function of physical status, electrode derivations, and other factors. Preliminary analysis of findings on 7 infants suffering from third degree malnutrition (marasmus) and 7 age-matched controls suggests that: (1) a click stimulus tends to evoke larger responses in the right hemisphere both in normal and in malnourished subjects; (2) a meaningful verbal stimulus evokes larger amplitude responses in the left hemisphere only in the case of normal subjects; and (3) subjects treated for marasmus fail to lateralize speech sounds to the left hemisphere even after their physical symptoms have been ameliorated. The speculation that "the failure of the marasmic infant to show a left" (hemisphere) "shift to his name may be related to dysfunction in cortical processes related to language" seems eminently justified. However, the extent to which that failure may have related to auditory processes per se remains to be determined.

These unconfirmed, but presumably valid, data on functional asymmetries in auditory processing during the first year of life are enormously important. In light of the recent Witelson and Paillie (1973) findings on anatomic asymmetry, they clearly support the notion that sensory or other specializations prerequisite to language acquisition may exist at birth. If, in fact, this is the case and the Barnet et al. (1974) data are confirmed and clarified by follow-up studies under better controlled conditions, the clinical and research implications relative to hemispheric asymmetry in early life are almost staggering: measures relative to lateralized brain wave responses to sound under matched speech and nonspeech conditions could turn out to be both predictive indicators of communicative problems and tools for monitoring recovery processes in the central nervous system.

CHAPTER 7
The Organization of
Hearing Functions

". . . false views, if supported by some
evidence, do little harm, for everyone
takes a salutary pleasure in proving their
falseness; and when this is done, one
path towards error is closed and the road
to truth is often at the same time
opened."
Charles Darwin, *The Descent of Man* (1871)

In an effort to present current information on infant hearing abilities in an
organized way, discussion thus far has centered on the functional properties
of specific signals that bear in some way upon verbal communication.
These signals have been grouped into two general classes, constant and
patterned, on the basis of their physical properties and their presumed
manner of coding in the central nervous system. Before considering what
current data imply for the organization of auditory behavior, then, it is
useful to summarize the functional properties of constant and patterned
signals to see how they relate to the theoretical constructs discussed in
Chapter 3.

THE PROPERTIES OF CONSTANT AND PATTERNED
SIGNALS AS A CLUE TO NEURONAL ORGANIZATION

From the experimental results reviewed in this volume, it is evident that all
of the acoustic signals explored so far have at least some functional
properties in common. These shared properties clearly bear upon organization in the CNS in that they have to do with state-related effects that are

seemingly independent of developmental status. Whatever the stimulus conditions employed, the incidence of neonatal responses to sound varies with arousal level much as adult detection scores vary during vigilance experiments. The curve describing these relations, like that showing the distribution of OQ responses during habituation, assumes an inverted U "cue function" predicted by activation theory. Except perhaps in the case of speechlike sounds, modes of response to any given signal seem to vary systematically according to an "awake-alert-aware" continuum often postulated for the RAS. It seems entirely likely, then, that mechanisms governing attentive behavior are operational at birth, at least in the term baby (Eisenberg, 1970a, 1970b, 1974a, and 1975a).

Constant and patterned signals have a number of differential functional properties that bear upon the organization of eighth nerve mechanisms. These differential properties are both varied and suggestive; and they are demonstrable both in overt behavior and in electrophysiologic measures.

Functional Properties of Constant Signals as a Class

During early infancy, the outstanding functional property of constant signals is *nonspecificity*. As a matter of fact, the auditory behavior evoked by such signals as pure tones and noisebands differs so little from nonstimulus behavior or from other kinds of perceptual behavior that reliable differentiation of response events poses serious problems. Overt reactions consist mostly of gross body movements, cessation of such movements, or components of the startle reflex. Although decelerative HR changes occasionally may be evoked during waking states, cardiac responses to a wide variety of constant signals almost uniformly have been found to be accelerative (Clifton, 1974b; Graham and Jackson, 1970; and Lewis, 1974). Relations between response magnitude and prestimulus indices of arousal agree with the so-called law of initial values (LIV), which holds that stimulus-bound activity is directed toward homeostasis. Large HR changes and intense motor responses characteristically occur during sleep states. Smaller cardiac changes and minor body movements usually are found during wakeful states. The effectiveness of pure tones or noisebands is a function of specific parameter variables and, within limits bearing upon the characteristics of spoken language, can be enhanced by increases in one or more of those parameters. Vocal responses almost never can be elicited, however, and the most sophisticated visual reaction found is a kind of wide-eyed "what-is-it?" look usually considered to be orienting behavior.

The response to constant signals is highly dependent upon the frequency characteristics of those signals, and high frequency stimuli have been shown to have at least three unique functional properties during the first year of life. Whatever the conditions of arousal under which they are presented, they prove singularly ineffective. Unlike lower frequency signals, which are most effective during doze states, reactions to sounds in the range above 4,000 Hz or thereabouts, like Moro reflexes and other responses that wane during development, can be best elicited during wakeful states. The behaviors most frequently evoked are strikingly similar to the freezing reactions described for infrahuman organisms.

Functional Properties of Patterned Signals as a Class

As Chapter 6 suggests, work with patterned signals is in its early stages and few investigators have been concerned with auditory operations per se. To consider the functional properties of patterned signals as a class, then, one is heavily dependent upon exploratory studies conducted at the Bio-acoustic Laboratory. The stimuli employed so far include matched pairs of ascending and descending tonal sequences[1] as well as a few synthetic speech sounds in addition to the vowel discussed in Chapter 5. Few of our data on the former have been reported in print and, as noted earlier, most of our data on the latter are so new that they remain to be processed. However, all of the signals explored seem to have similar happy properties.

In newborn life, as in later infancy, the effects of multidimensional signals are so distinctive that naive observers can detect response reliably. Overt reactions consist mainly of arousals or orienting behavior. Motor reflexes, which are relatively few, usually take such differentiated forms as facial grimacing or displacement of a single digit. What perhaps is more significant, the response repertoire associated with patterned signals includes such discriminative behavior as responsive crying or cessation of crying, pupillary dilatation, and, on rare occasions, a turning of the head in association with visual search.

Response magnitude, however measured, shows no systematic relation with prestimulus indices of arousal and, whatever the state of arousal, both tonal sequences and synthetic speech sounds seem remarkably effective. In some newborns studied, anticipatory HR and brain wave changes have been found after only 3 or 4 trials with either kind of stimulus. The average newborn responds overtly to at least 3 consecutive trials with these signals, even in deep sleep; the quiet-wakeful infant may respond to as many as 8 or 10. Both types of patterned stimuli are associated with longer latencies than any we have found for constant signals and, as noted in Chapter 5, the overt behaviors evoked by speechlike sounds are indistinguishable from those evoked by tonal sequences.

---

[1] 2,000 → 500 Hz vs. 500 → 2,000 Hz; 5,000 → 200 Hz vs. 200 → 5,000 Hz; and 250 → 75 Hz vs. 75 → 250 Hz.

The cardiac reactions evoked by patterned signals appear to differ according to whether the pattern presented is a tonal sequence or a synthetic speech sound. All of the tonal sequences explored thus far have been associated primarily with diphasic HR changes, that is, deceleration followed by acceleration, or the reverse. Sequences having an overall duration in excess of 2 sec seem to be associated with *on* and *off* effects and also with differences reflecting the direction of the sequence. Synthetic speech sounds, on the other hand, are associated mainly with decelerative responses and, insofar as present data constitute a valid index, such responses are characterized by longer latencies and more prolonged response activity. Moreover, the mode of response to synthetic speech signals appears to be not only quite specific, but also independent of a subject's state of arousal.

Data on infant brain wave responses to patterned signals are too sparse to permit either strong statements or secure inferences. All that can be said at present is that speechlike sounds seem to be extremely potent and associated with longer latencies than have been reported for constant signals.

Correlative Information on Adult Responses to Patterned Stimuli How these infant responses to different kinds of patterned signals related to language processing later in life is far from clear. However, given the results of some preliminary fishing expeditions conducted at the Bioacoustic Laboratory, it seems evident that the manner in which energy is dispersed among frequencies over time is a critical determinant of perceptual experiences.

All of the tonal sequences used thus far have proved not only intensely arresting for adult hearers, but also psychologically "softer" than constant signals. Trained listeners, who usually can guess presentation levels for constant signals within ± 5 dB, consistently underestimate sequences by 15 or 20 dB, or approximately the difference between pure tone and speech-hearing thresholds (Katz, 1972). Untrained listeners will judge an 80-dB tonal pattern to be no louder than a matched-spectrum band-limited noise of 60–65 dB.

All listeners, trained or untrained, seem to perceive a tonal sequence differently according to whether the amount of time consumed by the frequency sweep exceeds 200 msec or so: depending upon starting frequency and how much longer than 200 msec the signal is, it will be described alternatively as a sort of "whoop" or "siren;" when the signal is shorter than 200 msec, it is perceived in much the manner of isolated transitions (Lehiste, 1972; and Mattingly et al., 1971), that is, as the "yip of a dog," a "chirp," a glissando, or the like. It would appear, then, that the manner in which *any* short-duration frequency sweep is perceived reflects some basic feature detector mechanism in the auditory system.

From a functional standpoint, perhaps the most interesting difference between patterned and constant signals is that adult listeners tend to attribute meaning to the former but not to the latter. Just as a tonal sequence is perceived as having some referent in experience, the prolonged synthetic vowel considered in Chapter 5 is described as sounding like "the moo of a cow," "somebody wounded on the battlefield," and so on. On the other hand, although these same listeners may be prodded to assign loudness or frequency attributes to pure tones and noisebands, they never seem to report such sounds as anything other than tones or noises.

All things considered, current data suggest that the various kinds of selective behavior evoked by tonal patterns and synthetic speech sounds during early life may reflect relatively plastic mechanisms and relatively high levels of neuronal organization.

Implications of Current Data for a Developmental Model

As one considers the findings reviewed in this volume, it seems clear that the organizational principles outlined in Chapter 3 have a fair amount of face validity. The burden of the data is that the human organism emerges from the womb rather neatly equipped to organize his auditory world. Nonspecific mechanisms governing attentive behavior seem to be operational. Functionally differentiated channels for processing acoustic information according to discrete parameters, and also according to the organization of a stimulus envelope, seem to exist. The auditory behavior of the newborn seems to follow orderly rules that can be related to a stimulus hierarchy, and different rules, that evidently refer to different biologic determinants and surely must reflect differential coding mechanisms for sound, apply to high frequencies, constant signals, and patterned stimuli.

There is good reason to suppose that the biologic determinants in fact do cover a past to future time span. Frequency-bound behavior, which in the newborn period has correlates in the performance of lower animals, bears upon qualitative judgments of sound in adult life. Intensity-bound behavior, as measured by threshold and loudness functions, seems to have species-specific characteristics that are independent of developmental status. Pattern-bound behavior, although lacking clear-cut correlates either in adult or in animal performance, is uniquely selective in the newborn period and associated with vocal activity. Furthermore, since it seems possible that the rules governing such behavior may vary according to whether or not the evoking stimuli are speechlike in nature, certain aspects of pattern-bound behavior may bear directly upon the development of communicative functions.

TOWARD A DEVELOPMENTAL MODEL

Given the correlates summarized above, it seems useful, and perhaps even important, to make some general inferences about the intrinsic architecture of auditory pathways and the possibilities for developmental change. The inferences naturally are limited by a paucity of data and by substantial gaps in our understanding of how multidimensional signals in particular are processed. However, within current limitations, and without reference to anatomic or physiologic specifics, it certainly is possible to work out a preliminary framework within which developmental studies in hearing can be pursued systematically.

At the Bioacoustic Laboratory, we have postulated a hierarchy of functionally differentiated channels that reflects the presumed evolutionary order of coding mechanisms for sound (Eisenberg, 1967, 1970*b*, 1974*a*, and 1975*a*). In line with current data, which are summarized briefly in Table 8, each of these channels relates to specified stimulus conditions and primary modes of response behavior detailed in the various sections of this book.

In line with current thinking, lateral organization in the model incorporates a number of specific notions. First, as shown in Figure 20, both direct and indirect pathways are involved in the decoding of acoustic information. Second, centrifugal controls act at all levels of the nervous system. Third, additional channel capacity for coding acoustic information

Table 8. Stimulus Variables as a Determinant of Neonatal Responses to Sound

Input	Processing Level	Most Frequently Observed Outputs	
		Overt Behavior	Cardiac Pattern
High frequency tones and noisebands	I	Freezing; startle	Very shortlasting; accelerative
Low frequency tones and noisebands	II	Undifferentiated movements	Relatively shortlasting; accelerative
Tonal sequences and other non-speech ensembles	III	Differentiated movements; utterance	Somewhat prolonged; diphasic
Speech and speech-like sounds	IV	Differentiated movements; utterance	Very prolonged; decelerative

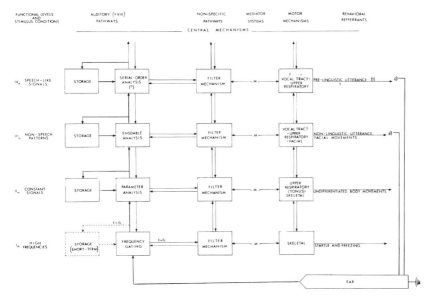

Figure 20. Schematic showing systems involved in auditory processing (from Eisenberg, 1970*b*).

is provided in nonspecific systems. Fourth, mechanisms for ensemble processing serve to increase the resolving power of the auditory system. Fifth, mechanisms for storage, processing, and encoding are found at all levels of the CNS. Finally, it is assumed, although not shown diagrammatically, that auditory mechanisms have their counterparts in motor specializations required for speech and in central specializations required for language (Kavanagh and Cutting, in press; and Lhermitte et al., 1973)

The auditory channels are shown schematically in Figure 21. Each of the four levels in the model refers to an indeterminate series of neuronal networks which, under the influence of normal growth and environmental forces, are incorporated into organized feedback systems.

Implicit in this organizational scheme is the idea that the degree of correspondence with peripheral input decreases at successive levels of the hierarchy, each processing operation yielding a product that is some derivative of the transmitted signal. In a sense, then, what is postulated is a form of "neural funneling" (v. Békésy, 1958) having specific functional consequences: acoustic information that is stored or processed at a given level of the system cannot be retrieved or processed in the same form at a higher level and processing may proceed in parallel at several levels of the hierarchy.

The lowest level in the hierarchy is essentially a *frequency-dependent gating circuit* which, given current evidence on structural and biochemical

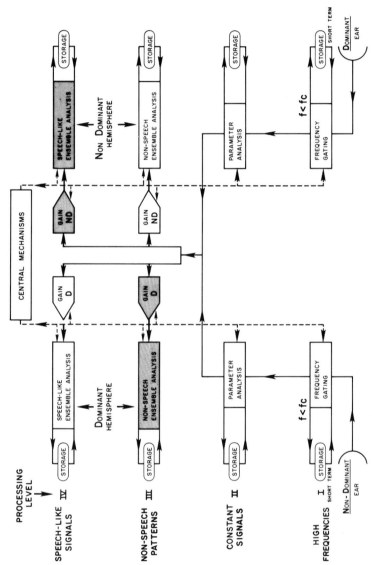

Figure 21. A model for the intrinsic organization of hearing mechanisms (from Eisenberg, 1974a).

specializations (Dayal, 1972; and Gleisner, Flock, and Wersäll, 1973) as well as frequency-dependent inhibitory controls (Buno et al., 1966; Fex, 1967; Sohmer, 1965; and Wiederhold and Kiang, 1970), one would be inclined to place at the cochlear level. Assuming some critical cut-off point, a gated network provides a mechanism whereby low frequencies can be funneled upward for specific coding while high frequencies can be filtered through nonspecific pathways for low-level storage and/or processing. The circuit, present at birth as a phylogenetic relic of approach-withdrawal behavior, is elaborated into an organized "affective" system as shunt mechanisms become operational during development. Considering the various kinds of background information provided in Chapter 1, it seems reasonable to speculate that this lowest channel might involve old brain mechanisms, and particularly the limbic system.

Whether long-term storage normally is possible at this lowest level seems debatable. Signals that are psychologically annoying when first heard remain annoying upon repetition (Kryter, 1966 and 1968) and recollections of pleasant or unpleasant sounds tend to be as ephemeral as memories of pain. Whether long-term storage is possible under *pathologic* conditions may be an important area for study since high frequencies evoke peculiarly interesting behavior in at least two clinical groups. Psychotics, for instance, tend to be vastly disturbed by such sounds (Coleman and Eisenberg, 1973), and children with developmental disorders of communication sometimes respond to high frequencies when they seem totally insensitive to other portions of the sound spectrum (unpublished Bioacoustic Laboratory observations).

The second level in the diagram represents a series of parameter-coding circuits which collectively serve as a kind of *species-specific adaptor.* Inasmuch as the eighth nerve system is tonotopographically organized, such circuits must be time-locked. Therefore, assuming critical limits for individual parameters, they provide a mechanism whereby, through successive recoding operations, incoming signals can be refined: significant perceptual elements can be extracted for further resolution at higher levels in the system; insignificant elements, filtered through nonspecific channels, can be stored or processed in a variety of ways. The circuits, present at birth in the form of "grading" or "scaling" mechanisms, are elaborated into an organized subceptor system as new networks become operational during development. Although the mechanisms clearly must be subcortical (Masterton and Berkeley, 1974; Møller, 1973; and Sachs, 1971), it seems likely that acoustic information serving life-long purposes would be stored permanently. As noted earlier, humans, like many other vertebrates, rely upon intensity cues for orienting themselves in space.

In light of the strong possibility that many parameter-coding mechanisms may be preadapted, it seems probable that operations on this second level bear, at least indirectly, upon language acquisition. Selective tuning to the carrier frequencies of language, for instance, would lead to selective reinforcement of language cues. A graded response to intensity would permit the developing child to orient himself preferentially toward language sounds. Hierarchal mechanisms, affording a time base for related decoding and encoding operations, might serve in toning up units of the speech apparatus for articulatory tasks. By the same token, as data on the effects of delayed auditory feedback (DAF) suggest (Cullen et al., 1968; and Timmons and Boudreau, 1972), defective operations at this level may be implicated in dysfluency and related speech problems. Under normal conditions, however, it seems highly unlikely that the processing of intensity per se—and perhaps any other discrete parameter except duration—bears directly upon the acquisition of language skills: normal loudness curves can be measured for severely aphasic adults who are unable to distinguish one nonsense syllable from another (unpublished Bioacoustic Laboratory observations).

The organization of higher levels must remain largely speculative until substantive information on neonatal responses to patterned stimuli of various kinds has been accumulated. All we have now is some sparse preliminary evidence (Barnet et al., 1974; Crowell et al., 1973; and Molfese, 1972) to suggest that functional asymmetries in perceptual processing may be present during the newborn period. Figure 21, then, sketches out a first guess notion (Eisenberg, 1974a) that mechanisms for processing speechlike and nonspeech ensembles are present at birth in both hemispheres. A differential exists, however, such that one hemisphere, usually the left, is specialized for processing speechlike signals, while the other hemisphere is specialized for processing other kinds of ensembles. This is shown schematically by the introduction of "gain" elements, to control the distribution of coding processes: the shaded gain areas in each hemisphere represent "inhibitory" mechanisms of one kind or another, so that functional asymmetry is achieved. The asymmetry could result from a differential distribution of short- and long-time constant cells, from differential projections of short- and long-time constant systems, from differential convergence patterns at one or more levels of the auditory pathway (Repp, 1975), from differential storage processes, from enhanced sensitivity in particular neuronal arrays (Saunders, 1967), or indeed from almost any combination of these and other unconsidered functional specializations.

Whatever the neurophysiologic and biochemical bases of functional asymmetry in man, their disclosure lies far outside the field of our inquiries. The model, in its current skeletal form, postulates only that some sort of "fourth level" specializations for processing speech sounds contribute differentially to hemispheric dominance in language functions. These specializations are normally present at birth as part of man's species-specific endowment, and they facilitate the establishment of specific neuronal connections which, during the normal course of development, become elaborated into an organized "communicative" network. However, since such mechanisms, like the proposed third level specializations for processing nonspeech ensembles, are represented redundantly, the schema allows for certain eventualities. For instance, the effects of central auditory damage theoretically should vary according to the stage of development at which pathology occurs (Miller, Goldman, and Rosvold, 1973): the earlier damage appears, the greater the chance that either hemisphere can assume dual functions and/or that alternate neuronal connections can be established (Basser, 1962; and Krashin, 1972). By the same token, assuming the best possible outcome of central auditory damage early in life, one must suppose that a major reduction in the channel and storage capacities of eighth nerve systems would be reflected not only in reduced auditory abilities of some kinds, but also perhaps in more generalized sensory-motor dysfunction.

Our present working hypothesis is that third level mechanisms, here tentatively placed in the nondominant hemisphere, somehow act collectively as a kind of *species-specific "ensemble-discriminator."* Since all of the tonal patterns explored thus far have evoked some amount of vocal utterance, it is assumed that certain of the individual networks may serve in the development and reinforcement of motor-speech plans. Similarly, since matched pairs of ascending and descending sequences have been associated with differential response patterns, it is assumed that some networks may bear upon perceptions of musical form, intonation, and the like. Purely as a guess, we are inclined to think that race-specific differences in language structure (Goto, 1971; and Van Lancker and Fromkin, 1973), as well as judgments relative to the spectral quality of sounds, may be contingent upon combined operations at the second and third levels of the hierarchy.

Whatever precise operations might be performed at the third level, we have no strong feelings that these relate directly to the processing of ensembles that ultimately carry linguistic information. As has been noted elsewhere, various kinds of experimental manipulations have yielded data showing that animals can discriminate among tonal sequences (Katsuki, 1965; and Neff, 1968) and even among format transitions (Sinnott, 1974), and difference detection may be quite another thing than differential responding (Trehub, 1973*a*).

Some Buttressing Information

The model considered here, first advanced some years ago (Eisenberg, 1966*b*, 1967, 1970*b*, 1974*a*, and 1975*a*), must be viewed simply as an attempt to reduce enormously complicated events to manageable conceptual dimensions. It accords with the general constructs outlined in Chapter 3, with the data reviewed in Chapter 6, with the concepts proposed by other investigators (Abbs and Sussman, 1971; Berlyne, 1960; Bronson, 1965 and 1974; Desmedt, Debecker, and Manil, 1965; Elliott and Trahoitis, 1972; Erickson, 1965; Flanagan, 1965; Froeschels, 1951; Kavanagh and Cutting, in press; and Osgood, 1964) and with information that has become available only recently.

Data Supporting the Possibility of a Communicative (Aural-Oral) Network Only within the past year, it has been shown experimentally (Crain and Peterson, 1975) that, in lower animals than man, some neuraxons can be induced to make selective synaptic connections with specific types of "target" neurons in nearby and not necessarily adjacent sites.

Functional Information Relevant to a Gating Circuit Corliss (1973), reporting data to show that adults with absolute pitch forget set pitches of high frequency at much the same rate as listeners who lack this ability, has related the findings to asynchronous firing of auditory neurons in the 4,000- to 8,000-Hz range. Her speculation that all listeners may have poor precision for high frequencies is consonant with the notion of a peripheral gating circuit associated with short-term memory mechanisms.

League and Bzoch (1970) have reported preliminary data suggesting the existence of a rudimentary "affective" system even in earliest life: infants exposed to five conditions of recorded human voice seem to attend more frequently to friendly (pleasant) utterances and the babbling of their peers than they do to angry utterances.

Haggard and Parkinson (1971), who stimulated adult listeners with a distracting babble in one ear and sentences spoken in four emotional tones in the other, found a significant left ear (right hemisphere) advantage for emotional tones.

Functional Information Relevant to Parameter-Coding Circuits Cullen and his colleagues (1974), in a systematic series of dichotic listening studies, have shown that when constant signals are paired along such dimensions as intensity and band width, performance is "qualitatively similar" in the left and the right ear.

Concepts and Data Relevant to Higher Level Processing Bartlett and John (1973) have presented electrophysiologic data suggesting a hierarchy of storage mechanisms, and a good many investigators working with adult subjects have reported findings to support a schema of the kind shown in Figure 21. Cutting (1973), Stevens and House (1972), and others (Berlin et al., 1973; Klatt, 1974; and Pisoni and Lazarus, 1974) have suggested that the processing of language sounds ultimately must depend upon prior auditory coding. Day and her colleagues (Day, 1973; and Day and Wood,

1972) showed that variations along a nonlinguistic dimension impeded performance on a task involving linguistic decisions, whereas linguistic variations had little or no effect on the performance of nonlinguistic listening tasks. Similarly, Martin and Strange (1968) demonstrated that listening for pauses disrupts linguistic performance. Thompson and his co-workers (1973) have suggested that the results of dichotic listening experiments can be explained on the basis of a functional "gating out" of information transmitted by two independent channels. Sinnott (1974), in attempting to explain the fact that humans, despite their greater sensitivity to formant transitions, require more time than monkeys to react to intraphonemic differences, has proposed a model in which a "timbre discriminator" operates after a "phoneme discriminator." In her schema, as in the Bioacoustic Laboratory model, it is assumed that each discriminatory operation involves both coding and storage phenomena in such a way that categorical perception reflects both sensory and memory processes. Kent (1974) has explained the ability of phonetically trained adults to imitate synthetic speech sounds in terms of sensory memory stores that vary according to whether the acoustic information is "primitive" or language specific. Steinheiser and Burrows (1973), who studied relations between phonologic and semantic properties of speech sounds in adult life, felt that syllable perception could not result from synthesis of "lower order" units such as phonemes, but rather must be processed as ensembles. Webster, Woodhead, and Carpenter (1970) have noted that speechlike signals have a high degree of "perceptual constancy" in that they can be identified more easily than musical sounds or noises when subjected to distortion or degradation.

Zaidel (1974) has come up with the "radical conclusion" that suppression of the ipsilateral pathway in dichotic listening is itself a function of hemispheric specialization, so that "left ear suppression in the left hemisphere is greater for dichotic signals whose processing involves greater left hemisphere specialization." The conclusion, in fact, is not very radical since there is increasing reason to suppose that functional asymmetries in the processing of speech and nonspeech ensembles relate to time-differentiated systems in eighth nerve channels. Despite conflicting earlier findings (Shankweiler and Studdert-Kennedy, 1967; and Studdert-Kennedy and Shankweiler, 1970), recent dichotic listening studies with children (Goodglass, 1973) and adults (Spellacy and Blumstein, 1970) suggest that speech sounds as a class are right ear (left hemisphere) dominant, provided that duration factors are taken into account. Short (50 msec) vowels are perceived differently from long (300 msec) ones by adults (Crowder, 1973). Stimuli with formant transitions yield a significant right ear advantage in dichotic listening whether or not they are speechlike in nature (Cutting, 1973). Steady state vowels can produce a right ear advantage in dichotic listening when they are reduced below 100 msec (Godfrey, 1974). Language dysfunction in adult patients with temporal lobe lesions (Speaks et al., 1974) and in school-aged children with "developmental aphasia" (Tallal, 1974) has been associated with inability to process onset transients in the range of 40 msec.

FUTURE DIRECTIONS IN THE STUDY OF DEVELOPMENTAL AUDITORY BEHAVIOR

From both research and clinical standpoints, there is an urgent need for some sort of organized framework in which to think about developmental auditory processes. Whether the schema proposed here is partially or even wholly correct, then, is secondary to whether it is useful as it stands.

We have found it eminently useful for Bioacoustic Laboratory purposes because it affords a concrete, yet flexible, approach to questions with which our program is mainly concerned. Stimulus-bound behavior refers to specified perceptual operations and specified functional levels. The stimulus, as a trigger for underlying events and a common denominator for comparative studies, has become the key determinant of strategy. The planning problem has reduced itself to selecting stimulus conditions applicable to predetermined lines of inquiry.

Major lines of inquiry have been discussed in preceding sections of this book and possibilities for related studies have been remarked in passing. Given the facts and constructs now provided, however, it may be worthwhile to review the kinds of questions that can cast light upon auditory processing, whether in healthy states or under pathologic conditions.

Frequency, for example, is one of many parameters that warrants further investigation and, as noted elsewhere, it can be explored at the behavioral level with many different ends in view. Psychoacoustically or linguistically oriented studies profitably might examine rates of frequency change as a function of starting frequency, the direction of a sequence, the range encompassed, the derivatives associated with second and third formants drawn from like or unlike phonemic categories, and so on. Anthropologically oriented studies might be directed toward comparing frequency discrimination functions in racial groups having very differently structured languages, as for example, Indo-European vs. Mandarin-speaking natives. Psychiatrically oriented studies perhaps might focus upon the differential effects of low and high frequencies as a function of diagnostic category, chemotherapeutic interventions, or other selected factors. By the same token, studies concerned more generally with the substrates of emotion might be geared to the disclosure of frequency-related affect as measured by somatic patterns, verbal associations, or other indices.

There is no need to spell our the ways in which additional aspects of human hearing can be explored. The gaps in our knowledge have been stressed throughout this book, and the directions research can take are limited only by the interests and ingenuity of investigators who are willing to work at the job of filling them in.

At the basic research level, the model suggested here has the virtue of providing a biologic frame of reference that is subject to experimental testing in complementary ways. Specifically, the organizing principles can be validated by studying the effects of age, phyletic, or other differences on the functional properties of a given signal or, alternatively, by studying the effects of signal differences on the response patterns of a given population. Therefore, it is encouraging that many of the supporting data reviewed in this book were accumulated after the model first was advanced and, in most cases, without reference to it. These supporting data are extremely limited, however, and it is clear that many questions need to be answered before the skeleton diagrammed in Figure 21 can be fleshed out or modified.

Whether the basic questions can be posed in complementary ways by investigators with traditionally divergent interests remains to be seen. The recent explosion of neurophysiologic data on hearing has had few repercussions at the clinical level, mainly because scientists concerned with behavior and scientists concerned with the mechanisms underlying that behavior seem unable to communicate adequately with each other. This is decidedly unfortunate since both groups stand to gain much from a sharing of experience and ideas. In any event, one of the most pressing needs now faced by all groups concerned with audition is for information on the neuronal and biochemical specializations associated with the coding of species-specific acoustic patterns. The question of whether and how pharmacologic interventions that alter the concentration of transmitter substances affects responsivity at given cellular levels may be directly relevant to the diagnosis and management of developmental disorders of communication. The question of whether primates or other infrahumans process species-specific vocalizations in the left hemisphere bears directly upon the question of whether man possesses a unique mechanism for the processing of speechlike ensembles. The question of whether functional asymmetries in human hearing relate to the existence of a short-time constant system bears directly upon the question of whether diagnostic tests predictive of developmental communicative dysfunction can be devised.

TOWARD A BONA FIDE PEDIATRIC AUDIOLOGY

Whatever the validity of the model presented here, the biologic "apportionment" of hearing functions has specific implications for clinical studies with the pediatric aged. It means that auditory competence, or the ability to code and organize acoustic information normally, cannot be measured solely in terms of threshold acuity or an ability to respond overtly to sound. It means that adequate indices of auditory competence must include measures bearing upon the integrity of specified coding and organizing mechanisms. It means that developmental abnormalities of hearing must be defined operationally, with respect to developmental norms for specific hearing functions. It means, in short, that connections must be made between the functions being measured at different age levels and the status of underlying mechanisms at those age levels.

Such connections can be made because, as pointed out in one way or another throughout this book, functional properties of sound reflect specialized eighth nerve mechanisms for coding physical properties of sound. Such connections regularly are made when older children and adults are evaluated audiologically. The term "differential diagnosis" attains validity precisely because the test battery includes a variety of measures bearing upon the site of a lesion, the nature of an auditory abnormality, and the extent to which that abnormality affects the communicative process. Moreover, since the battery includes both speech and pure tone signals, test procedures routinely take into account differences between constant and patterned stimuli.

Connections between physical and functional properties of sound almost regularly are ignored when newborns and infants are evaluated. For this reason, terminology such as differential diagnosis cannot properly apply to our labeling of young subjects. Indeed, as things now stand, the pediatric-aged patient can fall only between two stools—that is, he can be either "deaf" or "not deaf." If he is deaf, we can measure how deaf he is, tell his parents how to help him at home, recommend amplification as indicated, and provide appropriate schooling or other special assistance. If he is not deaf and not old enough to talk, we can say that he responds at normal levels, but *we cannot say that he hears normally.* If he is not deaf, old enough to talk, but unable to deal normally with acoustic information, his management will be guided by threshold measures that cannot disclose his problems, and by behavioral observations that reflect and sometimes obscure it (Eisenberg, 1966*a*).

In effect, our entire approach toward auditory problems in the pediatric-aged patient is geared to deafness rather than to hearing. There seems to be a general lack of interest in how hearing functions normally develop, and a corresponding lack of insight into the nature of childhood abnormalities. These lacks are reflected in the many numerous textbooks and journal articles that discuss hearing disorders without reference to normal developmental functions. They are reflected too in current audiologic procedures for young patients. Despite an alphabet of tests for studying pitch, loudness, and other functions in adult life (Katz, 1972), there are no techniques, standardized or unstandardized, for studying coding processes in early life. There has been no systematic attempt to design a battery of tests specific to infancy. Somehow or other, threshold measurements alone, and more frequently, only threshold approximations, have become accepted as a reasonable index of eighth nerve integrity, and "screening" of newborn infants has become stylish.

Perhaps the time has come for thoughtful clinicians to take a long, hard look at what passes for "pediatric audiology." Standardized procedures almost uniformly involve the use of abstract input signals such as clicks, pure tones, and band-limited noises; and the associated output measures reflect relatively low level activity in the nervous system (Field et al., 1967). Unstandardized procedures, which frequently involve the use of spoken voice or other meaningful signals, almost uniformly entail behavioral observations which may or may not be valid. EEG work, mainly involving vertex placements and the use of clicks or pure tones, has emphasized early AER components referable to low level auditory mechanisms (Hecox, and Galambos, 1974; and Stillman, Moushegian, and Rupert, in press) and, thus far, such work has not been especially productive (Lowell, 1971; Mitrinowicz-Modrzejewska, 1970; and Shephard and McCarren, 1972). Screening procedures for newborns, adopted enthusiastically and uncritically by hundreds of facilities only a few years ago, already have been characterized as "misleading" (Miller, 1971). So-called high-risk registers, which have been proposed as a replacement, have been said to combine the twin evils of high cost and dubious benefit (Altman and Shenhav, 1971).

It is neither realistic nor productive to ascribe limitations in current clinical practice to difficulties inherent in dealing with the pediatric aged or to lack of information. The problems, although they have historical roots (Eisenberg, 1971 and 1975a), stem mainly from inertia. The fact is that the audiologic focus has remained essentially static over the past 30 years or so while the nature of the clinical population has altered radically. Medical advances leading to a relative decline in the incidence of deafness among all age groups have been accompanied by a startling increase in the incidence of CNS disorders among the youngest and the oldest age groups. Developmental disorders of communication, which either did not exist or could not be defined when audiology emerged as a discipline in the 1940's, now constitute a substantial proportion of the clinical population. These are disorders for which there are no adequate diagnostic labels, no ade-

quate techniques for measurement, testing, or intervention, and no therapies based upon hard facts about hearing operations. They create enormous emotional and practical problems for families and they impose heavy
financial burdens upon communities as well as families.

We badly need new ideas that are pertinent to these disorders. We need
normative information in order to define which functions are affected and
in what ways. We need new clinical measures that refer quantitatively to
specific coding operations. Most of all, we must attack these needs in
rational order and ask critical questions about current priorities. Do we
need to use pure tones or other abstract signals when speech and speechlike sounds are more effective elicitors of response? Do we need monaural
studies of hearing in early life or would we be better advised to define the
conditions under which functional asymmetry is demonstrable? Do we
need to examine early AER components which tell us about the integrity
of low level auditory mechanisms or would it be preferable to concentrate
upon later components which may yield information on the status of
higher level mechanisms and the integrity of CNS organization? Do we
require mass infant screening programs to ferret out 2 cases of middle ear
disease among 3,000 newborn infants (Reddell and Calvert, 1969) or do
we require selective public health programs geared to the needs of indigent
groups who are known to have a high incidence of such problems (Current
Estimates from the Health Interview Survey, 1971; and Schein and Delk,
1974)? Do we need to find one case of congenital deafness among 5,000
newborn infants (Ling, Ling, and Doehring, 1970) or do we need to
differentiate an infant group of unknown dimensions who may be congenitally unable to process biologically significant sounds? As a matter of
fact, do we need infant case finding at all when we are unsure of what to
look for and how best to go about it?

These are very largely rhetorical questions, the answers to which are
implicit in the contents of this book. For the moment, pediatric audiology
is a myth, and differential diagnosis of the pediatric aged is all too often an
exercise in futility. It will become a reality when we have obtained
information of the kind that permits physicians to prescribe drugs according to the age and electrolytic balance of young patients, and for this we
will need to accumulate a sizable body of normative information on the
nature and sequence of developmental auditory processes. Such information will not be forthcoming either easily or cheaply and, in these difficult
days for research, the funding issue looms large (see Appendix B). Developmental research with human subjects is, of its nature, expensive and
time consuming. Most, if not all, of the easy questions that can be posed
relatively cheaply already have been answered. The difficult questions still
confronting us very probably will have to be asked in sophisticated ways,

that is, using EEG and/or other electrophysiologic measures. This is not to say that the future is bleak, however. Indeed, there is good reason to suppose that, given a concerted attack on the nature of developmental auditory processes and reasonable funding support for the effort, answers to fundamental questions might be forthcoming in relatively short order.

Part IV

Epilogue

"He who moves not forward goes backward."
Johann Wolfgang von Goethe, *Herman and Dorothea* (1797)

This book represents an effort to view infant hearing in biologic perspective and, toward that end, it considers a great many facts from a great many sources. The major concern is not with the facts per se, but with the ways in which they can be brought to bear upon current clinical and research issues. For this reason, the focus has been mainly upon new methods, new data, and new ideas. In the first section, the determinants of human hearing were discussed and the practical and theoretical issues guiding research strategy at the Bioacoustic Laboratory were detailed. The second section dealt with representative laboratory studies that cast light upon the nature of auditory processing operations during early life. The final section, which was partly a state-of-the-art report, reviewed current data, evaluated their implications, and proposed a frame of reference for further inquiry.

The book as a whole reflects a progression from total to relative ignorance that has taken place largely within the past decade, and the stage now is set for further gains. It is known, for instance, that even a newborn baby has well-developed hearing capacities that are susceptible to measurement. It seems indisputable that the disclosure of hearing capacities, whatever a subject's age or clinical status, depends upon the kinds of signals used for study and the ways in which these are employed. Thus, present data, however limited, have important implications for both clinical and laboratory inquiries. They suggest that pure tones and band noises, although used routinely in developmental work, are relatively ineffective because they are abstract and lack biologic significance. Similarly, they suggest that tonal patterns and synthetic speech sounds, although barely explored, have enormous potential. How quickly and how well that potential can be exploited depends upon the resolution of basic questions,

157

many of which remain totally unexplored. The extent to which the very tentative schema of intrinsic hearing mechanisms advanced in the last section of this book depends upon educated guesswork is merely one index of how far we are from productive applied research.

There can be little question that applied research is needed. Clinicians in almost every discipline today are faced with a substantial group of pediatric-aged patients presenting developmental disorders of communication. The questions posed by this spectrum of hearing, speech, and reading disabilities are not being answered by threshold measures and related indices of peripheral eighth nerve integrity. Nor can the underlying problems be disclosed by behavioral observations and performance tests that, in some cases, serve merely to obscure the problems.

There is a pressing need for new concepts leading to broader based studies in hearing. At the laboratory level, we need to fit our notions to the infant instead of fitting the infant to our notions. At the clinical level, we need to face the fact that current methods of evaluating developmental disorders of communication are woefully inadequate: except for a few procedures now in the developmental stage (Barnet et al., 1974; Bradford, 1975; Eisele, Berry, and Shriner, 1975; Jerger et al., 1974; and Tallal, 1974), standardized hearing tests in common use are neither specific to the developing human organism nor pertinent to today's major problems.

Questions about the nature of high level eighth nerve mechanisms, the integrity of auditory coding operations, and the effects of other CNS systems upon mechanisms and operations alike have been neglected by too many for too long. They are not only important questions, but exciting ones. Perhaps, then, this book best can be concluded with a plea for some kind of concerted attack upon the puzzles beyond the ears. If that attack can be mounted, we stand to gain not only a bona fide pediatric audiology, but also a rational basis for the treatment, and perhaps even prevention, of developmental disorders of communication.

"Now voyager, sail thou forth to seek and find."
*Walt Whitman, **The Untold Want** (1871)*

References

Abbs, J. H., and G. R. Eilenberg. 1975. Peripheral mechanisms of speech motor control. *In* N. J. Lass (ed.), Current Issues in Experimental Phonetics. Charles C Thomas, Publisher, Springfield, Ill.

Abbs, J. H., and H. M. Sussman. 1971. Neurophysiological feature detectors and speech perception: A discussion of theoretical implications. J. Speech & Hearing Res. 14:23–36.

Adams, F. H., T. Fujiwara, R. Spears, and J. Hodgman, 1964. Temperature regulation in premature infants. Pediatrics 33:487–495.

Ades, A. E. 1974. Bilateral component in speech perception? J. Acoust. Soc. Am. 56:610–616.

Adrian, H. O., J. M. Goldberg, and J. F. Brugge. 1966. Auditory evoked cortical potentials after lesions of brachium of inferior colliculus. J. Neurophysiol. 29:456–466.

Aeserinsky, E. 1965. Periodic respiratory pattern occurring in conjunction with eye movements during sleep. Science 150:763–766.

Aeserinsky, E., and N. Kleitman. 1955. A motility cycle in sleeping infants as manifested by ocular and gross bodily activity. J. Appl. Physiol. 8:11–25.

Aitkin, L. M., and W. R. Webster. 1972. Medial geniculate body of the cat: Organization and responses to tonal stimuli of neurons in ventral division. J. Neurophysiol. 35:365–380.

Akiyama, Y., F. J. Schulte, M. A. Schultz, and A. H. Parmalee, Jr. 1969. Acoustically evoked responses in premature and full-term newborn infants. Electroencephalog. & Clin. Neurophysiol. 26:371–380.

Albert, M. L., R. Sparks, T. von Stockert, and D. Sax. 1972. A case study of auditory agnosia: Linguistic and nonlinguistic processing. Cortex 8:427–443.

Aldrich, C. A. 1928. A new test for hearing in the new-born. Am. J. Dis. Child. 35:36–37.

Allen, G. D. 1971. Acoustic level and vocal effort as cues for the loudness of speech. J. Acoust. Soc. Am. 49:1831–1841.

Allport, F. H. 1924. Social Psychology. Houghton Mifflin. Boston.

Altman, J. A. 1968. Are there neurons detecting direction of sound source motion? Exper. Neurol. 22:13–25.

Altman, M. M., and R. Shenhav. 1971. Methods for early detection of hearing loss in infants. J. Laryng. & Otolaryng. 85:35–42.

Anders, T. F., R. Emde, and A. H. Parmalee, Jr. (eds.). 1971. A Manual of Standardized Terminology, Techniques and Criteria for Scoring of States of Sleep and Wakefulness in Newborn Infants. UCLA Brain Information Service, BRI Publications Office, NINDS Neurological Information Network, Los Angeles.

Anderson, D. E. 1973. Averaged electroencephalographic responses of infants to speech related stimuli. Ph.D. dissertation, University of Washington, Seattle.

Anderson, R. B., and J. F. Rosenblith. 1964. Light sensitivity in the neonate: A preliminary report. Biol. Neonat. 7:83−94.

Ando, Y., and H. Hattori. 1970. Effects of intense noise during fetal life upon postnatal adaptability (Statistical study of the reactions of babies to aircraft noise). J. Acoust. Soc. Am. 47:1128−1130.

Andreeva, V. A., Y. G. Kratin, and S. H. Kurbanov. 1972. Auditory stimulus duration effects on discrimination and brain activity. Neurosci. & Behav. Physiol. 5:10−23.

Annett, M. 1973. Laterality of childhood hemiplegia and the growth of speech and intelligence. Cortex 9:4−33.

Anokhin, P. K. 1961. A new conception of the physiological architecture of the conditioned reflex. In J. F. Delafresnaye (ed.), Brain Mechanisms and Learning, pp. 189−227. Blackwell Scientific Publications, Oxford, Eng.

Anson, B. J., D. G. Harper, and J. R. Hanson. 1962. Vascular anatomy of the auditory ossicles and petrous part of the temporal bone in man. Ann. Otol. Rhin. & Laryng. 71:622−631.

Anson, B. J., and T. R. Winch. 1974. Vascular channels in the auditory ossicles in man. Ann. Otol. Rhin. & Laryng. 83:142−158.

Apgar, V. A. 1953. A proposal for a new method of evaluating the newborn infant. Current Res. in Anesth. & Analg. 32:260−266.

Appleby, S. 1964. The slow vertex maximal sound response in infants. Acta Oto-laryng. 206 (Suppl.):146−152.

Arey, L. B. 1965. Developmental Anatomy. 7th Ed. W. B. Saunders Company, Philadelphia.

Armington, J. C. 1974. The Electroretinogram. Academic Press, Inc., New York.

Arnold, W. R., and S. W. Porges. 1972. Heart rate components of orientation in newborns as a function of age and experience. Presented at the Eastern Psychological Association, Boston.

Aronson, E., and S. Rosenbloom. 1971. Space perception in early infancy: Perception within a common auditory-visual space. Science 172:1161−1163.

Ashton, R. 1971a. The effects of the environment upon state cycles in the human newborn. J. Exper. Child Psychol. 12:1−9.

Ashton, R. 1971b. State and the auditory responsivity of the human neonate. J. Exper. Child Psychol. 12:339−346.

Ashton, R. 1973. The influence of state and prandial condition upon the reactivity of the newborn to auditory stimulation. J. Exper. Child Psychol. 15:315−327.

Athavale, V. B. 1963. Some observations on temperature in the newborn. Indian J. Child Health 12:381−410.

Bailey, P. J., and M. P. Haggard. 1973. Perception and production: Some correlations on voicing of an initial stop. Lang. & Speech 16:189—195.

Bar-Adon, A., and W. F. Leopold. 1971. Child Language: A Book of Readings. Prentice-Hall, Inc. Englewood Cliffs, N. J.

Barden, T. P., P. Peltzman, and J. T. Graham. 1968. Human fetal electro-encephalographic response to intrauterine acoustic signals. Am. J. Obst. & Gynec. 11:1128—1134.

Bargmann, W., and J. P. Schadé (eds.). 1963. The Rhinencephalon and Related Structures. Elsevier Press, Inc., New York.

Barnet, A. B. 1971. EEG audiometry in children under three years of age. Acta Oto-laryng. 72:1—13.

Barnet, A. B., M. Bazelon, and M. Zappella. 1966. Visual and auditory function in an hydranencephalic infant. Brain Res. 2:351—360.

Barnet, A. B., M. de Sotillo, and M. S. Campos. 1974. EEG sensory evoked potentials in early infancy malnutrition. Paper read at the Society for Neuroscience, St. Louis.

Barnet, A. B., and R. S. Goodwin. 1965. Averaged evoked electroencepha-lographic responses to clicks in the human newborn. Electro-encephalog. & Clin. Neurophysiol. 18:441—450.

Barnet, A. B., and A. B. Lodge. 1966. Diagnosis of deafness in infants with the use of computer-averaged electroencephalographic responses to sound. J. Pediat. 69:753—758.

Barnet, A. B., and A. B. Lodge. 1967a. Click evoked EEG responses in normal and developmentally retarded infants. Nature 214:252—255.

Barnet, A. B., and A. B. Lodge. 1967b. Diagnosis of hearing loss in infancy by means of electroencephalographic audiometry. Clin. Proc. Child. Hosp. (Wash.) 23:1—18.

Barnet, A. B., E. S. Ohlrich, and B. L. Shanks. 1971. EEG evoked responses to repetitive auditory stimulation in normal and Down's syndrome infants. Develop. Med. Child Neurol. 13:321—329.

Barnet, A. B., E. S. Ohlrich, I. P. Weiss, and B. Shanks. 1975. Auditory evoked responses in normal children from 10 days to 3 years of age. Electroencephalog. & Clin. Neurophysiol. (In press).

Barnett, S. A. 1971. The Human Species. Harper and Row, Publishers, New York.

Barrager, D. C. 1974. Responses of infants aged four and twelve weeks to speech and nonspeech stimuli. Ph.D. dissertation, Stanford University, Stanford, Calif.

Barrett, T. W. 1973. Information processing in the inferior colliculus of cat using high frequency acoustical stimulation and direct electrical stimu-lation of the osseons spiral laminae. Behav. Biol. 9:189—219.

Barrett-Goldfarb, M. S., and G. J. Whitehurst. 1973. Infant vocalization as a function of parental voice selection. Develop. Psychol. 8:273—276.

Barrie, H. 1962. The Apgar evaluation of the newborn infant. Develop. Med. Child Neurol. 4:128—132.

Bartholomeus, B. 1975. Effect of task requirements on ear superiority for sung speech. Cortex. (In press).

Bartlett, F., and E. R. John. 1973. Equipotentiality quantified: The anatomical distribution of the engram. Science 181:764—767.

Bartoshuk, A. K. 1962a. Human neonatal cardiac acceleration to sound: Habituation and dishabituation. Percept. Motor Skills 15:15—27.

Bartoshuk, A. K. 1962b. Response decrement with repeated elicitation of human neonatal cardiac acceleration to sound. J. Comp. & Physiol. Psychol. 55:9−13.

Bartoshuk, A. K. 1964. Human neonatal cardiac responses to sound: A power function. Psychonom. Sci. 1:151−152.

Baru, A. V. 1966. On the role of temporal parts of the cerebral cortex in the discrimination of acoustic signals of different duration. Zh. Vyssh. Nerv. Deyatel. Pavlova 16:655−665.

Bass, A. D. 1959. Evolution of Nervous Control from Primitive Organisms to Man. AAAS, Washington, D. C.

Basser, L. S. 1962. Hemiplegia of early onset and the faculty of speech with special reference to the effects of hemispherectomy. Brain 85:427−460.

Baumrin, J. M. 1974. Perception of the duration of a silent interval in nonspeech stimuli: A test of the motor theory of speech perception. J. Speech & Hearing Res. 17:294−309.

Beadle, K. R., and D. H. Crowell. 1962. Neonatal electrocardiographic responses to sound: Methodology. J. Speech & Hearing Res. 5:112−123.

Beer, C. G. 1969. Laughing gull chicks: Recognition of their parent's voices. Science 166:1030−1032.

Békésy, G. v. 1958. Funneling in the nervous system. J. Acoust. Soc. Am. 30:399−412; 609−619.

Békésy, G. v. 1963. Hearing theories and complex sounds. J. Acoust. Soc. Am 35:588−601.

Békésy, G. v. 1971. Localization of visceral pain and other sensations before and after anesthesia. Percept. & Psychophys. 9:1−4.

Bell, R. Q., and R. A. Haaf. 1971. Irrelevance of newborn waking states to some motor and appetitive responses. Child Develop. 42:69−77.

Bell, W. A. 1970. Muscle patterns of the late fetal tongue tip. Angle Orthodont. 40:262−265.

Bench, J. 1968. Sound transmission to the human fetus through the maternal abdominal wall. J. Genet. Psychol. 113:85−87.

Bench, J. 1969a. Audio-frequency and audio-intensity discrimination in the human neonate. Int. Audiol. 8:615−625.

Bench, J. 1969b. Some effects of audio-frequency stimulation on the crying baby. J. Aud. Res. 9:122−128.

Bench, J. 1970. The law of initial value: A neglected source of variance in infant audiometry. Int. Audiol. 9:314−322.

Bench, J. 1973. Square wave stimuli and neonatal auditory behavior: Some comments on Ashton (1971), Hutt et al (1968) and Lenard et al (1969). J. Exper. Child Psychol. 16:521−527.

Bench, J., Y. Collyer, C. Langford, and R. Toms. 1972. A comparison between the neonatal sound-evoked startle response and the head-drop (Moro) reflex. Develop. Med. Child. Neurol. 14:308−317.

Bench, J., E. Hoffman, and I. Wilson. 1974. A comparison of live and videorecorded viewing of infant behavior under sound stimulation. I. Neonates. Develop. Psychobiol. 7:455−464.

Bench, J., and A. Parker. 1971. Hyper-responsivity to sounds in the short-gestation baby. Develop. Med. Child Neurol. 13:15−19.

Bench, J., and A. Vass. 1970. Fetal audiometry. Lancet 1:91−92.

Berg, K. M. 1973. Elicitation of acoustic startle in the human. Ph.D. dissertation, University of Wisconsin, Madison.

Berg, K. M., W. K. Berg, and F. K. Graham. 1971. Infant heart rate response as a function of stimulus and state. Psychophysiology 8:30–44.

Berg, W. K. 1972. Habituation and dishabituation of cardiac responses in 4-month-old alert infants. J. Exper. Child Psychol. 14:92–107.

Berg, W. K. 1974. Cardiac orienting responses of 6- and 16-week-old infants. J. Exper. Child Psychology 17:303–312.

Berg, W. K., C. D. Adkinson, and B. D. Strock. 1973. Duration and frequency of periods of alertness in neonates. Develop. Psychol. 9:434.

Berger, H. 1929. Uber das Elektrenkephalogramm des menschen. Arch. Psychiat. Nervenkr. 87:527–570.

Bergman, T., and J. Shultz. 1972. Speech perception in infants. Unpublished study, Harvard Graduate School of Education, Cambridge, Mass.

Beritoff, J. S. 1965. Neural Mechanisms of Higher Vertebrate Behavior. Little, Brown, & Company, Boston.

Berkson, G., G. A. Wasserman, and R. E. Behrman. 1974. Heart rate responses to an auditory stimulus in premature infants. Psychophysiology 11:244–246.

Berlin, C. I., S. S. Lowe-Bell, J. K. Cullen, Jr., C. L. Thompson, and C. F. Loovis. 1973. Dichotic speech perception: An interpretation of right-ear advantage and temporal offset effects. J. Acoust. Soc. Am. 53:699–709.

Berlin, C. I., D. A. Majeau, and S. Steiner. 1969. Hearing and vocal output in normal, deaf and infant mice. J. Aud. Res. 9:318–331.

Berlin, C. I., R. J. Porter, Jr., S. S. Lowe-Bell, H. L. Berlin, C. L. Thompson, and L. F. Hughes. 1973. Dichotic signs of the recognition of speech elements in normal, temporal lobectomees and hemispherectomees. IEEE Trans. Audio and Electroacoust. 21:189–195.

Berlyne, D. E. 1960. Conflict, Arousal, and Curiosity. McGraw-Hill Book Company, Inc., New York.

Bernard, J., and L. W. Sontag. 1947. Fetal reactivity to tonal stimulation: A preliminary report. J. Genet. Psychol. 70:205–210.

Bernstein, A. 1969. To what does the orienting response respond? Psychophysiology 6:338–350.

Bever, T. G., and R. J. Chiarello. 1974. Cerebral dominance in musicians and nonmusicians. Science 185:537–539.

Billone, M., and S. Raynor. 1973. Transmission of radial shear forces to cochlear hair cells. J. Acoust. Soc. Am. 54:1143–1156.

Birns, B. 1965. Individual differences in human neonates' responses to stimulation. Child Develop. 36:249–256.

Birns, B., M. Blank, and W. H. Bridger. 1966. The effectiveness of various soothing techniques on human neonates. Psychosom. Med. 28:316–322.

Birns, B., M. Blank, W. H. Bridger, and S. Escalona. 1965. Behavioral inhibition in neonates produced by auditory stimuli. Child Develop. 36:639–645.

Blair, W. F. 1958. Mating call in the speciation of the Anuran amphibians. Am. Natur. 92:27–51.

164   References

Bobbin, R. P., and T. Konishi. 1974. Action of cholinergic and anti-cholinergic drugs at the crossed olivocochlear bundle-hair cell junction. Acta Oto-laryng. 77:56–65.

Boehm, J. J., and J. L. Haynes. 1964. Interrelationships between sucking, swallowing and cardiac rate in early infancy. Presented at the American Pediatric Society, Seattle, Wash.

Bonin, G. von. 1962. Anatomical asymmetries of the cerebral hemispheres. *In* V. Mountcastle (ed.), Interhemispheric Relations and Cerebral Dominance, pp. 1–6. Johns Hopkins Press, Batimore.

Bonin, G. von. 1963. The Evolution of the Human Brain. University of Chicago Press, Chicago.

Bordley, J. E., J. Hardy, and W. G. Hardy. 1963. Report of Johns Hopkins unit of collaborative project on conservation of hearing in children. Tr. Am. Acad. Ophth. Otolaryng. 67:230–232.

Bosma, J. F. (ed.). 1973. Oral Sensation and Perception: Development in the Fetus and Infant. U. S. Dept. H. E. W., N. I. H., Bethesda, Md.

Brackbill, Y. 1970. Acoustic variation and arousal level in infants. Psychophysiology 6:517–526.

Brackbill, Y. 1971*a*. The role of the cortex in orienting: OR in an anencephalic human infant. J. Develop. Psychol. 5:195–201.

Brackbill, Y. 1971*b*. The cumulative effects of continuous stimulation on arousal level in infants. Child Develop. 42:17–26.

Brackbill, Y., G. Adams, D. H. Crowell, and M. L. Gray. 1966. Arousal level in neonates and preschool children under continuous auditory stimulation. J. Exper. Child Psychol. 4:178–188.

Brackbill, Y., and H. E. Fitzgerland. 1969. Development of the sensory analyzers during infancy. *In* L. P. Lipsitt and H. Reese (eds.), Advances in Child Development and Behavior, pp. 173–208. Vol. 4. Academic Press, Inc., New York.

Bradford, L. J. (ed.). 1975. Physiological Measures of the Audio-Vestibular System. Academic Press, Inc., New York.

Brain, R. 1961. Speech Disorders. Butterworth & Co., Ltd., Washington, D. C.

Brazelton, T. B. 1962. Observations of the neonate. J. Am. Acad. Child Psychiat. 1:38–58.

Brazelton, T. B., and D. G. Freedman. 1971. Manual to accompany Cambridge newborn behavior and neurological scales. *In* G. B. A. Stoelinga and J. J. Van Der Werff Ten Bosch (eds.), Normal and Abnormal Development of Brain and Behavior, pp. 104–131. Leiden Univ. Press, Leiden, the Netherlands.

Brazier, M. A. B. (ed.). 1960. The Central Nervous System and Behavior. Josiah Macy, Jr., Foundation, New York.

Bredberg, G. 1968. Cellular pattern and nerve supply of the human organ of Corti. Acta Otolaryng. 235 (Suppl.).

Bridger, W. H. 1961. Sensory habituation and discrimination in the human neonate. Am. J. Psychiat. 117:991–996.

Bridger, W. H. 1962*a*. Sensory discrimination and autonomic function in the newborn. J. Am. Acad. Child Psychiat. 1:67–82.

Bridger, W. H. 1962*b*. Ethological concepts and human development. *In* J. Wortis (ed.), Recent Advances in Biological Psychiatry, pp. 95–107. Vol. 4, Plenum Publ. Corp., New York.

Bridger, W. H., and B. Birns. 1963. Neonates' behavioral and autonomic responses to stress during soothing. *In* J. Wortis (ed.), Recent Advances in Biological Psychiatry, pp. 1–6. Vol. 5. Plenum, New York.

Bridger, W. H., B. Birns, and M. Blank. 1965. A comparison of behavioral and heart rate measurements in human neonates. Psychosom. Med. 27:123–134.

Britt, E. 1963. Hearing and Language Development in Infancy. Sc.D. dissertation, Johns Hopkins University, Baltimore.

Broadbent, D. E. 1971. Decision and Stress. Academic Press, Inc., New York.

Brodal, A. 1957. The Reticular Formation of the Brain Stem: Anatomical Aspects and Functional Correlates. Oliver & Boyd, Ltd., Edinburgh, Scotland.

Brodal, A. 1969. Neurological Anatomy. 2nd Ed. Oxford University Press, New York.

Bronshtein, A. I., T. G. Antonova, A. G. Kamenetskaya, N. N. Luppova, and V. A. Systova. 1960. On the development of the functions of analyzers in infants and some animals at the early state of ontogenesis. *In* Problems of Evolution of Physiological Functions, pp. 106–116. Office Technical Service, Report No. 60-61066, Washington, D. C.

Bronshtein, A. I., and E. P. Petrova. 1967. The auditory analyzer in young infants. *In* Y. Brackbill and G. G. Thompson (eds.), Behavior in Infancy and Early Childhood, pp. 163–172. Free Press, New York.

Bronson, G. 1965. The hierarchal organization of the central nervous system: Implications for learning processes and critical periods in early development. Behav. Sci.: 10:7–25.

Bronson, G. 1974. The postnatal growth of visual capacity. Child Develop. 45:873–890.

Brown, C. C. 1967. A proposed standard nomenclature for psychophysiologic measures. Psychophysiology 4:260–264.

Brown, J. L. 1964. States in newborn infants. Merrill-Palmer Quart. 10:313–327.

Bryan, E. S. 1930. Variations in the responses of infants during the first ten days of post-natal life. Child Develop. 1:56–77.

Buckley, W. (ed.). 1968. Modern Systems Research for the Behavioral Scientist. Aldine, Chicago.

Buckner, E., and J. McGrath (eds.). 1963. Vigilance, A Symposium. McGraw-Hill Book Company, Inc., New York.

Buno, W., R. Velluti, P. Handler, and E. G. Austt. 1966. Neural control of the cochlear input in the wakeful free guinea-pig. Physiol. & Behav. 1:23–35.

Burdick, C. K., and J. D. Miller. 1974. Discrimination of speech sounds by the chinchilla: Steady-state /i/ vs /a/. Presented at the Acoust. Society of America, St. Louis.

Busnel, R. G. (ed.). 1963. Acoustic Behavior of Animals. Elsevier Press, Inc., New York.

Butler, R. A., W. D. Keidel, and M. Spreng. 1969. An investigation of the human cortical evoked potential under conditions of monaural and binaural stimulation. Acta Otolaryng. 68:317–326.

Butterfield, E. C., and G. F. Cairns. 1974a. Discussion summary—Infant Reception Research, pp. 75–102. *In* R. L. Schiefelbusch and L. L.

Lloyd, Language Perspectives—Acquisition, Retardation, and Intervention. University Park Press, Baltimore.

Butterfield, E. C., and G. F. Cairns. 1974*b*. The infant's auditory environment. Paper presented at the Conference on Early Intervention with High Risk Infants and Young Children, University of North Carolina at Chapel Hill.

Butterfield, E. C., and G. N. Siperstein. 1972. Influence of contingent auditory stimulation upon nonnutritional suckle. *In* J. Bosma (ed.), Oral Sensation and Perception: The Mouth of the Infant. Charles C Thomas, Publisher, Springfield, Ill.

Cairns, G. F., and E. C. Butterfield. 1975. Assessing infants' auditory function. *In* B. F. Friedlander, G. M. Sterritt, and G. Kirk (eds.), The Exceptional Infant. Vol. 3: Assessment and Intervention. Brunner/Mazel, New York.

Cairns, G. F., and M. A. Karchmer. 1975. Assessment of infants at-risk for language dysfunction through the use of their speech productions. Paper presented at a meeting of the Council for Exceptional Children, Los Angeles.

Camacho-Evangelista, A., and F. Reinoso-Suarez. 1964. Activating and synchronizing centers in cat brain: Electroencephalograms after lesions. Science 146:268–270.

Campbell, B. G. 1966. Human Evolution. Aldine, Chicago.

Campbell, H. J. 1965. Correlative Physiology of the Nervous System. Academic Press, Inc., New York.

Campos, J. J., and Y. Brackbill. 1971. Infant state: Relationship to heart rate, behavioral response and response decrement. Develop. Psychobiol. 6:9–19.

Candia, O., G. F. Rossi, and T. Sekino. 1967. Brain stem structures responsible for the EEG patterns of desynchronized sleep. Science 155:720–722.

Candiollo, L., and A. C. Levi. 1969. Studies on the morphogenesis of the middle ear muscles in man. Arch. Klin. Exp. Ohr.-Nas. u. Kehlk. Heilk. 195:55–67.

Canestrini, S. 1913. Über das sinnesleben des neugeborenen (nach physiologischen experimentenen). Gesemtegebiete Neurol. Psychiat. 5:1–104.

Capranica, R. R. 1966. Vocal response of the bullfrog to natural and synthetic mating calls. J. Acoust. Soc. Am. 40:1131–1139.

Capranica, R. R., L. S. Frishkopf, and E. Nevo. 1973. Encoding of geographic dialects in the auditory system of the cricket frog. Science 182:1272–1275.

Carlson, A. J., and H. Ginsburg. 1915. Contributions to the physiology of the stomach. XXIV. The tonus and hunger contractions of the stomach of the new-born. Am. J. Physiol. 38:29–32.

Carmel, P. W., and A. Starr. 1963. Acoustic and nonacoustic factors modifying middle-ear muscle activity in waking cats. J. Neurophysiol. 26:598–616.

Carmichael, L. D. (ed.). 1960. Manual of Child Psychology. 2nd Ed. John Wiley & Sons, Inc. New York.

Caspary, D. M., A. L. Rupert, and G. Moushegian. 1974. Processing of simple and complex stimuli by the globular and multipolar cell areas of the kangaroo rat cochlear nuclei. Presented at the Society for Neuroscience, St. Louis.

Celesia, G. G., R. J. Broughton, T. Rasmussen, and C. Branch. 1968. Auditory evoked responses from the exposed human cortex. Electroencephalog. & Clin. Neurophysiol. 24:458—466.

Celesia, G. G., and F. Puletti. 1969. Auditory cortical areas of man. Neurology 19:211—220.

Chaney, R. B., and J. C. Webster. 1966. Information in certain multidimensional sounds. J. Acoust. Soc. Am. 40:447—455.

Chase, H. H. 1965. Habituation of an acceleratory cardiac response in neonates. M.A. thesis, University of Wisconsin, Madison.

Chase, R. A., S. Sutton, D. First, and J. A. Zubin. 1961. A developmental study of changes in behavior under delayed auditory feedback. J. Genetic Psychol. 99:101—112.

Cherry, C. 1961. On Human Communication. Science Editions, New York.

Chomsky, N., and M. Halle. 1968. The Sound Pattern of English. Harper & Row, Publishers, New York.

Chun, R. W. M., R. Pawsat, and F. M. Forster. 1960. Sound localization in infancy. J. Nerv. & Ment. Dis. 130:472—476.

Churchill, J. A., J. Grisell, and J. D. Darnley. 1966. Rhythmic activity in the EEG of newborns. Electroencephalog. & Clin. Neurophysiol. 21:131—139.

Clark, G. M., and C. W. Dunlop. 1971. A field potential study of inhibition in cat superior olivary complex. J. Aud. Res. 11:79—87.

Clarke, F. M. 1939. A developmental study of the bodily reaction of infants to an auditory startle stimulus. J. Genetic Psychol. 55:415—427.

Clemente, C. D., D. P. Purpura, and F. E. Mayer, (eds.). 1972. Sleep and the Maturing Nervous System. Academic Press, Inc., New York.

Clifton, R. K. 1971. Heart rate conditioning in the newborn infant. Presented at the Society for Psychophysiological Research, St. Louis.

Clifton, R. K., 1974a. Cardiac conditioning and orienting in the infant. In P. Obrist, A. H. Black, J. Brener, and L. DiCara (eds.), Cardiovascular Psychophysiology-Current Issues in Response Mechanisms, Biofeedback, and Methodology, pp. 479—504. Aldine, Chicago.

Clifton, R. K. 1974b. Heart rate conditioning in the newborn infant. J. Exper. Child Psychol. 18:9—21.

Clifton, R. K., and F. K. Graham. 1968. Stability of individual differences in heart rate activity during the newborn period. Psychophysiology 5:37—50.

Clifton, R. K., F. K. Graham, and H. M. Hatton. 1968. Newborn heart rate response and response habituation as a function of stimulus duration. J. Exper. Child Psychol. 6:265—278.

Clifton, R. K., and W. J. Meyers. 1969. The heart-rate response of four-month-old infants to auditory stimuli. J. Exper. Child Psychol. 7:122—135.

Cody, D. T. R., D. W. Klass, and R. G. Bickford. 1967. Cortical audiometry: An objective method of evaluating auditory acuity in awake and sleeping man. Tr. Am. Acad. Ophth. Otolaryng. Jan.-Feb.:81—90.

Cody, D. T. R., and G. L. Townsend. 1973. Some physiologic aspects of the averaged vertex response in humans. Audiology 12:1—13.

Cohen, B. D., C. D. Noblin, and A. J. Silverman. 1968. Functional asymmetry of the human brain. Science 162:475.

Cohen, L. P., and P. Salapatek (eds.). 1975. Infant Perception. Academic Press, Inc., New York.

Cohen, S. E. 1974. Developmental differences in infants' attentional responses to face-voice incongruity of mother and stranger. Child Develop. 45:1155–1158.

Cohen, Y. A. (ed.). 1968. Man in Adaptation. Aldine, Chicago.

Cohn, R. 1971. Differential cerebral processing of noise and verbal stimuli. Science 172:599–601.

Colavita, F. B. 1974. Insular-temporal lesions and vibrotactile temporal pattern discrimination in cats. Physiol. & Behav. 12:215–218.

Colavita, F. B., F. V. Szeligo, and S. D. Zimmer. 1973. Temporal pattern discrimination in cats with insular-temporal lesions. Presented to the Psychonomic Society, St. Louis.

Cole, M., and I. Maltzman. 1969. A Handbook of Contemporary Soviet Psychology. Basic Books, Inc., New York.

Cole, R., B. Sales, and N. Haber. 1969. Mechanisms of aural encoding. II. The role of distinctive features in articulation and rehearsal. Percept. & Psychophys. 6:343–348.

Cole, R. A., and B. Scott. 1974. The phantom in the phoneme: Invariant cues for stop consonants. Percept. & Psychophys. 15:101–107.

Coleman, M. (ed.). 1973. Serotonin in Down's Syndrome. Elsevier Press, Inc., New York.

Coleman, M., and R. B. Eisenberg. 1973. Correlative studies of auditory behavior in autistic children and their matched controls. Unpublished Bioacoustic Laboratory study.

Collyer, Y., J. Bench, and I. Wilson. 1974. Newborns' responses to auditory stimuli judged in relation to stimulus onset and offset. Brit. J. Audiol. 8:14–17.

Condon, W. S., and L. W. Sander. 1974. Neonate movement is synchronized with adult speech: Interactional participation and language acquisition. Science 183:99–101.

Conel, J. L. 1963. The Postnatal Development of the Human Cerebral Cortex. Vol. 1. The Cortex of the Newborn. Harvard University Press, Cambridge, Mass.

Connolly, K., and P. Stratton 1969. An exploration of some parameters affecting classical conditioning in the neonate. Child Develop. 40:431–441.

Cooke, R. E. 1952. The behavioral response of infants to heat stress. Yale J. Biol. Med. 24:334–340.

Coombs, C. F. (ed.). 1972. Basic Electronic Instrument Handbook. McGraw-Hill, New York.

Cooper, W. A. Jr., and H. O'Malley. 1974. Effects of dichotically presented simultaneous synchronous and delayed auditory feedback on key tapping performance. Presented at the Acoust. Society of America, New York.

Cooper, W. E. 1974. Adaptation of phonetic feature analyzers for place of articulation. J. Acoust. Soc. Am. 56:617–627.

Corliss, E. L. R. 1971. Estimate of the inherent channel capacity of the ear. J. Acoust. Soc. Am. 50:671–677.

Corliss, E. L. R., 1973. Remark on "fixed-scale mechanism of absolute pitch" (Brady, P. T., 1970. J. Acoust. Soc. Am. 48:883–887). J. Acoust. Soc. Am. 53:1737–1739.

Cornwall, P. 1967. Loss of auditory pattern discrimination following insular-temporal lesions in cats. J. Comp. & Physiol. Psychol. 63:165–168.

Crain, S. M., M. B. Bornstein, and C. S. Raine. 1974. Early formation of synaptic network in cultures of fetal mouse cerebral neocortex and hippocampus. Presented at Society for Neuroscience, St. Louis.

Crain, S. M., and E. R. Peterson. 1975. Development of specific sensory-evoked synaptic networks in fetal mouse cord-brainstem cultures. Science 188:275–278.

Cravioto, J., L. Hambraes, and B. Vahlquist (eds.). 1974. Early Malnutrition and Mental Development. Symposium of the Swedish Nutrition Foundation. XII. Almquist & Wiksells International Booksellers, Uppsala, Sweden.

Cromwell, L., F. J. Weibell, E. A. Pfeiffer, and L. B. Usselman. 1973. Biomedical Instrumentation and Measurements. Prentice-Hall, Inc., Englewood Cliffs, N.J.

Cromwell, R. L., A. Baumeister, and W. F. Hawkins. 1963. Research in activity level. In N. Ellis (ed.) Handbook of Mental Deficiency, pp. 632–663. McGraw-Hill Book Company, Inc., New York.

Crowder, R. G. 1973. Precategorical acoustic storage for vowels of short and long duration. Percept. & Psychophys. 13:502–506.

Crowell, D. H., C. M. Davis, B. J. Chun, and F. J. Spellacy. 1965. Galvanic skin reflex in newborn humans. Science 148:1108–1111.

Crowell, D. H., R. H. Jones, L. E. Kapuniai, and J. K. Nakagawa. 1973. Unilateral cortical activity in newborn humans: An early index of cerebral dominance? Science 180:205–208.

Cullen, J. K., N. Fargo, R. A. Chase, and P. Baker. 1968. The development of auditory feedback monitoring. I. Delayed auditory feedback studies on infant cry. J. Speech & Hearing Res. 11:85–93.

Cullen, J. K., C. L. Thompson, L. F. Hughes, C. I. Berlin, and D. S. Samson. 1974. The effects of varied acoustic parameters on performance in dichotic speech perception tasks. Brain & Lang. 1:307–322.

Current Estimates from the Health Interview Survey, U. S. 1971. Vital and Health Statistics—Data from the National Health Survey, Series 10, No. 79. DHEW Publication No. (HSM) 73-1505. U. S. Dept. HEW, PHS, Health Services and Mental, Health Administration, National Center for Health Statistics, Rockville, Md., Feb. 1973.

Curry, F. K. W. 1967. A comparison of left-handed and right-handed subjects on verbal and non-verbal listening tasks. Cortex 3:343–352.

Curthoys, I. S., C. H. Markham, and R. H. Blanks. 1970. The Orientation of Middle and Inner Ear Structures in Cat and Man. UCLA Brain Information Service, BRI Publications Office, NINDS Neurological Information Network, Los Angeles. (NIH 70-2063).

Curzi-Dascalova, N., N. Pajot, and C. Dreyfus-Brisac. 1974. Spontaneous skin potential responses during sleep: Comparative studies in newborns and babies between 2 and 5 months of age. Neuropädiatrie 5:250–257.

Cutting, J. E. 1973. Perception of speech and nonspeech, with speech-relevant and speech irrelevant transitions. Status Report on Speech Research (SR 35/36), July-Dec., 1973, pp. 55–63. Haskins Laboratories, New Haven.

Cutting, J. E. 1975. Two left-hemisphere mechanisms in speech perception. Percept. & Psychophys. (In press).

Cutting, J. E., and P. D. Eimas. 1975. Phonetic feature analyzers and the processing of speech in infants. *In* J. F. Kavanagh and J. E. Cutting (eds.), The Role of Speech in Language. MIT Press, Cambridge, Mass. (In press).

Dallos, P. 1972. Cochlear potentials. Audiology 11:29–41.

Dallos, P., M. C. Billone, J. D. Durrant, C-y. Wang, and S. Raynor. 1972. Cochlear inner and outer hair cells: Functional differences. Science 177:356–358.

Darrouzet, J. 1972. L'innervation de l'organe de Corti vue au microscope electronique. Rev. Laryng. 93:335–341.

Davis, H. 1961. Peripheral coding of auditory information. *In* W. A. Rosenblith (ed.), Sensory Communication, pp. 119–142. MIT Press, Cambridge, Mass.

Davis, H. 1973. Classes of auditory evoked responses. Audiology 12:464–469.

Davis, H., P. A. Davis, A. L. Loomis, N. Harvey, and G. A. Hobart. 1939. Electrical reactions of the brain to auditory stimulation during sleep. J. Neurophysiol. 2:500–514.

Davis, H., T. Mast, N. Yoshie, and S. Zerlin. 1966. The slow response of the human cortex to auditory stimuli: Recovery process. Electroencephalog. & Clin. Neurophysiol. 21:105–113.

Davis, H., and S. Onishi. 1969. Maturation of auditory evoked potentials. Int. Audiol. 8:24–33.

Davis, H., and S. Zerlin. 1966. Acoustic relations of the human vertex potential. J. Acoust. Soc. Am. 39:109–116.

Davis, P. A. 1939. Effects of acoustic stimuli on the waking human brain. J. Neurophysiol. 2:494–499.

Day, R. S. 1973. Digit span memory in language-bound and stimulus-bound subjects. Paper presented at a meeting of the Acoustical Society of America, Boston, Mass.

Day, R. S., and C. C. Wood. 1972. Mutual interference between two linguistic dimensions of the same stimuli (Abst.). J. Acoust. Soc. Am. 51:175.

Dayal, V. S. 1972. A study of crossed olivocochlear bundle on adaptation of auditory action potentials. Laryngoscope 82:693–711.

Dayal, V. S., J. Farkashidy, and A. Kokshanian. 1973. Embryology of the ear. Canad. J. Otolaryng. 2:136–142.

Dearborn, G. V. N. 1910. Moto-Sensory Development: Observations of the First Three Years of a Child. Warwick and York, Baltimore.

Dekaban, A. 1970. Neurology of Early Childhood. The Williams & Wilkins Company, Baltimore.

Dember, W. N., and R. W. Earl. (1957). Analysis of exploratory, manipulatory, and curiosity behaviors. Psychol. Rev. 64:91–96.

Demetriades, T. 1923. The cochleo-palpebral reflex in infants. Ann. Otol. Rhin. & Laryng. 32:894–903.

Denes, P. B., and E. N. Pinson. 1963. The Speech Chain. Waverly Press, Baltimore.

DeReuck, A. V. S., and J. Knight (eds.). 1968. Hearing Mechanisms in Vertebrates. Little, Brown, & Company, Boston.

Desmedt, J. E. 1965. Neurophysiologic Correlates of Sensory Perception. AD 617796, Clearinghouse for Federal Scientific and Technical Information, U. S. Dept. Comm., Springfield, Va.

Desmedt, J. E., J. Debecker, and J. Manil. 1965. Evidence of a brain-wave pattern associated with subject detection of a tactile stimulus. Bull. Acad. Roy. Med. Belg. 5:887—936.

Desmedt, J. E., and J. Manil. 1970. Somatosensory evoked potentials of the normal human neonate in REM sleep, in slow wave sleep, and in waking. Electroencephalog. & Clin. Neurophysiol. 29:113—126.

Desmedt, J. E., and K. Mechelese. 1958. Suppression of acoustic input by thalamic stimulation. Proc. Soc. Exper. Biol. & Med. 99:772—775.

Desmond, M. M., R. R. Franklin, H. Arnold, J. Watts, C. Vallbona, R. M. Hill, and R. Plumb. 1963. The clinical behavior of the newly born. I. The term baby. J. Pediat. 62:307—325.

Desmond, M. M., and A. J. Rudolph. 1965. Progressive evaluation of the newborn infant. Postgrad. Med. 2:207—212.

Dethier, V. G., and E. Stellar. 1961. Animal Behavior. Prentice-Hall, Inc., Englewood Cliffs, N. J.

Deutsch, D. 1969. Music recognition. Psychol. Rev. 76:300—307.

Deutsch, D. 1970. Tones and numbers: Specificity of interference in immediate memory. Science 168:1604—1605.

DeVore, I. (ed.). 1965. Primate Behavior. Holt, Rinehart and Winston, New York.

Dewson, J. H., III, and A. C. Burlingame. 1975. Auditory discrimination and recall in monkeys. Science 187:267—268.

Dewson, J. H., III, and A. Cowey. 1969. Discrimination of auditory sequences by monkeys. Nature 222:695—697.

Dewson, J. H., III, W. C. Dement, and F. B. Simmons. 1965. Middle ear muscle activity in cats during sleep. Exper. Neurol. 12:1—8.

Dewson, J. H., III, K. W. Nobel, and K. H. Pribram. 1966. Corticofugal influence at cochlear nucleus of the cat: Some effects of ablation of insular-temporal cortex. Brain Res. 2:151—159.

Dewson, J. H., III, K. H. Pribram, and J. C. Lynch. 1969. Effects of ablations of temporal cortex upon speech sound discrimination in the monkey. Exper. Neurol. 24:579—591.

Diamond, I. T., J. M. Goldberg, and W. D. Neff. 1962. Tonal discrimination after ablation of auditory cortex. J. Neurophysiol. 25:223—235.

Diamond, I. T., and W. C. Hall. 1969. Evolution of neocortex. Science 164:251—252.

DiCarlo, L. M., and W. H. Bradley. 1961. A simplified auditory test for infants and young children. Laryngoscope 71:628—646.

Dickson, R. C. 1968. The normal hearing of Bantu and Bushmen. J. Laryng. & Otolaryng. 82:505—521.

Dirks, D. 1964. Perception of dichotic and monaural verbal material and cerebral dominance for speech. Acta Otolaryng. 58:73—80.

Dittrichova, J., and I. Lapackova. 1964. Development of the waking state in young infants. Child Develop. 35:365–370.

Dittus, W., and R. Lemon. 1969. Effects of song tutoring and acoustic isolation on the song repertoires of cardinals. Anim. Behav. 17:523–533.

Divenyi, P. L., and I. J. Hirsh. 1974. Identification of temporal order in three-tone sequences. J. Acoust. Soc. Am. 56:144–151.

Dobie, R. A., and F. B. Simmons. 1971. A dichotic threshold test: Normal and brain-damaged subjects. J. Speech & Hearing Res. 14:71–81.

Dodgson, M. C. H. 1962. The Growing Brain. The Williams & Wilkins Company, Baltimore.

Doehring, D. G., and B. N. Bartholomeus. 1971. Laterality effects in voice recognition. Neuropsychol. 9:425–430.

Doehring, D. G., and R. W. Ross. 1972. Voice recognition by matching to sample. J. Psycholing. Res. 1:233–242.

Donshin, E., and D. B. Lindsley. 1969. Average Evoked Potentials. SP-191, NASA, Washington, D. C.

Dooling, D. G. 1975. Rhythm and syntax in sentence perception. J. Verb. Learn. Verb. Behav. (In press).

Dorfman, D. D., and R. Megling. 1966. Comparison of magnitude estimation of loudness in children and adults. Percept. & Psychophys. 1:239–241.

Dorman, M. F. 1974. Auditory evoked potential correlates of speech sound discrimination. Percept. & Psychophys. 15:215–220.

Dorman, M. F., and D. C. Geffner. 1973. Hemispheric specialization for speech perception in six-year-old black and white children from low and middle socioeconomic classes. Status Report on Speech Perception (SR 34), April-June. Haskins Laboratories, New Haven.

Dorman, M. F., and R. Hoffman. 1973. Short-term habituation of the infant auditory evoked response. J. Speech & Hearing Res. 16:637–641.

Dotson, E., and M. M. Desmond. 1964. The evaluation of muscle tonus in the newborn. Neurology 14:464–471.

Dougherty, A. L., and J. L. Cohen. 1961. Auditory screening for infants and preschoolers. Nursing Outlook 9:310–312.

Douglas, R. 1967. The hippocampus and behavior. Psychol. Bull. 67:416–442.

Douglas, W. W. 1973. The release of biologically active substances. Paper presented at the Society for Neuroscience, San Diego, Calif. (BIS Conference Rep. No. 36, March, 1974, pp. 11–16).

Dowling, W. J. 1967. Rhythmic fission and the perceptual organization of tone sequences. Ph.D. thesis, Harvard University, Cambridge, Mass.

Dowling, W. J. 1972. Recognition of melodic transformations: Inversion, retrograde, and retrograde inversion. Percept. & Psychophys. 12:417–421.

Downs, M. P., and W. G. Hemenway. 1969. Report on the hearing screening of 17,000 neonates. Int. Audiol. 8:72–76.

Downs, M. P., and G. M. Sterritt. 1964. Identification audiometry for neonates: A preliminary report. J. Aud. Res. 4:69–80.

Doyle, J. C., R. Ornstein, and D. Galin. 1974. Lateral specialization of cognitive mode. Psychophysiology 11:567–578.

Dreyfus-Brisac, C. 1964. The electroencephalogram of the premature and full-term newborn. *In* P. Kellaway and I. Peterson (eds.), Neurological and Electroencephalographic Correlative Studies in Infancy, pp. 186–207. Grune & Stratton, Inc., New York.

Dreyfus-Brisac, C. 1966. The bioelectric development of the CNS during early life. *In* F. Falkner (ed.), Human Development, pp. 386–405. W. B. Saunders Company, Philadelphia.

Dreyfus-Brisac, C. 1970. Ontogenesis of sleep in human prematures after 32 weeks of conceptional age. Develop. Psychobiol. 3:91–121.

Dubner, R., and Y. Kawamura (eds.). 1971. Oral-Facial Sensory and Motor Mechanisms. Appelton-Century-Crofts, Inc., New York.

Dubowitz, V., G. F. Whittaker, B. H. Brown, and A. Robinson. 1968. Nerve conduction velocity—An index of neurological maturity of the newborn infant. Develop. Med. Child Neurol. 10:741–749.

DuBrul, E. L. 1967. Pattern of genetic control of structures in the evolution of behavior. Perspect. Biol. Med. 10:524–538.

Duffy, E. 1957. The psychological significance of the concept of "arousal" or "activation." Psychol. Rev. 64:265–275.

Duffy, E. 1962. Activation and Behavior. John Wiley & Sons, Inc., New York.

Dunker, E., and G. Grubel. 1965. On the function of the efferent auditory system. II. Changes in the variability of spike intervals and in the inhibition of deafferentiated cochlear neurons after division of decussating pathways in the ventral pons. Pflügers Arch. Ges. Physiol. 283:270–284.

Dunlop, C. W., E. M. McLachlan, W. R. Webster, and R. H. Day. 1964. Auditory habituation in cats as a function of stimulus intensity. Nature 203:874–875.

Dunlop, C. W., W. R. Webster, and R. H. Day. 1964. Amplitude changes of evoked potentials at the inferior colliculus during acoustic habituation. J. Aud. Res. 4:159–169.

Dunlop, C. W., W. R. Webster, and R. S. Rodger. 1966. Amplitude changes of evoked potentials in the auditory system of unanesthetized cats during acoustic habituation. J. Aud. Res. 6:47–66.

Dwornicka, B., J. Jasienska, W. Smolarz, and R. Wawryk. 1964. Attempt of determining the fetal reaction to acoustic stimulation. Acta Otolaryng. 57:571–574.

Eagles, E. L., S. M. Wishik, and L. G. Doerfler. 1961. A study of hearing in children. Tr. Am. Acad. Ophth., May-June, Parts I and II, pp. 260–296.

Eccles, J. C., M. Ito., and J. Szentágothai. 1967. The Cerebellum as a Neuronal Machine. Springer-Verlag, New York.

Edwards, D. C. 1974. Stimulus intensity and recency contrasts and orienting response strength. Psychophysiol. 11:543–547.

Ehrlich, A. 1974. Infant development in two prosimian species. Develop. Psychobiol. 7:439–454.

Eichorn, D. H. 1951. Electrocortical and autonomic response in infants to visual and auditory stimuli. Ph.D. thesis, University of California, Los Angeles.

Eichorn, D. H. 1970. Physiological development. *In* P. H. Mussen (ed.), Carmichael's Manual of Child Psychology, pp. 157–293. Vol. 1. 3rd Ed. John Wiley & Sons, Inc., New York.

Eilers, R. E., and F. D. Minifie. 1975. Fricative discrimination in early infancy. J. Speech & Hear. Res. 18:158–167.

Eimas, P. D. 1975. Developmental studies in speech perception. *In* L. B. Cohen and P. Salapatek (eds.), Infant Perception. Academic Press, Inc., New York.

Eimas, P. D., W. E. Cooper, and J. D. Corbit. 1973. Some properties of linguistic feature detectors. Percept. & Psychophys. 13:247–252.

Eimas, P. D., and J. D. Corbit. 1973. Selective adaptation of linguistic feature detectors. Cognitive Psychol. 4: 99–109.

Eimas, P. D., E. R. Siqueland, P. Jusczyk, and J. Vigorito. 1971. Speech perception in infants. Science 171:303–306.

Eisele, W. A., and R. C. Berry. 1974. Frequency discrimination abilities in neonates. Paper presented to the American Speech and Hearing Association, Las Vegas, Nev.

Eisele, W. A., R. C. Berry, and T. H. Shriner. 1975. Infant sucking response patterns as a conjugate function of changes in the sound pressure level of auditory stimuli. J. Speech & Hearing Res. 18:296–307.

Eisenberg, R. B. 1956. A study of the auditory threshold in normal and in hearing impaired persons, with special reference to the factors of the duration of the stimulus and its sound pressure level; and a discussion of the implications, clinical and physiological, of the reciprocal relationship between these factors. Sc.D. thesis, The Johns Hopkins University, Baltimore.

Eisenberg, R. B. 1963a. A practical method for screening visual-perceptual-motor performance. J. Speech & Hearing Dis. 28:87–90.

Eisenberg, R. B. 1963b. Integration of speech and hearing into a basic research program. ASHA 5:627–628.

Eisenberg, R. B. 1964. Critical age periods and their relation to developmental disorders of communication. J. Pa. Speech & Hearing Assn. 5:7–11.

Eisenberg, R. B. 1965a. Auditory behavior in the human neonate. I. Methodologic problems and the logical design of research procedures. J. Aud. Res. 5:159–177.

Eisenberg, R. B. 1965b. Auditory behavior in the human neonate. Int. Audiol. 4:65–68.

Eisenberg, R. B. 1965c. Auditory behavior in the human neonate. Paper presented to the Society for Research in Child Development, Minneapolis.

Eisenberg, R. B. 1966a. Electroencephalography in the study of developmental disorders of communication. J. Speech & Hearing Dis. 31:183–186.

Eisenberg, R. B. 1966b. Auditory behavior in the human neonate: Functional properties of sounds and their ontogenetic implications. Paper presented to the American Speech & Hearing Association, Washington, D. C.

Eisenberg, R. B. 1967. Stimulus significance as a determinant of infant responses to sound. Paper presented to the Society for Research in Child Development, New York.

Eisenberg, R. B. 1970a. The development of hearing in man: An assessment of current status. ASHA 12:199–123.

Eisenberg, R. B. 1970b. The organization of auditory behavior. J. Speech & Hearing Res. 13:454–471.

Eisenberg, R. B. 1970c. Developmental processes in hearing: A report from no man's land. Paper presented at Wayne State University, Detroit.

Eisenberg, R. B. 1971. Pediatric audiology: Shadow or substance? J. Aud. Res. 11:148–153.

Eisenberg, R. B. 1972. Human hearing: Development's undeveloped territory. Develop. Psychobiol. 5:97–99.

Eisenberg, R. B. 1974a. The ontogeny of auditory behavior in humans. In L. Jílek and S. Trojan (eds.), Ontogenesis of the Brain, pp. 307–315. Vol. 2. Universitas Carolina Pragensis, Prague, Czech.

Eisenberg, R. B. 1974b. Measurements of sensory capabilities. In R. E. Stark (ed.), Sensory Capabilities of Hearing-Impaired Children, pp. 20–33. University Park Press, Baltimore.

Eisenberg, R. B. 1975a. Auditory sensory processes: Some gleanings from the developmental lode. In J. F. Prescott, M. S. Read, and D. B. Coursin (eds.), Malnutrition and Brain Function: Neurophysiological Methods of Assessment, pp. 381–392. John Wiley & Sons, Inc., New York.

Eisenberg, R. B. 1975b. Cardiotachometry. In L. J. Bradford (ed.), Physiological Measures of the Audio-Vestibular System, pp. 319–347. Academic Press, Inc., New York.

Eisenberg, R. B., D. B. Coursin, and N. Rupp. 1966. Habituation to an acoustic pattern as an index of differences among human neonates. J. Aud. Res. 6:239–248.

Eisenberg, R. B., E. J. Griffin, D. B. Coursin, and M. A. Hunter. 1964. Auditory behavior in the human neonate: A preliminary report. J. Speech & Hearing Res. 7:245–269.

Eisenberg, R. B., A. Marmarou, and P. Giovachino. 1973. Heart rate changes to a synthetic vowel: The validity of response measures at various developmental stages. Unpublished Bioacoustic Laboratory report to NICHHD, Bethesda, Md.

Eisenberg, R. B., A. Marmarou, and P. Giovachino. 1974a. Infant heart rate changes to a synthetic speech sound. J. Aud. Res. 14:20–28.

Eisenberg, R. B., A. Marmarou, and P. Giovachino. 1974b. Heart rate changes to a synthetic speech sound as an index of individual differences. J. Aud. Res. 14:45–50.

Eisenberg, R. B., A. Marmarou, and P. Giovachino. 1974c. Electroencephalographic responses to a synthetic speech sound: A preliminary report. J. Aud. Res. 14:29–43.

Elkonin, D. B. 1957. The physiology of higher nervous activity and child psychology. In B. Simon (ed.), Psychology in the Soviet Union, pp. 47–68. Routledge & Kegan Paul, Ltd., London.

Ellingson, R. J. 1964. Cerebral electrical responses to auditory and visual stimuli in the human infant (human and subhuman studies). In P. Kellaway and I. Petersen (eds.), Neurological and Electroencephalographic Correlative Studies in Infancy, pp. 78–116. Grune & Stratton, Inc., New York.

Ellingson, R. J., T. Danahy, B. Nelson, and G. H. Lathrop. 1974. Variability of auditory evoked potentials in human newborns. Electroencephalog. & Clin. Neurophysiol. 36:155–162.

Ellingson, R. J., S. J. Deutch, and M. S. McInteir. 1974. EEG's of prematures: 3–8 year follow up study. Develop. Psychobiol. 7: 529–538.

Elliott, D. N., and C. Trahiotis. 1972. Cortical lesions and auditory discrimination. Physiol. Bull. 77:198–222.

Elliott, G. B., and K. A. Elliott. 1964a. Some pathological, radiological and clinical implications of the precocious development of the human ear. Laryngoscope 79:1160–1171.

Elliott, G. B., and K. A. Elliott. 1964b. Observations on the constitution of the petrosa. Am. J. Roentgenol. Radium Ther. Nucl. Med. 91:633–639.

Elliott, L. L., and A. F. Niemoeller. 1971. The role of hearing in controlling voice fundamental frequency. Int. Audiol. 9:47–52.

Elliott, R. 1972. The significance of heart rate for behavior: A critique of Lacey's hypothesis. J. Personality Soc. Psychol. 22:398–409.

Emmanouilides, G. C., A. J. Moss, E. K. Duffie, and F. H. Adams. 1964. Pulmonary arterial pressure changes in human newborn infants from birth to three days of age. J. Pediat. 65:327–333.

Engel, R. 1961. Evaluation of electroencephalographic tracings of newborns. Lancet 81:523–532.

Engel, R., and V. Milstein. 1971. Evoked response stability in tracé alternant. Electroencephalog. & Clin. Neurophysiol 31:377–382.

Engel, R., and N. B. Young. 1969. Calibrated pure tone audiograms in normal neonates based on evoked electroencephalographic responses. Neuropädiatrie 1:149–160.

Engen, T., L. P. Lipsitt, and H. Kaye. 1963. Olfactory response and adaptation in the human neonate. J. Comp. & Physiol. Psychol. 56:73–77.

Epstein, S., L. Boudreau, and S. Kling. 1975. Magnitude of the heart rate and electrodermal response as a function of stimulus input, motor output, and their interaction. Psychophysiology 12:15–24.

Erickson, R. 1965. Stimulus coding in topographic and nontopographic afferent modalities: On the significance of the activity of individual sensory neurons. Psychol. Rev. 75:447–464.

Erulkar, S. D., R. A. Butler, and G. L. Gerstein. 1968. Excitation and inhibition in cochlear nucleus. II. Frequency modulated tones. J. Neurophysiol. 31:637–648.

Erulkar, S. D., and P. G. Nelson. 1963. Synaptic mechanisms of excitation and inhibition in the central auditory pathway. J. Neurophysiol. 26:908–923.

Escalona, S. K. 1968. The Roots of Individuality. Aldine, Chicago.

Evans, C. R., and T. B. Mulholland (eds.). 1969. Attention in Neurophysiology. Appleton-Century-Crofts, Inc., New York.

Evans, W., and J. Bastian. 1969. Marine mammal communication: Social and ecological factors. In H. Anderson (ed.), The Biology of Marine Mammals. Academic Press, Inc., New York.

Ewing, A. 1969. The genetic basis of sound production in drosophila pseudoobscura and D. persimilis. Anim. Behav. 17:555–560.

Ewing, I. R., and A. W. G. Ewing. 1944. The ascertainment of deafness in infancy. J. Laryng. & Otol. 59:309–333.

Faglioni, P., H. Spinnler, and L. A. Vignolo. 1969. Contrasting behavior of right and left hemisphere-damaged patients on a discriminative and a semantic task of auditory recognition. Cortex 5:366–388.

Fairbanks, G. 1942. An acoustical study of the pitch of infant hunger wails. Child Develop. 13:227–232.

Falkner, F. (ed.). 1966. Human Development. W. B. Saunders Company, Philadelphia.

Fantz, R. L. 1963. Pattern vision in newborn infants. Science 140:296–297.

Fargo, N., D. Kewley-Port, R. Mobley, and V. E. Goodman. 1973. The development of auditory feedback monitoring: Delayed auditory feedback studies on the vocalization of children aged six months to 19 months. J. Speech & Hearing Res. 16:709–720.

Fay, R. R. 1974. Auditory frequency discrimination in vertebrates. J. Acoust. Soc. Am. 56:206–209.

Feldman, S. 1962. Neurophysiological mechanisms modifying afferent hypothalamo-hippocampal conduction. Exper. Neurol. 5:269–291.

Fex, J. 1965. The olivocochlear feedback systems. In A. B. Graham (ed.), Sensorineural Hearing Processes and Disorders. Little, Brown & Company, Boston.

Fex, J. 1967. Efferent inhibition in the cochlea related to hair-cell dc activity: Study of postsynaptic activity of the crossed olivocochlear fibers in the cat. J. Acoust. Soc. Am. 41:666–675.

Field, H., P. Copack, A. J. Derbyshire, G. J. Driessen, and R. E. Marcus. 1967. Responses of newborns to auditory stimulation. J. Aud. Res. 7:271–285.

Field, J. (ed.). 1960. Handbook of Physiology. Section I. Neurophysiology. Vol. II. Am. Physiol. Soc., Wash., D. C.

Filogama, G., L. Candiollo, and G. Rossi. 1967. The morphology and function of auditory input control. Beltone Inst. Hearing Res. (translation No. 20), Chicago.

Finck, A. 1968. Analysis of single unit response areas in the cochlear nerve. J. Aud. Res. 8:207–213.

Finck, A., and M. Sofouglu. 1966. Auditory sensitivity of the Mongolian gerbil. J. Aud. Res. 6:313–319.

Fior, R. 1972. Physiological maturation of auditory function between 3 and 13 years of age. Audiology 11:317–321.

Fiorentino, M. R. 1963. Reflex Testing Methods for Evaluating C. N. S. Development. Charles C Thomas, Publisher, Springfield, Ill.

Fischer, G. J. 1966. Auditory stimuli in imprinting. J. Comp. & Physiol. Psychol. 61:271–273.

Fisischelli, V. R. 1966. The phonetic content of the cries of normal infants and those with brain damage. J. Psychol. 64:119–126.

Fisichelli, V. R., and S. Karelitz. 1966. Frequency spectra of the cries of normal infants. Psychonom. Sci. 6:195–196.

Fitzgerald, H. E., L. M. Lintz, Y. Brackbill, and G. Adams. 1967. Time perception and conditioning of autonomic response in human infants. Percept. Motor Skills 24:479–486.

Flanagan, G. L. 1962. The First Nine Months of Life. Simon and Schuster, New York.

Flanagan, J. L. 1965. Speech Analysis, Synthesis and Perception. Academic Press, Inc., New York.

Flavell, J. H. 1963. The Developmental Psychology of Jean Piaget. Van Nostrand, New York.

Fletcher, S. G. 1973. Maturation of the speech mechanism. Folia Phoniat. (Basel) 25:161–172.

Flynn, W. E., and D. N. Elliott. 1965. Role of the pinna in hearing. J. Acous. Soc. Am. 38:104–105.

Forbes, H. S., and H. B. Forbes. 1927. Fetal sense reaction: Hearing. J. Comp. Psychol. 7:353–355.

Foss, B. M. (ed.). 1961. Determinants of Infant Behavior. John Wiley & Sons, Inc., New York.

Fox, M. W. 1966. Neuro-behavioral ontogeny. A systhesis of ethological and neurophysiological concepts. Brain Res. 2:3–20.

Freedman, D. G. 1961. The infant's fear of strangers and the flight response. J. Child Psychol. Psychiat. 4:242–248.

Freeman, G. L. 1940. The relationship between performance level and bodily activity level. J. Exper. Psychol. 26:602–608.

French, J. D. 1960. The reticular formation. In J. Field (ed.), Handbook of Physiology, pp. 1281–1305. Sect. 1. Vol. II. Am. Physiol. Soc., Washington, D. C.

French, J. D., R. Hernández-Péon, and R. B. Livingston. 1955. Projections from cortex to cephalic brain stem (reticular formation) in monkey. J. Neurophysiol. 18:74–95.

Frey, H. H., and W. Relke. 1965. Contributions to testing the hearing of newborn children. HNO 10:294–295.

Friedlander, B. Z. 1968. The effect of speaker identity, voice inflection, vocabulary, and message redundancy on infants' selection of vocal reinforcement. J. Exper. Child Psychol. 3:443–459.

Friedlander, B. Z. 1970. Receptive language development in infancy: Issues and problems. Merrill-Palmer Quart. 16:7–52.

Friedlander, B. Z., D. A. Silva, and M. S. Knight. 1973. Selective responses to auditory and auditory-vibratory stimuli by severely retarded deaf-blind children. J. Aud. Res. 13:105–112.

Friedlander, B. Z., and D. Whitten. 1970. Effects of regulated loudness and sound frequency on an 18-month "deaf" infant's discriminative self-selected listening with an automatic operant game in the home. Paper presented to the American Speech and Hearing Association, New York.

Frishkopf, L. S., and M. H. Goldstein. 1963. Responses to acoustic stimuli from single units in the eighth nerve of the bullfrog. J. Acoust. Soc. Am., 35:1219–1228.

Froding, C. 1960. Acoustic investigation of newborn infants. Acta Oto-laryng. 52:31–40.

Froeschels, E. 1951. What is hearing? The Nervous Child 9:2–7.

Froeschels, E., and H. Beebe. 1946. Testing the hearing of newborn infants. Arch. Oto-laryng. 44:710–714.

Fry, D. B. 1973. Acoustic cues in the speech of the hearing and the deaf. Proc. Roy. Soc. Med. 66:959–969.

Fujisaki, H., and T. Kawashima. 1969. On the modes and mechanisms of speech perception. Sogoshikenjo-Nenpo 28:67–73.

Fujisaki, H., and T. Kawashima. 1970. Some experiments on speech perception and a model for the perceptual mechanism. Ann. Rep. Eng. Res. Inst. Univ. Tokyo 29:207–214.

Fujisaki, H., and T. Kawashima. 1971. A model of the mechanisms for speech perception: Quantitative analysis of categorical effects in discrimination. Ann. Rep. Eng. Res. Inst. Univ. Tokyo, 30:59–68.

Funkenstein, H. H., P. G. Nelson, P. Winter, Z. Wollberg, and J. D. Newman. 1971. Unit responses in auditory cortex of awake squirrel monkeys to vocal stimulation. *In* M. B. Sachs (ed.), Physiology of the Auditory System, pp. 307–315. Nat. Ed. Consult., Baltimore.

Funkenstein, H. H., and P. Winter. 1973. Responses to acoustic stimuli of units in the auditory cortex of awake squirrel monkeys. Exper. Brain Res. 18:464–488.

Gacek, R. R. 1965. Afferent auditory neural system. *In* A. B. Graham (ed.), Sensorineural Processes and Disorders. Little, Brown & Company, Boston.

Gaddum, J. 1965. The neurological basis of learning. Perspect. Biol. Med. 8:436–474.

Galambos, R. 1954. Neural mechanisms of audition. Physiol. Rev. 34:497–528.

Galambos, R., R. E. Myers, and G. C. Sheatz. 1961. Extralemniscal activation of auditory cortex in cats. Am. J. Physiol. 200:23–28.

Galin, D. 1964a. Auditory nuclei: Distinctive response patterns to white noise and tones in unanesthetized cats. Science 146:270–272.

Galin, D. 1964b. Effects of conditioning on auditory signals. *In* W. S. Fields and B. R. Alford (eds.), Neurological Aspects of Auditory and Vestibular Disorders, pp. 61–76. Charles C Thomas, Publisher, Springfield, Ill.

Galin, D. 1965. Background and evoked activity in the auditory pathway: Effects of noise-shock pairing. Science 149:761–763.

Gates, G. R., J. C. Saunders, G. R. Bock, L. M. Aitkin, and M. A. Elliott. 1974. Peripheral auditory function in the platypus, Ornithorhynchus anatinus. J. Acoust. Soc. Am. 56:152–156.

Gates, H. W., J. J. Romba, and P. Martin. 1963. Response latencies in the Rhesus monkey as a function of tone intensity. U. S. Army Tech. Mem. 3–63., Aberdeen Proving Ground, Md.

Gazzaniga, M. S. 1972. One brain–two minds? Am. Sci. 60:311–317.

Gellhorn, E. 1967. The tuning of the nervous system: Physiological foundations and implications for behavior. Perspect. Biol. Med. 10:559–591.

Geniec, P., and D. K. Morest. 1971. The neuronal architecture of the human posterior colliculus. Acta Oto-laryng. (Suppl.) 295 (whole).

Gerber, S. E., and P. Goldman. 1971. Ear preference for dichotically presented verbal stimuli as a function of report strategies. J. Acoust. Soc. Am. 49:1163–1168.

Gersuni, G. V. (ed.). 1971. Sensory Processes at the Neuronal and Behavioral Levels. Academic Press, Inc., New York.

Gersuni, G. V., Y. A. Altman, I. A. Vartanian, A. M. Maruseva, E. A. Radionova, and G. I. Ratnikova. 1969. Temporal characteristics classifying neurons of inferior colliculus in the cat. Neurophysiol. 1:137–146.

Gersuni, G. V., and I. A. Vartanian. 1973. Time dependent features of adequate sound stimuli and the functional organization of central auditory neurons. *In* A. R. Møller (ed.), Basic Mechanisms in Hearing, pp. 623–674. Academic Press, Inc., New York.

Geschwind, N. 1964. The development of the brain and the evolution of language. *In* C. I. J. M. Stuart (ed.), Report of the 15th Ann. R. T. M. on Linguistic and Language Studies, pp. 155–169.

Geschwind, N. 1965. Disconnection syndromes in animal and man. Brain 88:237–294.

Geschwind, N. 1970. The organization of language and the brain. Science 170:940–944.

Geschwind, N. 1972. Language and the brain. Scient. Am. 226:76–83.

Geschwind, N., and W. Levitsky. 1968. Human brain: Left-right asymmetries in temporal speech region. Science 161:186–187.

Gilbert, J. H. (ed.). 1972. Speech and Cortical Functioning. Academic Press, Inc., New York.

Glanzer, M. 1953. Stimulation satiation: An explanation of spontaneous alternation and related phenomena. Psychol. Rev. 60:257–268.

Gleisner, L., A. Flock, and J. Wersäll. 1973. The ultrastructure of the afferent synapse on hair cells in the frog labyrinth. Acta Oto-laryng. 76:199–207.

Godfrey, J. J. 1974. Perceptual difficulty and the right ear advantage for vowels. Brain & Lang. 4:323–336.

Godovikova, D. B. 1973. Some characteristics of infants' reactions to "physical" and "social" auditory stimuli. Early Child Develop. & Care (Ireland) 2:291–306.

Goldberg, J. M., H. O. Adrian, and F. D. Smith. 1964. Response of neurons of the superior olivary complex of the cat to acoustic stimuli of long duration. J. Neurophysiol. 27:706–749.

Goldberg, J. M., and P. Brown. 1968. Functional organization of the dog superior olivary complex: An anatomical and electrophysiological study. J. Neurophysiol. 31:639–656.

Goldberg, J. M., and P. Brown. 1969. Response of binaural neurons of dog superior olivary complex to dichotic tonal stimuli: Some physiological mechanisms of sound localization. J. Neurophysiol. 32:613–635.

Goldberg, J., and D. D. Greenwood. 1966. Responses of neurons in the cochlear nucleus to tones and noise of long duration. J. Neurophysiol. 29:72–93.

Goldstein, M. H., J. L. Hall, and B. O. Butterfield. 1968. Single-unit activity in the primary auditory cortex of unanesthetized cats. J. Acoust. Soc. Am. 43:444–455.

Goldstein, R., and D. Kendall. 1963. Electroencephalographic audiometry in young children. J. Speech & Hearing Dis. 28:331–354.

Goldstein, R., C. C. McRandle, and M. A. Smith. 1973. Early and late AERs to clicks in neonates. Paper presented at a meeting of the American Electroencephalographic Society, Boston.

Goodglass, R. 1973. Developmental comparison of vowels and consonants in dichotic listening. J. Speech & Hearing Res. 16:744–752.

Goodman, W. S., S. V. Appleby, J. W. Scott, and P. E. Ireland. 1964. Audiometry in newborn children by electroencephalography. Laryngoscope 74:1316–1328.

Goto, H. 1971. Auditory perception by normal Japanese adults of the sounds "l" and "r." Neuropsychologia 9:317–323.

Gottlieb, G. 1965. Imprinting in relation to parental and species identification by avian neonates. J. Comp. & Physiol. Psychol. 59:345–356.

Gottlieb, G. 1966. Species identification by avian neonates: Contributory effects of perinatal auditory stimulation. Anim. Behav. 14:282–290.

Gottlieb, G. 1968. Prenatal behavior of birds. Quart. Rev. Biol. 43:148–174.

Gottlieb, G., and P. H. Klopfer. 1962. The relation of developmental age to auditory and visual imprinting. J. Comp. & Physiol. Psychol. 55:821–826.

Gottlieb, G., and M. L. Simner. 1966. Relationship between cardiac rate and nonnutritive sucking in human infants. J. Comp. & Physiol. Psychol. 61:128–131.

Grabow, J. D., and F. W. Elliott. 1974. The electrophysiologic assessment of hemispheric asymmetries during speech. J. Speech & Hearing Res. 17:64–72.

Graham, F. K. 1973. Habituation and dishabituation of responses innervated by the autonomic nervous system. *In* H. V. S. Peeke and M. J. Herz (eds.), Habituation: Behavioral Studies and Physiological Substrates, pp. 163–218. Academic Press, Inc., New York.

Graham, F. K., K. M. Berg, W. K. Berg, J. C. Jackson, H. M. Hatton, and S. R. Kantowitz. 1970. Cardiac orienting responses as a function of age. Psychonom. Sci. 19:363–365.

Graham, F. K., and R. K. Clifton. 1966. Heart-rate change as a component of the orienting response. Psychol. Bull. 65:305–320.

Graham, F. K., R. K. Clifton, and H. M. Hatton. 1968. Habituation of heart rate response to repeated auditory stimulation during the first five days of life. Child Develop. 39:35–52.

Graham, F. K., and J. C. Jackson. 1970. Arousal systems and infant heart rate responses. *In* L. P. Lipsitt and H. W. Reese (eds.), Advances in Child Development and Behavior, pp. 60–118. Vol. 5. Academic Press, Inc., New York.

Gray, M. L., and D. H. Crowell. 1968. Heart rate changes to sudden peripheral stimuli in the human during early infancy. J. Pediat. 72:807–814.

Graziani, L. J., E. D. Weitzman, and M. S. A. Velasco. 1968. Neurologic maturation and auditory evoked responses in low birth weight infants. Pediatrics 41:483–494.

Green, J. D. 1964. The hippocampus. Physiol. Rev. 44:561–608.

Greenberg, H. J. 1974. Averaged encephalic response of aphasics to linguistic and nonlinguistic auditory stimuli. J. Speech & Hearing Res. 17:113–121.

Greenberg, H. J., and J. T. Graham. 1970. EEG changes during learning of speech and nonspeech stimuli. J. Verb. Learn. Verb. Behav. 9:274–281.

Greenberg, J. H. 1966. Universals of Language. 2nd Ed. MIT Press, Cambridge, Mass.

Greenwood, D. D., and J. M. Goldberg. 1970. Response of neurons in the cochlear nuclei to variations in noise bandwidth and to tone-noise combination. J. Acoust. Soc. Am. 47:1022–1040.

Gregory, A. H., J. C. Harriman, and L. D. Roberts. 1972. Cerebral dominance for the perception of rhythm. Psychonom. Sci 28:75–76.

Griffiths, J. D. 1968. A comparison of vowel and consonant perception. Paper presented to the Acoustic Society of America, Ottawa, Canada.

Grimwade, J. C., D. W. Walker, M. Bartlett, S. Gordon, and C. Wood. 1971. Human fetal heart rate change and movement in response to sound and vibration. Am. J. Obst. & Gynec. 109:86–90.

Groth, H., D. H. Crowell, A. Salamy, and D. Jardine. 1967. An exploratory study of neonatal pitch perception. Paper presented to the Western Psychological Association, San Francisco.

Haggard, M. P. 1971. Encoding and the REA for speech signals. Quart. J. Exper. Psychol. 23:34–45.

Haggard, M. P., S. Ambler, and M. Callow. 1970. Pitch as a voicing cue. J. Acoust. Soc. Am. 47:613–617.

Haggard, M. P., and A. M. Parkinson. 1971. Stimulus and task factors as determinants of ear advantages. Quart. J. Exper. Psychol. 23:168–177.

Haller, M. W. 1932. The reactions of infants to changes in the intensity and pitch of pure tone. J. Genet. Psychol. 40:162–180.

Halperin, Y., I. Nachson, and A. Carmon. 1973. Shift of ear superiority in dichotic listening to temporally patterned non-verbal stimuli. J. Acoust. Soc. Am. 53:46–50.

Halverson, H. M. 1942. The differential effects of nudity and clothing on muscular tonus in infancy. J. Genet. Psychol. 61:55–67.

Hamm, C. L. 1971. Exposure learning of auditory stimuli by rats. Psychonom. Sci. 23:81–82.

Hannah, J. E. 1971. Phonetic and temporal titration of the dichotic right ear effect. Ph.D. thesis, Louisiana State University, New Orleans, La.

Hardy, J. B., A. Dougherty, and W. G. Hardy. 1959. Hearing responses and audiologic screening in infants. J. Pediat. 55:382–390.

Hardy, W. G., and J. E. Bordley. 1951. Evaluation of hearing in young children. Acta Oto-laryng. 40:346–360.

Hardy, W. G., J. B. Hardy, C. H. Brinker, T. M. Frazier, and A. Dougherty. 1962. Auditory screening in infants. Ann. Otol. Rhin. & Laryng. 71:759–766.

Harker, L. A., and R. Van Wagoner. 1974. Application of impedance audiometry as a screening instrument. Acta Oto-laryng. 77:198–201.

Harlow, H. F., and C. N. Woolsey (eds.). 1965. Biological and Biochemical Bases of Behavior. University of Wisconsin Press, Madison.

Harris, G., and J. Seigel. 1975. Categorical perception and absolute pitch. Paper presented at a meeting of the Acoustical Society of America, Austin, Texas.

Harris, J. D. 1943. Habituatory response decrement in the intact organism. Psychol. Bull. 40:385–422.

Harrison, J. M., and M. D. Beecher. 1967. Medial superior olive and sound localization. Science, 155:1696–1697.

Harrison, J. M., and R. E. Irving. 1964. Nucleus of the trapezoid body: Dual afferent innervation. Science 143:473–474.

Harrison, J. M., and R. E. Irving. 1966. Visual and nonvisual auditory systems in mammals. Science 154:738–743.

Harrison, J. M., and W. B. Warr. 1962. A study of the cochlear nuclei and ascending auditory pathways of the medulla. J. Comp. Neurol. 119:341–380.

Harrison, J. M., W. B. Warr, and R. E. Irving. 1962. Second order neurons in the acoustic nerve. Science 138:893–895.

Hatton, H. M., W. K. Berg, and F. K. Graham. 1970. Effects of acoustic rise time on heart rate response. Psychonom. Sci. 19:101–103.

Haugan, G. M., and R. W. McIntire. 1972. Comparisons of vocal imitation, tactile stimulation and food as reinforcers for infant vocalizations. Develop. Psychol. 6:201−209.

Haydon, S. P., and F. J. Spellacy. 1973. Monaural reaction time asymmetries for speech and nonspeech sounds. Cortex 9:288−294.

Haynes, H., B. L. White, and R. Held. 1965. Visual accommodation in human infants. Science 148:528−530.

Hebb, D. O. 1955. Drives and the C. N. S. (conceptual nervous system). Psychol. Rev. 62:243−254.

Hecox, K., and R. Galambos. 1974. Brain stem auditory evoked responses in human infants and adults. Arch. Oto-laryng. 99:30−33.

Heilman, K., D. Pandya, E. Karol, and N. Geschwind. 1971. Auditory inattention. Arch. Neurol. 24:323−325.

Heilman, K., and E. Valenstein. 1972a. Auditory neglect in man. Arch Neurol. 26:32−35.

Heilman, K., and E. Valenstein. 1972b. Frontal lobe neglect in man. Neurobiology 22:660−664.

Hendry, L. S., and W. Kessen. 1964. Oral behavior of newborn infants as a function of age and time since feeding. Child Develop. 35:201−208.

Herman, S. 1972. The right ear advantage for speech processing. Presented to the Acoustic Society of America, Miami, Fla.

Hernández-Péon, R. 1966. Physiological mechanisms in attention. In R. W. Russell (ed.), Frontiers in Physiological Psychology, pp. 121−148. Academic Press, Inc., New York.

Hess, W. R. 1957. The Functional Organization of the Diencephalon. Grune & Stratton, Inc., New York.

Hess, W. R. 1964. The Biology of Mind. University of Chicago Press, Chicago.

Hewes, G. W. 1973. Primate communication and the gestural origin of language. Current Anthropol. 14:5−24.

Hicks, R. E. 1975. Intrahemispheric response competition between vocal and unimanual performance in normal adult human males. J. Comp. & Physiol. Psychol. (In press).

Hillyard, S. A. 1969. The CNV and the vertex evoked potential during signal detection: A preliminary report, pp. 349−353. In E. Donshin and D. B. Lindsley (eds.), Average Evoked Potentials. NASA, Washington, D. C.

Himwich, W. A., and H. E. Himwich (eds.). 1964. The Developing Brain. Elsevier Press, Inc., New York.

Hind, J. E., J. M. Goldberg, D. D. Greenwood, and J. E. Rose. 1963. Some discharge characteristics of single neurons in the inferior colliculus of the cat. II. Timing of discharges and observations on binaural stimulation. J. Neurophysiol. 26:321−341.

Hinde, R. E. 1970. Animal Behavior. McGraw-Hill Book Company, Inc., New York.

Hinde, R. E. (ed.). 1972. Non-verbal Communication. University Press, Cambridge, England.

Hirsh, I. J. 1959. Auditory perception of temporal order. J. Acoust. Soc. Am. 31:759−767.

Hirsh, I. J. 1974. Temporal order and auditory perception. In H. R. Moskowitz et al. (eds.), Sensation and Measurement, pp. 251−258. D. Reidel Publ. Co., Dordrecht, The Netherlands.

Hirsh, I. J., and C. E. Sherrick. 1961. Perceived order in different sense modalities. J. Exper. Psychol. 62:423–432.

Hochberg, I. 1965. Effect of previous listening experience upon semantic perception of simple and complex tones. Percept. Motor Skills 20:1201–1208.

Holliday, R., and J. E. Pugh. 1975. DNA modification mechanisms and gene activity during development. Science 187:226–232.

Holstein, S. B., J. S. Buchwald, and J. A. Schwafel. 1969. Tone response patterns of the auditory nuclei during normal wakefulness, paralysis, and anesthesia. Brain Res. 15:483–499.

Horenstein, S., R. LeZak, and W. Pitts. 1966. Temporal tone discrimination in auditory agnosia and aphasic states. Tr. Am. Neurol. A. 251–253.

Horowitz, A. B. 1972. Habituation and memory: Infant cardiac responses to familiar and discrepant auditory stimuli. Child Develop. 43:43–53.

House, A. S., K. N. Stevens, T. T. Sandel, and J. B. Arnold. 1962. On the learning of speechlike vocabularies. J. Verb. Learn. Verb. Behav. 1:133–143.

Hoversten, G. H., and J. P. Moncur. 1969. Stimuli and intensity factors in testing infants. J. Speech & Hearing Res. 12:687–702.

Hughes, J. B., B. Ehemann, and U. A. Brown. 1948. Electroencephalography of the newborn. Am. J. Dis. Child. 76:503–512.

Hulse, F. S. 1963. The Human Species. Random House, New York.

Humphrey, G. L., and J. S. Buchwald. 1972. Response decrements in the cochlear nucleus of decerebrate cats during repeated acoustic stimulation. Science 175:1488–1491.

Humphrey, T. 1970. The development of fetal activity and its relation to postnatal behavior. In L. P. Lipsitt and H. W. Reese (eds.), Advances in the Study of Behavior, pp. 1–57. Vol. 5. Academic Press, Inc., New York.

Hursh, J. B. 1939. The properties of growing nerve fibers. Amer. J. Physiol. 127:140–153.

Hutchinson, B. B. 1973. Performance of aphasics on a dichotic listening task. J. Aud. Res. 13:64–70.

Hutt, C., H. v. Bernuth, H. Lenard, S. J. Hutt, and H. F. R. Prechtl. 1968a. Habituation in relation to state in the human neonate. Nature 220:618–620.

Hutt, C., and S. J. Hutt. 1970. The neonatal evoked heart rate response and the law of initial value. Psychophysiology 6:661–668.

Hutt, S. J. 1973. Square-wave stimuli and neonatal auditory behavior: Reply to Bench. J. Exper. Child Psychol. 16:530–533.

Hutt, S. J., C. Hutt, H. G. Lenard, H. v. Bernuth, and W. J. Muntjewerff. 1968b. Auditory responsivity in the human neonate. Nature 218:888–890.

Hutt, S. J., H. G. Lenard, and H. F. R. Prechtl. 1969. Psychophysiological studies in newborn infants. In L. P. Lipsitt and H. W. Reese (eds.), Advances in Child Development and Behavior, pp. 127–172. Vol. 4. Academic Press, Inc., New York.

Huttenlocher, P. R. 1960. Effects of state of arousal on click responses in the mesencephalic reticular formation. Electroencephalog. & Clin. Neurphysiol. 12:819–827.

Hyden, H., and P. W. Lange. 1965. Rhythmic enzyme changes in neurons and glia during sleep. Science 149:654–656.

Inglis, J. 1965. Dichotic listening and cerebral dominance. Acta Oto-laryng. 60:231–238.

Irwin, O. A. 1930. The amount and nature of activities of newborn infants under constant external stimulating conditions during the first ten days of life. J. Gen. Psychol. Monogr. 8:1–92.

Irwin, O. A. 1932. The latent time of the body startle in infants. Child Develop. 3:104–107.

Irwin, O. A. 1933. Motility in young infants. Am. J. Dis. Child. 45:534–537.

Irwin, O. A. 1941. Effects of strong light on the body activity of newborns. J. Comp. Psychol. 32:233–236.

Irwin, O. A. 1946. Infant psychology. In P. L. Harriman (ed.), Encyclopedia of Psychology. Philosophical Library, New York.

Irwin, O. A., and L. A. Weiss. 1934a. Differential variations in the activity and crying of the newborn infant under different intensities of light: A comparison of observational with polygraphic findings. Univ. Iowa Stud. Child Welf. 9:137–147.

Irwin, O. A., and L. A. Weiss. 1934b. The effect of darkness on the activity of newborn infants. Univ. Iowa Stud. Child Welf. 9:164–175.

Irwin, R. J., and A. W. Mills. 1965. Matching loudness and vocal level: An experiment requiring no apparatus. Brit. J. Psychol. 56:143–146.

Isaacson, R. L. 1974. The Limbic System. Plenum Press, New York.

Jackson, J. C., S. R. Kantowitz, and F. K. Graham. 1971. Can newborns show cardiac orienting? Child Develop. 42:107–121.

Jacobson, A. G. 1966. Inductive processes in embryonic development. Science 152:25–34.

Jacobson, M. 1969. Development of specific neuronal connections. Science 163:543–547.

Jakobson, R., C. G. Fant, and M. Halle. 1967. Preliminaries to Speech Analysis–The Distinctive Features and Their Correlates. MIT Press, Cambridge, Mass.

Jane, J. A., R. B. Masterton, and I. T. Diamond. 1965. The function of the tectum for attention to auditory stimuli in the cat. J. Comp. Neurol. 125:165–191.

Jane, J. A., D. Yashon, and I. T. Diamond. 1968. An anatomic basis for multimodal thalamic units. Exper. Neurol. 22:464–471.

Jarvis, J. F., and H. G. Heerden. 1967. The acuity of hearing in the Kalahari Bushmen. J. Larying. & Otol. 81:63–68.

Jeffress, L. A. 1964. Stimulus-oriented approach to detection. J. Acoust. Soc. Am. 36:766–774.

Jeffrey, W. E. 1968. The orienting reflex and attention in cognitive development. Psychol. Rev. 75:323–334.

Jeffrey, W. E., and L. B. Cohen. 1971. Habituation in the human infant. In H. W. Reese (ed.), Advances in Child Development and Behavior, pp. 123–176. Vol. 6. Academic Press, Inc., New York.

Jennings. J. R., J. C. Stringfellow, and M. Graham. 1974. A comparison of the statistical distributions of beat-by-beat heart rate and heart period. Psychophysiology 11:207–210.

Jerger, J. (ed.). 1963. Modern Developments in Audiology. Academic Press, Inc., New York.

Jerger, J., P. Burney, L. Mauldin, and B. Crump. 1974. Predicting hearing loss from the acoustic reflex. J. Speech & Hearing Dis. 39:11–22.

Jerger, S., J. Jerger, L. Mauldin, and P. Segal. 1974. Studies in impedance audiometry II. Children less than 6 years old. Arch. Otolaryng. 99: 1–9.

Johansson, B., E. Wedenberg, and B. Westin. 1964. Measurement of tone response by the human foetus: A preliminary report. Acta Oto-laryng. 57:188–192.

Johnson, C. S. 1968. Relation between absolute threshold and duration of tone pulses in the bottlenosed porpoise. J. Acoust. Soc. Am. 43:757–763.

Johnson, E. F. 1962. Automatic process control. Science 135:403–407.

Johnson, L. C. 1970. A psychophysiology for all states. Psychophysiology 6:501–516.

Johnson, L. C., and W. E. Karpan. 1968. Autonomic correlates of the spontaneous K-complex. Psychophysiology 4:444–452.

Johnson, L. C., and A. Lubin. 1967. The orienting reflex during waking and sleeping. Electroencephalog. & Clin. Neurophysiol. 22:11–21.

Johnsson, L.-G. 1971. Reissner's membrane in the human cochlea. Ann. Otol. Rhin. & Laryng. 80:425–439.

Jones, R. H., D. H. Crowell, and L. E. Kapuniai. 1969. Change detection model for serially correlated data. Psychol. Bull. 71:352–358.

Kaas, J., S. Axelrod, and I. T. Diamond. 1967. An ablation study of the auditory cortex in the cat using binaural tonal patterns. J. Neurophysiol. 30:710–724.

Kaas, J., and I. T. Diamond. 1969. Corpus callosum section and selective attention to one ear. Presented at the 10th Annual Meeting of the Psychonomic Society.

Kagan, J., and M. Lewis. 1965. Studies of attention in the human infant. Merrill-Palmer Quart. 11:95–127.

Kakizaki, I., and F. Altmann. 1970. The interglobular spaces in the human labyrinthine capsule. Ann. Otol. Rhin. & Laryng. 79:666–679.

Kaneko, Y., and J. Daly. 1968. Acetylcholinesterase on the nerve endings of outer hair cells and the tunnel radial fibers. Laryngoscope 78:1566–1581.

Kaplan, E. L. 1970. Intonation and language acquisition. In Papers and Reports on Child Language Development. Committee on Linguistics, Stanford University 1:2–21.

Karlin, I. W., D. B. Karlin, and L. Gurren. 1965. Development and Disorders of Speech in Childhood. Charles C Thomas, Publisher, Springfield, Ill.

Karlovich, R., and B. Luterman. 1970. Application of the TTS paradigm for assessing sound transmission in the auditory system during speech production. J. Acoust. Soc. Am. 47:510–517.

Kasatkin, N. I. 1957. Ranii ontogenez reflektornoi deiatelnosti rebenka. Zh. Vyssh. Nerv. Deiat. Pavlov 7:805–818.

Kasatkin, N. I., and A. M. Levikova. 1935. On the development of early conditioned reflexes and differentiations of auditory stimuli in infants. J. Exper. Psychol. 18:1–19.

Katsuki, Y. 1965. Comparative neurophysiology of hearing. Physiol. Rev. 45:380–423.

Katsuki, Y., N. Suga, and Y. Kanno. 1962. Neural mechanisms of the peripheral and central auditory system in monkeys. J. Acoust. Soc. Am. 34:1396–1410.

Katsuki, Y., and T. Watanabe. 1966. Cortical efferent flow influencing responses of geniculate and collicular auditory neurons. Int. Audiol. 5:82–85.

Katz, J. (ed.). 1972. Handbook of Clincal Audiology. The Williams & Wilkins Company, Baltimore.

Kavanagh, J. F. 1971. The genesis and pathogenesis of speech and language. In J. Hellmuth (ed.), Exceptional Infant, pp. 211–247. Vol. 2. Bruner/Mazel, New York.

Kavanagh, J. F., and J. E. Cutting (eds.). 1975. The Role of Speech in Language. MIT Press, Cambridge, Mass. (In press).

Kavanagh, J. F., and I. G. Mattingly (eds.). 1972. Language by Ear and by Eye. MIT Press, Cambridge, Mass.

Kaye, H. 1964. Skin conductance in the human neonate. Child Develop. 35:1297–1305.

Kaye, H. 1966. The effects of feeding and tonal stimulation on nonnutritive sucking in the human newborn. J. Exper. Child Psychol. 3:131–145.

Kaye, H., and G. R. Levin. 1963. Two attempts to demonstrate tonal suppression of non-nutritive sucking in neonates. Percept. Motor Skills 17:521–522.

Kaye, H., and L. P. Lipsitt. 1964. Relation of electrotactual threshold to basal skin conductance. Child Develop. 35:1307–1312.

Kearsley, R. B. 1973. The newborn's response to auditory stimulation: A demonstration of orienting and defensive behavior. Child Develop. 44:582–590.

Keen, R. E. 1964. Effects of auditory stimuli on sucking behavior in the human neonate. J. Exper. Child Psychol. 1:348–354.

Keen, R. E., H. Chase, and F. K. Graham. 1965. Twenty-four hour retention by neonates of an habituated heart rate response. Psychonom. Sci. 2:265–266.

Keith, R. W. 1973. Impedance audiometry with neonates. Arch. Otolaryng. 97:465–467.

Keith, R. W. 1974. The application of impedance measurement techniques to neonates. Presented at Regional Audiology Research Unit, Royal Berkshire Hospital, Reading, England.

Keith, R. W. 1975. Middle ear function in neonates. Arch. Oto-laryng. (In press).

Kelly, J. B. 1974. The acquisition of three types of auditory pattern discrimination in the cat. Physiol. Psychol. 2:481–483.

Kent, R. D. 1974. Auditory-motor formant tracking: A study of speech imitation. J. Speech & Hearing Res. 17:203–222.

Kessen, W., M. M. Haith, and P. H. Salapatek. 1970. Infancy. In P. H. Mussen (ed.)., Carmichael's Manual of Child Psychology, pp. 287–445. Vol. 1. 3rd Ed. John Wiley & Sons, Inc., New York.

Kessen, W., E. J. Williams, and J. P. Williams. 1961. Selection and test of response measures in the study of the human newborn. Child Develop. 32:7–24.

Khachaturian, Z. S., J. Kerr, R. Kruger, and J. Schachter. 1972. A methodological note: Comparison between period and rate data in studies of cardiac function. Psychophysiology 9:539–545.

Khanna, S. M., R. E. Sears, and J. Tonndorf. 1968. Some properties of longitudinal shear waves: A study by computer simulation. J. Acoust. Soc. Am. 43:1077–1084.

Kiang, N. Y-S. 1965. Discharge Patterns of Single Fibers in the Cat's Auditory Nerve. MIT Press, Cambridge, Mass.

Kiang, N. Y-S., M. B. Sachs, and W. T. Peake. 1967. Shapes of tuning curves for single auditory-nerve fibers. J. Acoust. Am. 42:1341–1342.

Kilmer, W., and W. S. McCulloch. 1969. The reticular formation command and control system. *In* K. N. Leibovic (ed.), Information Processing in the Nervous System, pp. 297–307. Springer-Verlag, New York.

Kimble, D. P. 1968. Hippocampus and internal inhibition. Psychol. Bull. 70:285–295.

Kimura, D. 1961a. Some effects of temporal-lobe damage on auditory perception. Canad. J. Psychol. 15:156–165.

Kimura, D. 1961b. Cerebral dominance and the perception of verbal stimuli. Canad. J. Psychol. 15:166–171.

Kimura, D. 1963. Speech lateralization in young children as determined by an auditory test. J. Comp. & Physiol. Psychol. 56:899–902.

Kimura, D. 1964. Left-right differences in the perception of melodies. Quart. J. Exper. Psychol. 14:355–358.

Kimura, D., and S. Folb. 1968. Neural processing of backwards-speech sounds. Science 161:395–396.

Kimura, R. S. 1966. Hairs of the cochlear sensory cells and their attachment to the tectorial membrane. Acta Oto-laryng. 61:55–72.

Kincaid, J. P., and F. Cooper. 1972. Release from proactive inhibition as a function of pleasantness of verbal materials. Psychonom. Sci. 27:214–216.

King, F. L., and D. Kimura. 1972. Left-ear superiority in dichotic perception of vocal nonverbal sounds. Canad. J. Psychol. 26:111–116.

Klasen, E. 1972. The Syndrome of Specific Dyslexia. University Park Press, Baltimore.

Klatt, D. 1974. The duration of /s/ in English words. J. Speech & Hearing Res. 17:51–63.

Klatzky, R. L., and R. C. Atkinson. 1971. Specialization of the cerebral hemispheres in scanning for information in short-term memory. Percept. & Psychophys. 10:335–338.

Kleitman, N. 1965. Sleep and Wakefulness. 2nd Ed. University of Chicago Press, Chicago.

Knox, C., and D. Kimura. 1970. Cerebral processing of nonverbal sounds in boys and girls. Neuropsychologica 8:227–237.

Kobrak, H. G. 1959. The Middle Ear. University of Chicago Press, Chicago.

Konishi, M. 1969. Time resolution by single auditory neurones in birds. Nature 222:566–567.

Konishi, T., and J. Z. Slepian. 1971a. Effects of the electrical stimulation of the crossed olivocochlear bundle on cochlear potentials recorded with intracochlear electrodes in guinea pigs. J. Acoust. Soc. Am. 49:1762–1769.

Konishi, T., and J. Z. Slepian. 1971b. Summating potential with electrical stimulation of crossed olivocochlear bundle. Science 172:483–484.

Kopp, C. 1970. Inhibition of infant crying: A comparison of stimuli. Presented at Western Psychological Association, Los Angeles.

Korner, A. F. 1964. Some hypotheses regarding the significance of individual differences at birth for later development. Psychoanal. Stud. Child 19:58–72.

Korner, A. F. 1968. REM organization in neonates. Theoretical implications for development and the biological function of REM. Arch. Gen. Psychiat. (Chicago) 19:330–341.

Korner, A. F. 1973. Early stimulation and maternal care as related to infant capabilities and individual differences. Early Child Develop. & Care (Ireland) 2:307–327.

Kósa, F., and I. Fazekas. 1973. Emberi magzatok hallócsontjainak méretei. (Size of the auditory ossicles of human fetuses). Fülorrgégegyogyaszat 19:153–159.

Kosyagina, E. B. 1967. Alteration of the weight, form and size of the human incus. Vestn. Otorinolaring. 19:35–38.

Krashin, S. D. 1972. Lateralization, language learning, and the critical period: Some new evidence. Lang. Learning 23:630–674.

Kron, R. E., J. Ipsen, and K. E. Goddard. 1968. Consistent individual differences in the nutritive sucking behavior of the human newborn. Psychosom. Med. 30:151–161.

Krushinskii, L. V. 1962. Animal Behavior. Consultant Bureau, New York.

Kryter, K. D. 1966. Psychological reactions to aircraft noise. Science 151:1346–1355.

Kryter, K. D. 1968. Concepts of perceived noisiness, their implementation and application. J. Acoust. Soc. Am. 43:344–361.

Kubovy, M., J. E. Cutting, and R. M. McGuire. 1974. Hearing with the third ear: Dichotic perception of a melody without monaural familiarity cues. Science 186:272–274.

Kuhl, P. K., and J. D. Miller. 1974. Discrimination of speech sounds by the chinchilla: /t/ vs /d/ in CV syllables. Presented at the Acoustic Society of America, St. Louis.

Kupperman, R. 1972. Cochlear adaptation, central influences. Acta Otolaryng. 73:130–140.

Lacey, J. I., J. Kagan, B. C. Lacey, and H. A. Moss. 1963. In P. H. Knapp (ed.), Expressions of the Emotions in Man, pp. 161–196. International Universities Press, New York.

Lacey, J. I., and B. C. Lacey. 1970. Some autonomic-central nervous system interrelationships. In P. Black (ed.), Physiological Correlates of Emotion, pp. 205–228. Academic Press, Inc., New York.

Lamper, C., and C. Eisdorfer. 1971. Prestimulus activity level and responsivity in the neonate. Child Develop. 42:465–473.

Lane, H. 1965. The motor theory of speech perception: A critical review. Psychol. Rev. 72:275–309.

Lane, H. 1968. On the necessity of distinguishing between speaking and listening. Studies in Language Behavior. Progress Report VI, Center for

Research on Language and Language Behavior. University of Michigan, Ann Arbor.

Lane, H., and B. Tranel. 1971. The Lombard sign and the role of hearing in speech. J. Speech & Hearing Res. 14:677–709.

Lane, H., B. Tranel, and C. Sisson. 1970. Regulation of voice communication by sensory dynamics. J. Acoust. Soc. Am. 47:618–624.

Langford, C., and J. Bench. 1973. Neonatal auditory responses assessed by trained and untrained observers: A preliminary study. Brit. J. Audiol. 7:29–37.

Langworthy, O. R. 1928. A correlated study of the development of reflex activity in fetal and young kittens and the myelinization of tracts in the nervous system. Contrib. Embryol. 20:127–138.

Langworthy, O. R. 1933. Development of behavior patterns and myelinization of the nervous system in the human fetus and infant. Contrib. Embryol. 24:139–143.

Lanyon, W. E., and W. N. Tavolga (eds.). 1960. Animal Sounds and Communication. American Institute of Biological Sciences, Washington, D. C.

Lapham, L. W., and W. R. Marksbery. 1971. Human fetal cerebellar cortex: Organization and maturation of cells in vitro. Science 173:829–832.

Laughlin, W. S. 1963. Eskimos and Aleuts: Their origins and evolution. Science 142:633–645.

Lawrence, D. G., and H. G. J. M. Kuypers. 1965. Pyramidal and non-pyramidal pathways in monkeys: Anatomical and functional correlation. Science 148:973–975.

Lazarus, R. S., and R. A. McCleary. 1951. Autonomic discrimination without awareness: A study of subception. Psychol. Rev. 58:113–122.

League, R., and K. R. Bzoch. 1970. Affective dimensions of voice and infant awareness. Presented at 123rd Annual Meeting of the American Psychiatric Association, Miami.

Leavy, A., and J. H. Geer. 1967. The effect of low levels of stimulus intensity upon the orienting response. Psychonom. Sci. 9:105–106.

Lehiste, I. 1972. The units of speech perception. In J. H. Gilbert (ed.), Speech and Cortical Functioning, pp. 187–235. Academic Press, Inc., New York.

Leibovic, K. N. 1969. Information Processing in the Nervous System. Springer-Verlag, New York.

Leibrecht, B. C. 1974. Habituation: Supplemental bibliography. Physiol. Psychol. 2:401–419.

Lenard, H. G., H. v. Bernuth, and S. J. Hutt. 1969. Acoustic evoked responses in newborn infants: The influence of pitch and complexity of the stimulus. Electroencephalog. & Clin. Neurophysiol. 27:121–127.

Lenard, H. G., H. v. Bernuth, and H. F. R. Prechtl. 1968. Reflexes and their relationship to behavioral state in the newborn. Acta Pädiat. Scand. 57:177–185.

Lenneberg, E. H. 1967. Biological Foundations of Language. John Wiley & Sons, Inc., New York.

Lenneberg, E. H. 1974. Language and brain: Developmental aspects. Neurosci. Res. Program Bull. 12:513–656.

Lentz, W. E., and G. A. McCandless. 1971. Averaged electroencephalic audiometry in infants. J. Speech & Hearing Dis. 36:19−28.

Lesak, J. 1970. Results of and experience with audiometric examination of normally hearing children. Pract. Otorhinolaryng. 32:74−89.

Leventhal, A., & L. P. Lipsitt. 1964. Adaptation, pitch discrimination and sound localization in the neonate. Child Develop. 35:759−767.

Levin, H., and J. Williams (eds.). 1970. Basic Studies on Reading. Basic Books, Inc. New York.

Lewis, M. 1971. A developmental study of the cardiac response to stimulus onset and offset during the first year of life. Psychophysiology 8:689−698.

Lewis, M. 1974. The cardiac response during infancy. In R. F. Thompson and M. M. Patternson (eds.), Recording of Bioelectric Activity. Academic Press, Inc., New York.

Lewis, M., B. Bartels, H. Campbell, and S. Goldberg. 1967. Individual differences in attention: The relation between infants condition at birth and attention distribution within the first year. Am. J. Dis. Child. 113:461−465.

Lewis, M., B. Bartels, and S. Goldberg. 1967. State as a determinant of infants' heart rate response to stimulation. Science 155:486−488.

Lewis, M., J. Kagan, F. Zavala, and R. Grossberg. 1964. Behavioral and cardiac responses to auditory stimulation in the infants. Presented at the Eastern Psychological Association, Philadelphia.

Lewis, M., and S. J. Spaulding. 1967. Differential cardiac response to visual and auditory stimulation in the young child. Psychophysiology 3:229−237.

Lewis, M. M. 1941. Infant Speech: A Study of the Beginning of Language. Harcourt, Brace, and Company, Inc., New York.

Lhermitte, F., A. R. Lecours, B. Ducarne, and R. Escourolle. 1973. Unexpected anatomical findings in a case of fluent jargon aphasia. Cortex 9:433−446.

Liberman, A. M. 1970. Some characteristics of perception in the speech mode. In D. A. Hamburg et al. (eds.), Perception and Its Disorders. Proc. A. Res. Nerv. & Ment. Dis. 58:238−254.

Liberman, A. M., F. S. Cooper, K. S. Harris, and P. F. MacNeilage. 1963. A motor theory of speech perception. In C. G. M. Fant (ed.), Proceedings of the Speech Comm. Seminar, Stockholm, 1962. Speech Transmission Lab. Roy. Inst. Tech., Stockholm.

Liberman, A. M., F. S. Cooper, D. P. Shankweiler, and M. Studdert-Kennedy. 1967. Perception of the speech code. Psychol. Rev. 74: 431−461.

Licklider, J. C. R. 1951. Basic correlates of the auditory stimulus. In S. S. Stevens (ed.), Handbook of Experimental Psychology, pp. 985−1039. John Wiley & Sons, Inc., New York.

Lidén, G., and A. Kankkunen. 1969. Visual reinforcement audiometry. Arch. Oto-laryng. 89:87−94.

Lieberman, P. 1967. Intonation, Perception and Language. MIT Press, Cambridge, Mass.

Lieberman, P. 1968. Primate vocalizations and human linguistic ability. J. Acoust. Soc. Am. 44:1574−1584.

Lieberman, P. 1969. Methods and designs on the acoustic analysis of primate vocalizations. Behav. Res. Methods Instrum. 1:169−174.

Lieberman, P. 1971. The evolution of human speech anatomy. Haskins Laboratories Status Report on Speech Research (SR-28), pp. 205–222.

Lieberman, P. 1975. The evolution of speech and language. In J. F. Kavanagh and J. E. Cutting (eds.), The Role of Speech in Language. MIT Press, Cambridge, Mass. (In press).

Lieberman, P., and E. S. Crelin. 1971. On the speech of Neanderthal man. Linguistic Inquiry 2:203–222.

Lieberman, P., E. S. Crelin, and D. H. Klatt. 1972. Phonetic ability and related anatomy of the newborn and adult human, Neanderthal man, and the chimpanzee. Am. Anthrop. 74:287–307.

Lieberman, P., K. S. Harris, P. Wolff, and L. H. Russell. 1971. Newborn infant cry and nonhuman primate vocalization. J. Speech & Hearing Res. 14:718–727.

Lieberman, P., D. H. Klatt, and W. H. Wilson. 1969. Vocal tract limitations on the vowel repertoires of Rhesus monkey and other nonhuman primates. Science 164:1185–1187.

Lind, J. (ed.). 1965. Newborn Infant Cry. Almqvist & Wiksells, Stockholm.

Lindsley, D. B. 1951. Emotion. In S. S. Stevens (ed.), Handbook of Experimental Psychology, pp. 473–516. John Wiley & Sons, Inc., New York.

Ling, D. 1972a. Response validity in auditory tests of newborn infants. Laryngoscope 82:376–380.

Ling, D. 1972b. Acoustic stimulus duration in relation to behavioral responses of newborn infants. J. Speech & Hearing Res. 15:567–571.

Ling, D., C. Heaney, and D. G. Doehring, 1971. The use of alternated stimuli to reduce response decrement in the auditory testing of newborn infants. J. Speech & Hearing Res. 14:531–534.

Ling, D., A. Ling, and D. G. Doehring. 1970. Stimulus, response, and observer variables in the auditory screening of newborn infants. J. Speech & Hearing Res. 13:9–18.

Lintz, L. M., H. E. Fitzgerald, and Y. Brackbill. 1967. Conditioning the eyeblink response to sound in infants. Psychonom. Sci. 7:405–406.

Lipsitt, L. P. 1963. Learning in the first year of life. In L. P. Lipsitt and C. C. Spiker (eds.), Advances in Child Development and Behavior, pp. 147–195. Vol. 1. Academic Press, Inc., New York.

Lipsitt, L. P., T. Engen, and H. Kaye. 1963. Developmental changes in the olfactory threshold of the neonate. Child Develop. 34:371–376.

Lipsett, L. P., and H. Kaye. 1964. Conditioned sucking in the human newborn. Psychonom. Sci. 1:29–30.

Lipsitt, L. P., and N. Levy. 1959. Electrotactual threshold in the neonate. Child Develop. 30:547–554.

Lipton, E. L., and A. Steinschneider. 1964. Studies on the psychophysiology of infancy. Merrill-Palmer Quart. 10:103–117.

Lipton, E. L., A. Steinschneider, and J. B. Richmond. 1960. Autonomic function in the neonate. II. Physiologic effects of motor restraint. Psychosom. Med. 22:57–64.

Lipton, E. L., A. Steinschneider, and J. B. Richmond. 1961a. Autonomic function in the neonate. III. Methodological Considerations. Psychosom. Med. 23:461–471.

Lipton, E. L., A. Steinschneider, and J. B. Richmond. 1961b. Autonomic function in the neonate. IV. Individual differences in cardiac reactivity. Psychosom. Med. 23:472−484.

Lipton, E. L., A. Steinschneider, and J. B. Richmond. 1963. Auditory discrimination in the newborn infant. Presented at the Society for Research in Child Development, Berkeley, Calif.

Lipton, E. L., A. Steinschneider, and J. B. Richmond. 1964. Autonomic function in the neonate. VIII. Cardio-pulmonary observations. Pediatrics 33:212−215.

Lipton, E. L., A. Steinschneider, and J. B. Richmond. 1965a. The autonomic nervous system in early life. New England J. Med. 273:147−154.

Lipton, E. L., A. Steinschneider, and J. B. Richmond. 1965b. Swaddling, a child chare practice: Historical, cultural and experimental observations. Pediatrics 35:521−567.

Lipton, E. L., A. Steinschneider, and J. B. Richmond. 1966. Autonomic function in the neonate. VII. Maturational changes in cardiac control. Child Develop. 37:1−16

Lisker, L., and A. S. Abramson. 1964. A cross-language study of voicing in initial stops: Acoustical Measurements. Word 20:384−422.

Locke, S., and L. Kellar. 1973. Categorical perception in a non-linguistic mode. Cortex 9:355−369.

Loe, P. R., and L. A. Benevento. 1969. Auditory-visual interaction in single units in the orbito-insular cortex of the cat. Electroencephalog. & Clin. Neurophysiol. 26:395−398.

Loomis, A. L., N. Harvery, and G. A. Hobart. 1938. Distribution of disturbance patterns in the human electroencephalogram, with special reference to sleep. J. Neurophysiol. 1:413−430.

Lorenz, K. 1965. Evolution and Modification of Behavior. University of Chicago Press, Chicago.

Low, M. D. (ed.). 1973. The Beckman EEG Handbook. Beckman Instruments, Fullerton, Calif.

Lowell, M. 1971. Recent research developments in pediatric audiometry. Aust. Teacher of the Deaf 12:40−53.

Lumio, J. S., and T. Laukola. 1968. Hearing tests for neonates. Monatsschr. Ohrenheilkunder 6:353.

Lykken, D. T., and A. Tellegen. 1974. On the validity of the preception hypothesis. Psychophysiology 10:125−132.

Lynn, G. E., and J. Gilroy. 1972. Neuro-audiological abnormalities in patients with temporal lobe tumors. J. Neurol. Sci. 17:167−184.

Lynn, R. 1966. Attention, Arousal and the Orienting Reaction. Pergamon Press, Ltd., New York.

Madonia, T., F. Modica, and G. Cali. 1963. Several interesting aspects of the ampullar crests in the human fetus. Clin. Otorhinolaryng. 15:272−291.

Maezawa, K. 1965. Hearing tests by use of startling reactions with pure tone stimulation. Otolaryng. (Tokyo) 37:5−7.

Magoun, H. W. 1963. The Waking Brain. 2nd Ed. Charles C Thomas, Publisher, Springfield, Ill.

Mahaffey, R. B. 1970. Temporal aspects of audition as correlates of temporal aspects of speech. Presented at Acoustic Society of America, Houston, Tex.

Maiorana, V. A., and W. M. Schleidt. 1972. The auditory sensitivity of the turkey. J. Aud. Res. 12:203–207.

Mallard, A. R., and R. G. Daniloff. 1973. Glottal cues for parent judgment of emotional aspects of infant vocalizations. J. Speech & Hearing Res. 16:592–596.

Malmo, R. B. 1962. Activation. In A. J. Bachrach (ed.), Experimental Foundations of Clinical Psychology, pp. 386–422. Basic Books, Inc., New York.

Malmo, R. B., and D. Bélanger. 1967. Related physiological and behavioral changes: What are their determinants? Proc. A. Res. Nerv. & Ment. Dis. 45:288–318.

Maltzman, I., and D. C. Raskin. 1965. Effects of individual differences in the orienting reflex on conditioning and complex processes. J. Exper. Res. Personality 1:1–16.

Marler, P. 1961. The logical analysis of animal communication. J. Theor. Biol. 1:295–317.

Marler, P. 1967. Animal communication signals. Science 157:769–774.

Marler, P. 1969. Vocalizations of wild chimpanzees. In C. R. Carpenter (ed.), Recent Advances in Primatology, pp. 94–100. Vol. 1. S. Karger AG, Basel.

Marler, P., and W. J. Hamilton, III. 1966. Mechanisms of Animal Behavior. John Wiley & Sons, Inc., New York.

Marler, P., and P. Mundinger. 1971. Vocal learning in birds. In H. Moltz (ed.), Ontogeny of Vertebrate Behavior, pp. 389–450. Academic Press, Inc., New York.

Marler, P., and M. Tamura. 1964. Culturally transmitted patterns of vocal behavior in sparrows. Science 146:1483–1486.

Marquis, D. 1931. Can conditioned responses be established in the newborn infant? J. Genetic Psychol. 39:479–492.

Marsh, J. T., and F. G. Worden. 1964. Auditory potentials during acoustic habituation: Cochlear nucleus, cerebellum, and auditory cortex. Electroencephalog. & Clin. Neurophysiol. 17:685–692.

Martin, J. G., and W. Strange. 1968. The perception of hesitation in spontaneous speech. Percept. & Psychophys. 3:427–438.

Martinius, J. W., and H. Papousek. 1970. Responses to optic and exteroceptive stimuli in relation to state in the human newborn: Habituation of the blink reflex. Neuropädiatrie 1:452–460.

Maruyama, N., T. Kawasaki, J. Abe, I. Katoh, and H. Yamazaki. 1966. Unitary response to tone stimuli recorded from the medical geniculate body of cats. Int. Audiol. 5:184–188.

Mason, W. A. 1968. Early social deprivation in nonhuman primates. In D. C. Glass (ed.), Environmental Influences, pp. 70–101. Rockefeller University Press, New York.

Masterton, R. B., and M. A. Berkeley. 1974. Brain function: Changing ideas on the role of sensory, motor, and association cortex in behavior. Ann. Rev. Psychol. 25:218–312.

Matkin, N., E. Harford, and B. Murphy. 1968. A preliminary critique of an auditory test battery for pediatric cases. Presented at ASHA, Denver.

Matsumiya, Y., V. Tagliasco, C. T. Lombroso, and H. Goodglass. 1972. Auditory evoked response: Meaningfulness of stimuli and interhemispheric asymmetry. Science 175:790–792.

Mattingly, I. G. 1972. Speech cues and sign stimuli. Am. Sci. 60:327–337.

Mattingly, I. G. 1975. The human aspect of speech. *In* J. F. Kavanagh and J. E. Cutting (eds.), The Role of Speech in Language. MIT Press, Cambridge, Mass. (In press).

Mattingly, I. G., A. M. Liberman, A. K. Syrdal, and T. Halwes. 1971. Discrimination in speech and nonspeech modes. Cognitive Psychol 2:131–157.

Mavilya, M. P. 1969. Spontaneous vocalization and babbling in hearing impaired infants. Ph.D. dissertation, Columbia University, New York.

Maw, A. R. 1974. Synaptic contacts within the intra-ganglionic spiral bundle and other recent ultrastructural findings in relation to concepts of efferent cochlear innervation. Ann. Otol. Rhin. & Laryng. 83: 180–192.

Mayr, E. 1965. Animal Species and Evolution. Harvard University Press, Cambridge, Mass.

McAdam, D. W., and H. A. Whitaker. 1971. Language production: Electroencephalographic localization in the normal human brain. Science 172:499–502.

McCaffrey, A. 1971. Speech perception in infancy. Ph.D. thesis, Cornell University, Ithaca, New York.

McCall, R. B., and W. H. Melson. 1970. Amount of short-term familiarization and the response to auditory discrepancies. Child Develop. 41: 861–869.

McCallum, W. C., and J. R. Knott. 1973. Event-related slow potentials of the brain: Their relations to behavior. Suppl. 33. Electroencephalog. & Clin. Neurophysiol. Elsevier, New York.

McCandless, G. A. 1967. Clinical application of evoked response audiometry. J. Speech & Hearing Res. 10:468–478.

McCleary, R. A., and R. Y. Moore. 1956. Subcortical Mechanisms of Behavior. Basic Books, Inc., New York.

McFarland, W. H., and S. J. Kirksey. 1973. Ocular response to auditory stimulation during controlled, repetitive ocular movements. J. Aud. Res. 13:1–5.

McGurk, H., and M. Lewis. 1974. Space perception in early infancy: Perception within a common auditory-visual space. Science 186:649–650.

McKenzie, B. E., and R. H. Day. 1972. Object distance as a determinant of visual fixation in early infancy. Science 178:1108–1110.

McLellan, M. S., J. R. Brown, H. Rondeau, E. Shoughro, R. A. Johnson, and A. R. Hale. 1964. Embryonal connective tissue and exudate in ear. Am. J Dis. Child. 108:164–170.

McLellan, M. S., and A. Struck. 1965. Ear studies in the premature infant: A statistical description of otoscopic landmarks. J. Pediat. 67:122–124.

McNeill, D. 1970. The development of language. *In* P. H. Mussen (ed.), Carmichael's Manual of Child Development, pp. 1061–1161. Vol. 1. 3rd Ed. John Wiley & Sons, Inc., New York.

McNeil, J. D., and E. R. Keislar. 1963. Value of the oral response in beginning reading: An experimental study using programmed instruction. Brit. J. Educ. Psychol. 33:163–168.

McRandle, C. C., and M. A. Smith. 1973. Early AER components to monotic and diotic click stimuli in neonates. Presented at the American Speech and Hearing Association, Detroit.

Mencher, G. T., M. Kushner, and B. McCulloch. 1975. White noise as a pretest sensitizer for neonatal hearing screening. Audiology 14:152–163.

Mendel, M. I. 1968. Infant responses to recorded sounds. J. Speech & Hearing Res. 11:811–816.

Menyuk, P. 1971. The Acquisition and Development of Language. Prentice-Hall, Inc., Englewood Cliffs, N. J.

Mestyan, G., and F. Varga. 1960. Chemical thermoregulation of full-term and premature newborn infants. J. Pediat. 56:623–629.

Metcalf, D. R. 1970. EEG sleep spindle ontogenesis. Neuropädiatrie 1: 428–433.

Metcalf, D. R., J. Mondale, and F. K. Butler. 1972. Ontogenesis of spontaneous K-complexes. Psychophysiology 8:340–347.

Meyer, D. H., and V. I. Wolfe. 1974. Use of a high risk register in newborn hearing screening. Presented at ASHA, Las Vegas.

Milhorn, H. T. 1968. The Application of Control Theory to Physiological Systems. W. B. Saunders Company, Philadelphia.

Miller, E. A., P. S. Goldman, and H. E. Rosvold. 1973. Delayed recovery of function following orbital prefrontal lesions in infant monkeys. Science 182:304–306.

Miller, J., L. de Schweinitz, and C. P. Goetzinger. 1963. How infants three, four, and five months of age respond to sound. Exceptional Child. 30:149–154.

Miller, J. G. 1965. The organization of life. Perspect. Biol. Med. 9:107–125.

Miller, M. H. 1971. Neonatal and infant auditory screening programs. Clin. Pediat. 10:340–345.

Miller, M. H., and M. Rabinowitz. 1970. Conditioned orienting reflex audiometry with maternal rubella children. J. Commun. Dis. 3:59–64.

Mills, M., and E. Melhuish. 1974. Recognition of mother's voice in early infancy. Nature 252:123–124.

Milnarich, R. F. 1958. A Manual for EEG Technicians. Little, Brown & Company, Boston.

Milner, B., L. Taylor, and R. W. Sperry. 1968. Lateralized suppression of dichotically presented digits after commissural section in man. Science 161:184–186.

Mitrinowicz-Modrzejewska, A. 1970. New methods of auditory investigations in cases of connatal deafness. Ann. Med. Sect. Polish Acad. Sci. 15:99–114.

Moffitt, A. R. 1968. Speech perception by infants. Ph.D. thesis, University of Minnesota, Minneapolis.

Moffitt, A. R. 1971. Consonant cue perception by twenty- to twenty-four-week-old infants. Child Develop. 42:717–732.

Moffitt, A. R. 1973. Intensity discrimination and cardiac reaction in young infants. Develop. Psychol. 8:357–359.

Molfese, D. L. 1972. Cerebral asymmetry in infants, children and adults: Auditory evoked responses to speech and noise stimulus. Ph.D. thesis, Pennsylvania State University, University Park, Pa.

Møller, A. R. 1969. Unit responses in the cochlear nucleus of the rat to pure tones. Acta Physiol. Scand. 75:530–541.

Møller, A. R. 1971. Unit responses in the rat cochlear nucleus to tones of rapidly varying frequency and amplitude. Acta Physiol. Scand. 81: 540–556.

Møller, A. R. (ed.). 1973. Basic Mechanisms in Hearing. Academic Press, Inc., New York.

Møller, A. R. 1974. Coding of sounds with rapidly varying spectrum in the cochlear nucleus. J. Acoust. Soc. Am. 55:631–640.

Moncur, J. P. 1968. Judge reliability in infant testing. J. Speech & Hearing Res. 11:348–357.

Monod, N., J. Eliet-Flescher, and C. Dreyfus-Brisac. 1967. Sleep patterns in full-term and premature newborns: Polygraphic studies of sleep organization in the pathological newborn. Biol. Neonat. 11:216–247.

Monod, N., and L. Garma. 1971. Auditory responsivity in the human premature. Biol. Neonat. 17:292–316.

Monod, N., N. Pajot, and S. Guidasci. 1972. The neonatal EEG: Statistical studies and prognostic value in full-term and premature babies. Electroencephalog. & Clin. Neurophysiol. 32:529–544.

Moore, B. C. 1973. Frequency difference limens for narrow bands of noise. J. Acoust. Soc. Am. 54:888–896.

Moore, J. M., G. Thompson, and M. Thompson. 1975. Auditory localization of infants as a function of reinforcement conditions. J. Speech & Hearing Dis. 40:29–34.

Moore, T., and L. E. Ucko. 1957. Night waking in early infancy. Arch. Dis. Child. 32:333–342.

Moore, T. J., and J. L. Cashin, Jr. 1974. Response patterns of cochlear nucleus neurons to exerpts from sustained vowels. J. Acoust. Soc. Am. 56:1565–1576.

Moreau, T., H. G. Birch, and G. Turkewitz. 1970. Ease of habituation to repeated auditory and somesthetic stimulation in the human newborn. J. Exper. Child Psychol. 9:193–207.

Morrell, L. K., and D. A. Huntington. 1971. Electrocortical localization of speech production. Science 174:1359–1360.

Morrell, L. K., and J. G. Salamy. 1971. Hemispheric asymmetry of electrocortical responses to speech stimuli. Science 174:164–166.

Morse, P. A. 1972. The discrimination of speech and nonspeech stimuli in early infancy. J. Exper. Child Psychol. 14:477–492.

Morse, P. A. 1973. Infant speech perception: A preliminary model and review of the literature. Presented at the Conference on Language Intervention with the Mentally Retarded. Wisconsin Dells, Wisc.

Morse, P. A. 1974. Synthetic vowel discrimination abilities in young infants. Paper presented at meeting of the American Speech and Hearing Association, Las Vegas.

Morse, P. A., and C. T. Snowdon. 1975. An investigation of categorical speech discrimination by Rhesus monkeys. Percept. Psychophys. 17: 9–16.

Moruzzi, G., and H. W. Magoun. 1949. Brain stem reticular formation and activation of the EEG. Electroencephalog. & Clin. Neurophysiol. 1:455–473.

Moskowitz, H., and W. Lohmann. 1970. Auditory threshold for evoking an orienting reflex in mongoloid patients. Percept. Motor Skills 31:879–882.

Motta, G., G. M. Facchini, and E. D'Auria. 1970. Objective conditioned-reflex audiometry in children. Acta Otolaryng. (Suppl.) 273 (whole).

Moushegian, G., A. Ruppert, and R. Galambos. 1962. Microelectrode study of ventral cochlear nucleus of the cat. J. Neurophysiol. 25:515–529.

Moushegian, G., A. Rupert, and M. A. Whitcomb. 1964a. Brain-stem neuronal response patterns to monaural and binaural tones. J. Neurophysiol. 27:1174–1191.

Moushegian, G., A. Rupert, and M. A. Whitcomb. 1964b. Medial superior-olivary-unit response patterns to monaural and binaural clicks. J. Acoust. Soc. Am. 36:196–202.

Mukhina-Korotova, T. K. 1964. The formation of sound pitch differentiation. Vop. Psikhol. 1:61–71.

Munn, N. L. 1965. The Evolution and Growth of Human Behavior. 2nd Ed. Houghton Mifflin, Boston.

Murphy, E. H., and P. H. Venables. 1969. Effects of ipsilateral and contralateral shock on ear asymmetry in the detection of two clicks. Psychonom. Sci. 17:214–215.

Murphy, E. H., and P. H. Venables. 1970. The investigation of ear asymmetry by simple and disjunctive reaction-time tasks. Percept. & Psychophys. 8:104–105.

Murphy, K. P., and C. M. Smyth. 1962. Responses of fetus to auditory stimulation. Lancet 1:972–973.

Murray, B., and D. Campbell. 1970. Differences between olfactory thresholds in two sleep states in the newborn infant. Psychonom. Sci. 18:313–314.

Nabelik, I., and I. J. Hirsh. 1969. On the discrimination of frequency transitions. J. Acoust. Soc. Am. 45:1510–1519.

Nachson, I., and A. Carmon. 1974. Relationship between accuracy of report and ear-differences in dichotic listening. Percept. Motor Skills 37:653–654.

Naeser, M. A. 1970. Development of a non-phonemic feature in child speech-differential vowel duration in English. Presented at Acoustic Society of America, Atlantic City, N. J.

Naeser, M. A., and J. C. Lilly. 1970. Preliminary evidence for a universal feature detector system-perception of the repeating word. Presented at Acoustic Society of America, Atlantic City, N. J.

Nagafuchi, M. 1970. Development of dichotic and monaural hearing abilities in young children. Acta Oto-laryng. 69:409–414.

Nagafuchi, M., and J. Suzuki. 1973. Auditory agnosia due to incision of splenium corporis callosi. Acta Oto-laryng. 76:109–113.

Nakai, Y. 1970. An electron microscopic study of the human fetus cochlea. Pract. Otorhinolaryng. 32:257–267.

Namin, E. P., and R. A. Miller. 1974. The normal electrocardiogram and vectorcardiogram in children. In D. E. Cassels and R. F. Ziegler (eds.), Electrocardiography in Infants and Children, pp. 99–108. Grune & Stratton, Inc., New York.

Nash, J. 1970. Developmental Psychology: A Psychobiological Approach. Prentice-Hall, Inc., Englewood Cliffs, N. J.

Neff, W. D. 1964. Temporal pattern discrimination in lower animals and its relation to language perception in man. In A. B. S. de Reuck and M.

O'Connor (eds.), Ciba Foundation Symposium on Disorders of Language. pp. 183–193. J. & A. Churchill, Ltd., London.

Neff, W. D. (ed.). 1968. Contributions to Sensory Physiology. Vol. 3. Academic Press, Inc., New York.

Nelson, E. E. (ed.). 1975. Textbook of Pediatrics. W. B. Saunders Company, Philadelphia.

Nelson, P. G., and S. D. Erulkar. 1963. Synaptic mechanisms of excitation and inhibition in the central auditory pathway. J. Neurophys. 26:908–923.

Newman, J. D., and D. Symmes. 1974a. Vocal pathology in socially deprived monkeys. Develop. Psychobiol. 7:351–358.

Newman, J. D., and D. Symmes. 1974b. Arousal effects on unit responsiveness to vocalizations in squirrel monkey auditory cortex. Brain Res. 78:125–138.

Newman, J. D., and Z. Wollberg. 1973a. Multiple coding of species-specific vocalizations in the auditory cortex of squirrel monkeys. Brain Res. 54:287–304.

Newman, J. D., and Z. Wollberg. 1973b. Responses of single neurons in the auditory cortex of squirrel monkeys to variants of a single call type. Exper. Neurol. 40:821–824.

Newton, G., and S. Levine. (eds.). 1968. Early Experience and Behavior: The Psychobiology of Development. Charles C Thomas, Publisher, Springfield, Ill.

Nobel, K. W., and J. H. Dewson, III. 1966. A corticofugal projection from insular and temporal cortex to the homolateral inferior colliculus in cat. J. Aud. Res. 6:67–75.

Northern, J. L., and M. P. Downs. 1974. Hearing in Children. The Williams & Wilkins Company, Baltimore.

Nottebohm, F. 1970. Ontogeny of bird song. Science 167:950–956.

Nottebohm, F. 1972. Neural lateralization of vocal control in a passerine bird. II. Subsong, calls, and a theory of vocal learning. J. Exper. Zool. 179:35–49.

Nottebohm, F., and M. E. Nottebohm. 1971. Vocalizations and breeding behavior of surgically deafened ring doves. Anim. Behav. 19:313–327.

Obrist, P. A., R. A. Webb, and J. R. Sutterer. 1969. Heart rate and somatic changes during aversive conditioning and a simple reaction time task. Psychophysiol. 5:696–723.

Obrist, P. A., R. A. Webb, J. R. Sutterer, and J. C. Howard. 1970. The cardiac-somatic relationship: Some reformulations. Psychophysiology 6:569–587.

O'Connor, N. (ed.). 1961. Recent Soviet Psychology. Liveright, New York.

O'Doherty, N. 1968. A hearing test applicable to the crying newborn infant. Develop. Med. Child Neurol. 10:380–383.

Ohlrich, E. S., and A. B. Barnet. 1972. Auditory evoked responses during the first year of life. Electroencephalog. & Clin. Neurophysiol. 32:161–169.

Olson, G. M. 1975. An information processing analysis of visual memory and habituation in infants. In T. J. Tighe and R. N. Leaton (eds.), Habituation: Perspectives from Child Development, Animal Behavior, and Neurophysiology. Erlbaum Associates, Hillsdale, N. J.

Ornitz, E. M., E. R. Ritvo, Y. H. Lee, L. M. Panman, R. D. Walter, and A.

Mason. 1969. The auditory evoked response in babies during REM sleep. Electroencephalog. & Clin. Neurophysiol. 27:195—198.

Osgood, C. 1964. Semantic differential technique in the comparative study of cultures. Am. Anthrop. 66:171—200.

Ostwald, P. 1972. The sounds of infancy. Develop. Med. Child Neurol. 14:350—361.

Ostwald, P., R. Phibbs, and S. Fox. 1968. Diagnostic use of infant cry. Biol. Neonat. 13:68—82.

Oswald, I. 1962. Sleeping and Waking. Elsevier Press, Inc., New York.

Otellin, V. A. 1970. Projections of auditory cortex to caudate nucleus and possible role of the latter as a subcortical association area. Fiziol. SSSR Sechenov. 56:967—972. (In Neuroscience Trans. No. 16, 1970—1971).

Ottelin, V. A. 1972. Projections of the auditory cortex to the neostratum. Neurosci. & Behav. Psychol. 5:267—274.

Palmqvist, H. 1975. The effect of heartbeat sound stimulation on the weight development of newborn infants. Child Develop. 46:292—295.

Palva, T. 1970. Cochlear aqueduct in infants. Acta Oto-laryng. 70:83—94.

Papcun, G., S. Krashen, D. Terbeek, R. Remington, and R. Harshman. 1974. Is the left hemisphere specialized for speech, language, and/or something else? J. Acoust. Soc. Am. 55:319—327.

Papousek, H. 1961. Conditioned head rotation reflexes in the first months of life. Acta Pediat. 50:565—570.

Papousek, H. 1969. Elaborations of conditioned head-turning. Presented at the 19th Congress of Psychology, London.

Parker, M. V., S. W. Miller, and P. M. Groves. 1974. Neuronal habituation and sensitization in the reticular formation of the rat. Physiol. & Psychol. 2:464—470.

Parmalee, A. H., Jr. 1961. Sleep patterns in infancy: A study of one infant from birth to eight months of age. Acta Pädiatrica 50:160—170.

Parmalee, A. H., Jr. 1963a. The palmomental reflex in premature infants. Develop. Med Child Neurol. 5:381—387.

Parmalee, A. H., Jr. 1963b. The hand-mouth reflex of Babkin in premature infants. Pediatrics 31:734—740.

Parmalee, A. H., Jr. 1964. A critical evaluation of the Moro reflex. Pediatrics 33:773—788.

Parmalee, A. H., Jr., Y. Akiyama, E. Stern, and M. A. Harris. 1969. A periodic cerebral rhythm in newborn infants. Exper. Neurol. 25:575—584.

Parmalee, A. H., Jr., K. Brück, and M. Brück. 1962. Activity and inactivity cycles during the sleep of premature infants exposed to neutral temperatures. Biol. Neonat. 4:317—339.

Parmalee, A. H., Jr., F. J. Schulte, Y. Akiyama, W. H. Wenner, H. R. Schultz, and E. Stern. 1968. Maturation of EEG activity during sleep in premature infants. Electroencephalog. & Clin. Neurophysiol 24:319—329.

Parmalee, A. H., Jr., H. R. Schultz, and M. A. Disbrow. 1961. Sleep patterns of the newborn. J. Pediat. 58:241—250.

Parmalee, A. H., Jr., E. Stern, G. Chervin, and A. Minkowski. 1964. Gestational age and the size of premature infants. Biol. Neonat. 6:309—323.

Parmalee, A. H., Jr., E. Stern, and M. A. Harris. 1972. Maturation of respiration in prematures and young infants. Neuropädiatrie 3:294–304.

Parmalee, A. H., Jr., H. W. Waldemar, Y. Akiyama, H. R. Schultz, and E. Stern. 1967. Sleep states in premature infants. Develop. Med. Child Neurol. 9:70–77.

Parr, W. G. 1962. The ascertainment of deafness in infancy. Proceedings of the 8th Trien. Conference of Teachers of Deaf in Australia, pp. 25–47.

Peiper, A. 1963. Cerebral Function in Infancy and Childhood. Consultants Bureau of New York.

Penfield, W., and L. Roberts. 1959. Speech and Brain Mechanisms. Princeton University Press, Princeton, N. J.

Perl, N. 1968. The recall of dichotic stimuli–is order or laterality more important? Papers in Psychol. 2:25–27.

Perret, E., E. Grandjean, and A. Lauber. 1963. Evaluation subjective de la gene provoqué par des bruits d'avions. Helvet. Physiol. & Pharmacol. Acta 21:40–42.

Peters, R. 1967. Perceptual organization for speech and other auditory signals. Report No. AMRL-TR-68-31, Aerospace Medical Research Laboratory, Wright-Patterson Air Force Base, Ohio.

Peterson, E. A., W. E. Pate, and S. D. Wruble. 1966. Cochlear potentials in the dog. I. Differences with variations in external-ear structure. J. Aud. Res. 6:1–11.

Petrakis, N. L., K. T. Molohon, and D. J. Tepper. 1967. Cerumen in American Indians: Genetic implications of sticky and dry types. Science 158:1192.

Petre-Quadens, O. 1967. Ontogenesis of paradoxical sleep in the human newborn. J. Neurol. Sci. 4:153–157.

Pfeiffer, C. C., and J. R. Smythies (eds.). 1962. International Review of Neurobiology. Vol. 4. Academic Press, Inc., New York.

Phillips, M., and J. Olds. 1969. Unit activity: Motivation-dependent responses from midbrain neurons. Science 165:1269–1271.

Philips, S. J., F. J. Agate, W. A. Silverman, and P. Steiner. 1964. Autonomic cardiac reactivity in premature infants. Biol. Neonat. 6:225–249.

Picton, T. W., and T. W. Hillyard. 1974. Human auditory evoked potentials. II. Effects of attention. Electroencephalog. & Clin. Neurophysiol. 36:191–199.

Picton, T. W., T. W. Hillyard, H. I. Krausz, and R. Galambos. 1974. Human auditory evoked potentials. I. Evaluation of components. Electroencephalog. & Clin. Neurophysiol. 36:179–190.

Pinheiro, M. L. 1973. Auditory pattern perception in patients with left and right hemispheric lesions. Presented at ASHA, Detroit.

Pisoni, D. B. 1971. Very brief short-term memory in speech perception. Presented at Acoustic Society of America, Denver.

Pisoni, D. B. 1973. Auditory and phonetic memory codes in the discrimination of consonants and vowels. Percept. & Psycholphys. 13:253–260.

Pisoni, D. B., and J. H. Lazarus. 1974. Categorical and noncategorical modes of speech perception along the voicing continuum. J. Acoust. Soc. Am. 55:328–333.

Ploog, D., and T. Melnechuk. 1969. Primate communication. Neurosci. Res. Program Bull. 7, No. 5.

Podvoll, E. M., and S. J. Goodman. 1967. Averaged neural electrical activity and arousal. Science 155:223–225.

Polikanina, R. I. 1966. Extinction of the orienting reflex to an acoustic rhythmic stimulus in slightly premature babies (an electrophysiological study). Zh. Vyssh. Nerv. Deiat. Pavlov. 16:813–821.

Polikanina, R. I., and L. M. Sergeeva. 1967. Development of extinctive inhibition in children in early ontogenesis. Zh. Vyssh. Nerv. Deyatel. Pavlova 17:228–239.

Pollack, I. 1968. The apparent pitch of short tones. Am. J. Psychol. 81:165–169.

Pomerleau-Malcuit, A., and R. K. Clifton. 1973. Neonatal heart rate responses to tactile, auditory, and vestibular stimulation in different states. Child Develop. 44:485–496.

Poon, L. W., L. W. Thompson, R. B. Williams, Jr., and G. R. Marsh. 1974. Changes of antero-posterior distribution of CNV and late positive component as a function of information processing demands. Psychophysiology 11:660–673.

Porges, S. W. 1974. Heart rate indices of newborn attentional responsivity. Merrill-Palmer Quart. 20:231–254.

Porges, S. W., W. R. Arnold, and E. J. Forbes. 1973. Heart rate variability: An index of attentional responsivity in human newborns. Develop. Psychol. 8:85–92.

Post, R. H. 1964. Hearing acuity variation among negroes and whites. Eugen. Quart. 11:65–81.

Powers, W. T. 1973. Behavior: The Control of Perception. Aldine, Chicago.

Prather, E. M., D. L. Hedrick, and L. M. Winstead. 1971. Speech sound discrimination in children aged two to four years. Presented at ASHA, Chicago.

Pratt, K. C. 1930. Note on the relation of temperature and humidity to the activity of young infants. J. Genetic Psychol. 38:480–484.

Pratt, K. C. 1934. The effects of repeated auditory stimulation upon general activity of newborn infants. J. Genetic Psychol. 44:96–116.

Pratt, K. C. 1960. The neonate. *In* L. Carmichael (ed.), Manual of Child Psychology, pp. 215–291. John Wiley & Sons, Inc., New York.

Pratt, K. C., A. Nelson, and K. Sun. 1930. The behavior of the newborn infant. Ohio State University Studies in Psychology 10:79–104.

Prechtl, H. F. R. 1953. Stammesgeschichtliche rese in verhalten des sauglings. Umschau 21:656–658.

Prechtl, H. F. R. 1965. Problems of behavioral studies in the newborn infant. *In* D. S. Lehrman, R. A. Hinde and E. Shaw (eds.), Advances in the Study of Behavior, pp. 75–98. Academic Press, Inc., New York.

Prechtl, H. F. R. 1974. The behavioral states of the newborn infant. (A review). Brain Res. 76:185–212.

Prechtl, H. F. R., and D. Beintema. 1964. The Neurological Examination of the Full-term Newborn Infant. William Heinemann, Ltd., London.

Prechtl, H. F. R., V. Vlach, H. G. Lenard, and D. K. Grant. 1967. Exteroceptive and tendon reflexes in the newborn infant. Biol. Neonat. 11:159–175.

Prechtl, H. F. R., H. Weinmann, and Y. Akiyama. 1969. Organization of physiological parameters in normal and neurologically abnormal infants. Neurpädiat. 1:101–129.

Prescott, J. W., M. S. Read, and D. B. Coursin (eds.). 1975. Malnutrition and Brain Function. John Wiley & Sons, Inc., New York.

Prestrude, A. M. 1970. Sensory capacities of the chimpanzee, a review. Psychol. Bull. 7:47–67.

Pribram, K. H. 1969. The primate frontal cortex. Neuropsychologia 7: 259–266.

Price, R. L., and B. D. Smith. 1974. The $P_{3(00)}$ wave of the averaged evoked potential: A bibliography. Physiol. & Psychol. 2:387–391.

Proctor, L. D., and W. R. Adey (eds.). 1965. The Analysis of Central Nervous System and Cardiovascular Data Using Computer Methods. NASA, Washington, D.C.

Raab, D. H. 1971. Audition. Ann. Rev. Psychol. 22:95–118.

Rabinowicz, T. L. 1967. Techniques for the establishment of an atlas of the cerebral cortex of the premature. In A. Minkowski (ed.), Regional Development of the Brain in Early Life, pp. 71–128. F. A. Davis Company, Philadelphia.

Radionova, E. A., and A. V. Popov. 1966. Electrophysiological examination of neurons in cochlear nucleus of the cat. Fed. Proc. (Trans. Suppl.) 25: (no. II), T231–235.

Radionova, E. A., and I. A. Vartanian. 1971. Comparative description of some characteristics of the neuronal activity at different levels of the auditory system. J. Aud. Res. 11:195–217.

Raisman, G., W. Cowan, and T. Powell. 1965. The extrinsic, commissural and association fibers of the hippocampus. Brain 88:963–996.

Rapin, I., and L. J. Graziani. 1967. Auditory evoked responses in normal, brain damaged, and deaf infants. Neurol. 17:881–894.

Rapin, I., R. J. Ruben, and M. Lyttle. 1970. Diagnosis of hearing loss in infants using auditory evoked responses. Laryngoscope 80:712–722.

Rasmussen, G. L. 1964. Anatomic relationships of the ascending and descending auditory systems. In W. S. Fields and B. R. Alford (eds.), Neurological Aspects of Auditory and Vestibular Disorders, pp. 5–23. Charles C Thomas, Publisher, Springfield, Ill.

Ratliff, S. S. and H. Greenberg. 1972. The averaged encephalic response to linguistic and nonlinguistic auditory stimuli. J. Aud. Res. 12:14–25.

Rechtschaffen, A., and A. Kales (eds.). 1968. A Manual of Standardized Terminology Techniques and Scoring System for Sleep Stages of Human Subjects. United States Public Health Service No. 204, Washington, D. C.

Reddell, R. C., and D. R. Calvert. 1967. Conditioned audio-visual response audiometry. Voice 16:52–57.

Reddell, R. C., and D. R. Calvert. 1969. Factors in screening hearing of the newborn. J. Aud. Res. 9:278–289.

Regan, D. 1972. Evoked Potentials. Chapman & Hall, Ltd., London.

Reis, D. J., N. Doba, and M. A. Nathan. 1973. Predatory attack, grooming, and consummatory behaviors evoked by electrical stimulation of cat cerebellar nuclei. Science 182:845–847.

Reneau, J. P., and G. Z. Hnatiow. 1975. Evoked Response Audiometry: A Topical and Historical Review. University Park Press, Baltimore.

Repp, B. H. 1975. Dichotic masking of consonants by vowels. J. Acoust. Soc. Am. 57:724–735.

Rewey, H. H. 1973. Developmental change in infant heart rate response during sleeping and waking states. Develop. Psychol. 8:35–41.

Rheingold, H., J. L. Gewirtz, and H. W. Ross. 1959. Social conditioning of vocalizations in the infant. J. Comp. & Physiol. Psych. 52:68–73.

Ricciuti, H. N., and R. H. Poresky. 1972. Emotional behavior and development in the first year of life: An analysis of arousal, approach-withdrawal and affective responses. In A. D. Pick (ed.), Minnesota Symposium on Child Psychology, pp. 69–96. Vol. 6. University of Minnesota Press, Minneapolis.

Richmond, J. B., H. J. Grossman, and S. L. Lustman. 1953. A hearing test for newborn infants. Pediatrics 11:634–638.

Richmond, J. B., E. L. Lipton, and A. Steinschneider. 1962a. Observations on differences in autonomic nervous system function between and within individuals during early infancy. J. Am. Acad. Child Psychiat. 1:83–91.

Richmond, J. B., E. L. Lipton, and A. Steinschneider. 1962b. Autonomic function in the neonate. V. Individual homeostatic capacity in cardiac response. Psychosom. Med. 24:66–74.

Richter, C. P. 1966. A hitherto unrecognized difference between man and other primates. Presented at the National Academy of Science, Durham, North Carolina.

Roberts, B., and D. Campbell. 1967. Activity in newborns and the sound of a human heart. Psychom. Sci. 9:339–340.

Roberts, J. R., and B. W. Watson. 1973. The objective assessment of hearing in the young infant. Estratto Minerva Otorhinolaryng. 23:188–196.

Robertson, A. D., and J. Inglis. 1973. Cerebral asymmetry and electroconvulsive therapy. Presented at the American Psychological Association, New Orleans.

Robinson, R. J. 1966. Assessment of gestational age by neurological examination. Arch Dis. Child. 41:437–447.

Robson, J. 1971. Screening techniques in babies. Sound 4:91–94.

Roeder, K. D. 1966. Auditory system of noctuid moths. Science 154:1515–1521.

Roederer, J. G. 1973. Introduction to the Physics and Psychophysics of Music. Springer-Verlag, New York.

Roffwarg, H. P., J. N. Muzio, and W. C. Dement. 1966. Ontogenetic development of the human sleep-dream cycle. Science 152:604–609.

Rosenblith, J. F. 1961. The modified Graham behavior test for neonates: Test-retest reliability, normative data, and hypotheses for future work. Biol Neonat. 3:174–192.

Rosenblith, J. F. 1970. Are newborn auditory responses prognostic of deafness? Am. Acad. Ophthal. Otolaryng. 74:1215–1227.

Rosenblith, J. F. 1973. Prognostic value of neonatal behavioral tests. Early Child Develop. & Care (Ireland) 3:31–50.

Rosenblith, J. F., and L. P. Lipsitt. 1959. Interscorer agreement for the Graham behavior test for neonates. J. Pediat. 54:200–205.

Rosenblith, W. A. 1959. Some quantifiable aspects of the electrical activity of the mervous system (with emphasis upon responses to sensory stimuli). Rev. Mod. Physics 31:532–545.

Rosenthal, W. S. 1971. Auditory threshold-duration functions in aphasic subjects: Implications for the interaction of linguistic and auditory processing in aphasia. Presented at ASHA, Chicago.

Ross, M. D. 1971. Fluorescence and electron microscopic observations of the general visceral, efferent innervation of the inner ear. Acta Otolaryng. (Suppl.) 286:1–18.

Ross, M. D., and W. Burkel. 1973. Multipolar neurons in the spiral ganglion of the cat. Acta Otolaryng. 76:381–394.

Roth, W. T., and B. S. Kopell. 1969. The auditory evoked response to repeated stimuli during a vigilance task. Psychophysiology 6:301–309.

Rothman, H. W. 1970. Effects of high frequencies and intersubject variability on the auditory-evoked cortical response. J. Acoust. Soc. Am. 47:569–573.

Routh, D. 1969. Conditioning of vocal response differentiation in infants. Develop. Psychol. 1:219–225.

Rowell, T. E. 1962. Agonistic noises of the Rhesus monkey. Sympos. Zool. Soc.(London) 8:81–96.

Ruben, R. J. 1969. The synthesis of DNA and RNA in the developing inner ear. Laryngoscope 79:1546–1556.

Rupert, A., G. Moushegian, and R. Galambos. 1963. Unit responses to sound from auditory nerve of the cat. J. Neurophysiol. 26:449–465.

Russ, F. M., and F. B. Simmons. 1974. Five years of experience with electric response audiometry. J. Speech & Hearing Res. 17:184–193.

Ryugo, D. K., and H. P. Killackey. 1974. The differential telencephalic projections of the medial geniculate of the rat. Presented at the Society for Neuroscience, St. Louis.

Sachs, M. B. (ed.). 1971. Physiology of the Auditory System. Natl. Educ. Consult. Baltimore.

Sackett, G. P. 1966. Development of preference for differentially complex patterns by infant monkeys. Psychonom. Sci. 6:441–442.

Sakabe, N., T. Arayama, and T. Suzuki. 1969. Human fetal evoked response to acoustic stimulation. Acta Otolaryng. (Suppl.) 252:29–36.

Salk, L. 1960. The effects of the normal heartbeat sound on the behavior of the newborn infant: Implications for mental health. World Ment. Health 12:168–175.

Salk, L. 1961. The importance of the heartbeat rhythm to human nature: Theoretical, clinical and experimental observations. Proceedings of the 3rd World Congress on Psychiatry, pp. 740–746. Vol. 1.

Salk, L. 1962. Mothers' heartbeat as an imprinting stimulus. Acad. Sci. Trans. (Div. Psychol.), pp. 753–763

Sameroff, A. J. 1970. Respiration and sucking as components of the orienting reaction in newborns. Psychophysiology 7:213–222.

Sameroff, A. J. 1974. Early influences on development: fact or fancy? Presented at Merrill-Palmer Conference on Infancy, Detroit.

Sato, S., and H. E. Dreifuss. 1973. Electroencephalographic findings in a patient with developmental expressive aphasia. Neurology 23:181–185.

Saunders, J. C. 1967. Selective facilitation and inhibition of evoked potentials elicited by auditory and visual stimuli during avoidance conditioning. Ph. D. thesis, Princeton University, Princeton, N.J.

Savin, H. B. 1967. On the successive perception of simultaneous stimuli. Percept. & Psychophys. 2:479–482.

Schachter, J., L. Bickman, J. S. Schachter, J. Jameson, S. Lituchi, and T. A. Williams. 1966. Behavioral and physiologic reactivity in human neonates. Ment. Hyg. 50:516–521.

Schachter, J., J. L. Kerr, F. C. Wimberly, and J. M. Lachin. 1975. Heart rate levels of black and white newborns. Psychosom. Med. (In press).

Schachter, J., T. Williams, Z. Khachaturian, M. Tobin, R. Kruger, and J. Kerr. 1971. Heart rate responses to auditory clicks in neonates. Psychophysiology 8:163–179.

Scheibel, M., and A. Scheibel. 1964. Some structural and functional substrates of development in young cats, pp. 6–25. *In* W. A. Himwich and H. E. Himwich (eds.), The Developing Brain. American Elsevier Publishing Company, Inc., New York.

Scheich, H. 1974. Neuronal analysis of wave form in the time domain: Midbrain units in electric fish during social behavior. Science 185: 365–367.

Scheich, H., R. Koch, and G. Langner. 1974. Coding of species specific vocalization in the auditory midbrain nucleus of the guinea fowl. Presented at the Society for Neuroscience, St. Louis.

Schein, J. D., and M. T. Delk. 1974. The Deaf Population of the United States. National Association of the Deaf, Silver Spring, Md.

Schiller, C. H. (ed.). 1964. Instinctive Behavior. International Universities Press, Inc., New York.

Schmidt, K., S. A. Rose, and W. H. Bridger. 1974. The law of initial values and neonatal sleep states. Psychophysiology 11:44–52.

Schneider, B. A., A. J. Neuringer, and D. Ramsey. 1972. Magnitude estimation of loudness with a minimum 24-h interstimulus interval. Psychonom. Sci. 27:243–245.

Schrier, A. M., H. F. Harlow, and F. Stollnitz (eds.). 1965. Behavior of Nonhuman Primates. Vol. II. Academic Press, Inc., New York.

Schulman, C. A. 1970*a*. Heart rate response habituation in high-risk premature infants. Psychophysiology 6:690–694.

Schulman, C. A. 1970*b*. Effects of auditory stimulation on heart rate in premature infants as a function of level of arousal, probability of CNS damage, and conceptional age. Develop. Psychobiol. 2:172–183.

Schulman, C. A. 1973. Heart rate audiometry. Part I. An evaluation of heart rate response to auditory stimuli in newborn hearing screening. Neuropädiatrie 4:362–374.

Schulman, C. A., and R. Kreiter. 1970. Averaged heart rate change in response to auditory stimulation using a special-purpose computer. Presented at the Society for Psychophysiological Research, New Orleans.

Schulman, C. A., C. R. Smith, M. Weisinger, and T H. Fay. 1970. The use of heart rate in the audiological evaluation of nonverbal children. Part I. Evaluation of children at risk for hearing impairment. Neuropädiatrie 2:187–196.

Schulman, C. A., and G. Wade. 1970. The use of heart rate in the audiological evaluation of nonverbal children. Part II. Clinical trials on an infant population. Neuropädiatrie 2:197–205.

Schulte, F. J., G. Albert, and R. Michaelis. 1969. Gestational age and nerve-conduction velocity in normal and abnormal newborn babies. Deutsche Med. Wchnschr. 94:599–601.

Schulte, F. J., R. Michaelis, I. Linke, and R. Nolte. 1968. Motor nerve conduction velocity in term, preterm, and small-for-dates newborn infants. Pediatrics 42:17–26.

Schulte, F. J., and W. Schwenvel. 1965. Motor control and muscle tone in the newborn period. Biol. Neonat. 8:198–215.

Schusterman, R., R. Balliet, and S. St. John. 1970. Vocal displays under water by the grey seal, the harbor seal, and the stellar sea lion. Psychonom. Sci. 18:303–305.

Schwartz, A., D. Rosenberg, and Y. Brackbill. 1970. Analysis of the components of social reinforcement of infant vocalization. Psychonom. Sci. 20:323–325.

Schwartzkopf, J. 1967. Hearing. Ann. Rev. Physiol. 29:485–512.

Sebeok, T. A. 1965. Animal communication. Science 147:1006–1014.

Sebeok, T. A. (ed.). 1968. Animal Communication. Indiana University Press, Bloomington.

Sedlacek, K. 1971. Hearing and communication in birds. Acta Otolaryng. 71:194–196.

Segall, M. E. 1972. Cardiac responsivity to auditory stimulation in premature infants. Nursing Res. 21:15–19.

Semb, G., and L. P. Lipsitt. 1968. The effects of acoustic stimulation on cessation and initiation of non-nutritive sucking in neonates. J. Exper. Child. Psychol 6:585–597.

Semmel, M. I. 1963. Arousal theory applied to vigilance behavior of educable mentally retarded and average children. Ph.D. thesis, George Peabody College, Nashville, Tenn.

Shallop, J. K. 1974. The assessment of hearing in young children with the Murphy chair. Presented at ASHA, Las Vegas.

Shankweiler, D. 1966. Effects of temporal-lobe damage on perception of dichotically presented melodies. J. Comp. & Physiol. Psychol. 62: 115–119.

Shankweiler, D., and M. Studdert-Kennedy. 1967. Identification of consonants and vowels presented to left and right ears. Quart. J. Exper. Psychol. 19:59–63.

Shapiro, I. 1974. Newborn hearing screening in a county hospital. J. Speech & Hearing Dis. 39:89–92.

Sharpless, S., and H. Jasper. 1956. Habituation of the arousal reaction. Brain 79:655–80.

Shepherd, D. C., R. Goldstein, and Rosenblüt, B. 1964. Race difference in auditory sensitivity. J. Speech & Hearing Res. 7:389–393.

Shepherd, D. C., and K. McCarren. 1972. An averaged electroencephalographic audiometric sensitivity (AEA-S) procedure. J. Speech & Hearing Dis. 37:503–522.

Sherman, M., I. Sherman, and C. D. Flory. 1936. Infant behavior. Comp. Psychol. Monograph No. 59 (whole).

Shriner, T. H., C. C. Condron, and R. C. Berry. 1973. Infants sucking responses as a conjugate function of auditory stimuli. Presented at ASHA, Detroit.

Siegel, G. M., and H. L. Pick, Jr. 1974. Auditory feedback in the regulation of voice. J. Acoust. Soc. Am. 56:1618–1624.

Siegel, S. 1956. Nonparametric Statistics for the Behavioral Sciences. McGraw-Hill Book Company, Inc., New York.

Siegel, W., and R. Sopo. 1975. Tonal intervals are perceived categorically by musicians with relative pitch. Paper presented at a meeting of the Acoustical Society of America, Austin, Texas.

Silverio, J. 1964. Gastric emptying time in the newborn and the nursling. Am. J. Med. Sci. 247:732–738.

Silverman, W. A., and F. J. Agate. 1964. Variation in cold resistance among small newborn infants. Biol. Neonat. 6:113–127.

Silverman, W. A., F. J. Lucey, A. Beard, A. K. Brown, M. Cornblath, M. Grossman, J. A. Little, and L. O. Lubchenko. 1967. Nomenclature for duration of gestation, birth weight and intra-uterine growth. Pediatrics 39:935–939.

Simmons, F. B. 1964. Variable nature of the middle ear muscle reflex. Int. Audiol. 3:1–11.

Simmons, F. B., and F. N. Russ. 1974. Automated newborn hearing screening, the Crib-o-gram. Arch. Otolaryn. 100:1–7.

Simmons, J. A., E. G. Wever, and J. M. Pylka. 1971. Periodical cicada: Sound production and hearing. Science 171:212–213.

Simner, M. L. 1970. Auditory self-stimulative feedback and reflexive crying in human infants. Presented at the Eastern Psychological Association, Atlantic City, New Jersey.

Simner, M. L. 1971. Newborn's response to the cry of another infant. Develop. Psychol. 5:136–150.

Simner, M. L., and B. Reilly. 1969. Response of the newborn infant to the cry of another infant. Paper presented at a meeting of the Society for Research in Child Development, Santa Monica, Calif.

Simons, G. 1964. Comparisons of incipient music responses among very young twins and singletons. Music Educ. 12:212–226.

Simons, L. A., C. W. Dunlop, W. R. Webster, and L. M. Aitkin. 1966. Acoustic habituation in cats as a function of stimulus rate and role of temporal conditioning of the middle ear muscles. Electroencephalog. & Clin. Neurophysiol. 20:485–493.

Simpson, G. G. 1966. The biological nature of man. Science 152:472–478.

Singer, M. 1966. Emotional and psychiatric aspects of the limbic lobe. Dis. Nerv. System 27:309–317.

Singh, S. D. 1968. Effect of urban environment on visual curiosity behavior in Rhesus monkeys. Psychonom. Sci. 11:83–84.

Sinnott, J. M. 1974. A comparison of speech sound discrimination in humans and monkeys. Ph.D. thesis, University of Michigan, Ann Arbor.

Siqueland, E. R., and C. A. De Lucia. 1969. Visual reinforcement of nonnutritive sucking in human infants. Science 165:1144–1146.

Skinner, P. H. 1972. Electroencephalic response audiometry. In J. Katz (ed.), Handbook of Clinical Audiology, pp. 407–433. The Williams & Wilkins Company, Baltimore.

Smith, C. A. 1973. Anatomical correlates of deafness. J. Acoust. Soc. Am. 54:576–588.

Smith, D. and P. Strawbridge. 1969. The heart rate response to a brief auditory and visual stimulus. Psychophysiology 6:317–329.

Smith, H. W. 1953. From Fish to Philosopher. Little, Brown & Company, Boston.

Snapp, B. 1969. Recognition of maternal calls by parentally naive Gallus Gallus chicks. Anim. Behav. 17:440–445.

Soderquist, D. R., and M. J. Moore. 1970. Effect of training on frequency discrimination in primary school children. J. Aud. Res. 10: 185–192.

Sohmer, A. 1965. The effect of contralateral olivocochlear bundle stimulation on the cochlear potentials evoked by acoustic stimuli of various frequencies and intensities. Acta Otolaryng. 60:59–70.

Sohmer, H., M. Feinmesser, L. Bauberger-Tell, A. Lev, and S. David. 1972. Audiometry in infants with uncertain diagnosis. Ann. Otol. Rhinol. Laryng. 81:72–75.

Sokolov, E. N. 1960. Neuronal models and the orienting reflex. In M. A. B. Brazier (ed.), The Central Nervous System and Behavior, pp. 187–276. Josiah Macy, Jr., Foundation, New York.

Sokolov, E. N. 1963. Perception and the Conditioned Reflex. The Macmillan Company, New York.

Solomons, G., J. C. Hardy, and J. Melrose. 1965. Auditory reactions of the neonate. Lancet 85:17–21.

Sontag, L. W., W. G. Steele, and M. Lewis. 1969. The fetal and maternal cardiac response to environmental stress. Human Develop. 12:1–9.

Sontag, L. W., and R. F. Wallace. 1935. The movement response of the human fetus to sound stimuli. Child Develop. 6:253–258.

Sparks, R., and N. Geschwind. 1968. Dichotic listening in man after section of neocortical commissures. Cortex 4:3–16.

Speaks, C., T. Gray, J. Miller, A. Rubens, and M. Waller. 1974. Interference with processing dichotic pairs of CV syllables after temporal lobe lesions. Presented at Acoustic Society of America, New York.

Spellacy, F. 1970. Lateral preferences in the identification of patterned stimuli. J. Acoust. Soc. Am. 47:574–577.

Spellacy, F., and S. Blumstein. 1970. Perception of language and non-language sounds: Evidence for unilateral brain function. Presented to Acoustic Society of America, Houston.

Spielman, R. S., E. C. Migliazza, and J. V. Neel. 1974. Regional linguistic and genetic differences among Yanomama Indians. Science 184:637–644.

Spoendlin, H. 1972. Innervation densities of the cochlea. Acta Otolaryng. 73:235–248.

Spreen, O., F. J. Spellacy, and J. R. Reid. 1970. The effect of interstimulus interval and intensity on ear symmetry for nonverbal stimuli in dichotic listening. Neuropsychologia 8:245–250.

Springer, S. P. 1971. Ear asymmetry in a dichotic detection task. Percept. & Psychophys. 10:239–241.

Springer, S. P., and M. S. Gazzaniga. 1975. Dichotic testing of partial and complete split brain subjects. Neuropsychologia. (In press).

Sprunt, K., and W. M. Redman. 1964. Vernix caseosa and bacteria. Am. J. Dis. Child. 107:125–130.

Sroufe, A. L. 1971. Effects of depth and rate of breathing on heart rate and heart rate variability. Psychophysiology 8:648–655.

Sroufe, A. L., and D. Morris. 1973. Respiratory-cardiac relationships in children. Psychophysiology 10:377–382.

Stamps, L. E., and S. W. Porges. 1975. Heart rate conditioning in newborn infants: Relationships among conditionability, heart rate variability, and sex. Develop. Psychol. (In press).

Stark, R. E. (ed.). 1974. Sensory Capabilities of Hearing Impaired Children. University Park Press, Baltimore.

Starzl, T. E., C. W. Taylor, and H. W. Magoun. 1951a. Collateral afferent excitation of reticular formation of brain stem. J. Neurophysiol. 14: 479–496.

Starzl, T. E., C. W. Taylor, and H. W. Magoun. 1951b. Ascending conduction in reticular activating system with special reference to the diencephalon. J. Neurophysiol. 14:461–477.

Stebbins, W. C. 1966. Auditory reaction time and the derivation of equal loudness contours for the monkey. J. Exper. Anal. Behav. 9:135–142.

Stebbins, W. C. 1973. Hearing of old world monkeys (Cercopithecinae). Amer. J. Phys. Anthrop. 38:357–364.

Stebbins, W. C., S. Green, and F. L. Miller. 1966. Auditory sensitivity of the monkey. Science 153:1646–1647.

Stechler, G., S. Bradford, and H. Levy. 1966. Attention in the newborn: Effect on motility and skin potential. Science 151:1246–1248.

Stein, D. G., J. J. Rosen, and N. Butters. (eds.). 1974. Plasticity and Recovery of Function in the Central Nervous System. Academic Press, Inc., New York.

Steinschneider, A. 1968. Sound intensity and respiratory responses in the neonate. Psychosom. Med. 30:534–541.

Steinschneider, A. 1971. Determinants of an infant's cardiac response to simulation. In D. N. Walcher and D. L. Peters (eds.), Early Childhood: The Development of Self-Regulatory Mechanisms, pp. 73–105. Academic Press, Inc., New York.

Steinschneider, A., and E. L. Lipton. 1965. Individual differences in autonomic responsivity. Psychosom. Med. 27:446–456.

Steinschneider, A., E. L. Lipton, and J. B. Richmond. 1964. Autonomic function in the neonate. VI. Discriminability, consistency, and slope as measures of an individual's cardiac responsivity. J. Gen. Psychol. 105:295–310.

Steinschneider, A., E. L. Lipton, and J. B. Richmond. 1966. Auditory sensitivity in the infant: Effect of intensity on cardiac and motor responsivity. Child Develop. 37:233–252.

Stennett, R. G. 1957. The relationship of performance level to level of arousal. J. Exper. Psychol. 54:54–61.

Stern, L., M. H. Lees, and J. Leduc. 1965. Environmental temperature, oxygen consumption, and catecholamine excretion in newborn infants. Pediatrics 36:367–373.

Stevens, K. N. 1973. Potential role of property detectors in the perception of consonants. Massachusetts Institute of Technology Research Laboratory Electronics Quarterly Progress Report (No. 110).

Stevens, K. N., and A. S. House. 1972. Speech perception. In J. V. Tobias (ed.), Foundations of Modern Auditory Theory, pp. 1–62. Academic Press, Inc., New York.

Stevens, K. N., and D. H. Klatt. 1974. Role of formant transitions in the voiced-voiceless distinction for stops. J. Acoust. Soc. Am. 55:653–659.

Stevens, S. S. (ed.). 1951. Handbook of Experimental Psychology. John Wiley & Sons, Inc., New York.

Stevens, S. S. 1961. To honor Fechner and repeal his law. Science 133:80–86.

Stillman, R. D., G. Moushegian, and A. L. Rupert. 1975. Early tone-evoked responses in normal and hearing-impaired subjects. Audiology. (In press).

Stratton, P. M. 1970. The use of heart rate for the study of habituation in the neonate. Psychophysiology 7:44–56.

Stratton, P. M., and K. Connolly. 1973. Discrimination by newborns of the intensity, frequency and temporal characteristics of auditory stimuli. Brit. J. Psychol. 64:219–232.

Strickland, E. M., J. R. Hanson, and B. J. Anson. 1962. Branchial sources of auditory ossicles in man. Arch Otolaryng. 76:100–122.

Strong, O. S., and A. Elwyn. 1974. Human Neuroanatomy. The Williams & Wilkins Company, Baltimore. (6th Ed. edited by R. C. Truex and M. B. Carpenter.)

Stubbs, E. 1934. The effect of the factors of duration, intensity, and pitch of sound stimuli on the responses of newborn infants. Univ. Iowa Stud. Child Welf. 9:76–135.

Stubbs, E., and O. C. Irwin. 1934. A note on reaction times in infants. Child Develop. 5:291–292.

Studdert-Kennedy, M. 1975. From continuous signal to discrete message: Syllable to phoneme. In J. F. Kavanagh and J. E. Cutting (eds.), The Role of Speech in Language. MIT Press, Cambridge. (In press).

Studdert-Kennedy, M., and D. Shankweiler. 1970. Hemispheric specialization for speech perception. J. Acoust. Soc. Am. 48:579–594.

Suchman, R. G., and T. Trabasso. 1966. Stimulus preference and cue function in young children's concept attainment. J. Exper. Child Psychol. 3:188–198.

Suga, N. 1972. Analysis of information-bearing elements in complex sounds by auditory neurons of bats. Audiology 11:58–72.

Suga, N. 1973. Feature extraction in the auditory system of bats. In A. R. Møller (ed.), Basic Mechanisms of Hearing, pp. 675–744. Academic Press, Inc., New York.

Suga, N., and H. W. Campbell. 1967. Frequency sensitivity of single auditory neurons in the Gecko Coleonyx variegatus. Science 157:88–90.

Suga, N., and T. Shimozawa. 1974. Site of neural attenuation of responses to self-vocalized sounds in echolocating bats. Science 183:1211–1213.

Sullivan, R. F., I. A. Polisar, M. L. Ruffy, and M. H. Miller. 1973. Relative influence of the Lombard and delayed auditory feedback tests for functional hearing loss on phonation/time ratio. J. Aud. Res. 13:50–63.

Sussman, H. M. 1971. The laterality effect in lingual-auditory tracking. J. Acoust. Soc. Am. 49:1874–1880.

Sussman, H. M., P. F. MacNeilage, and J. Lumbley. 1974. Sensorimotor dominance and the right-ear advantage in mandibular-auditory tracking. J. Acoust. Soc. Am. 52:214–216.

Sutker, L. W., A. Altman, and P. Satz. 1974. Differential performance of right and left-handed subjects in response to verbal and non-verbal stimuli. Paper presented at a meeting of the American Psychological Association, New Orleans.

Sutton, S., P. Tueting, J. Zubin, and E. R. John. 1967. Information delivery and the sensory evoked potential. Science 155:1436–1439.

Suzuki, T. 1973. Problems in electric response audiometry (ERA) during sedation. Audiology 12:129–136.

Suzuki, T., T. Hirose, I. Asawa, N. Nishijima, and H. Sasaki. 1962. Evoked potential of waking human brain to acoustic stimulus. Pract. Otorhinolaryng. 24:217–224.

Suzuki, T., Y. Kamijo, and S. Kiuchi. 1964. Auditory test of newborn infants. Ann. Otolaryng. 73:914–923.

Suzuki, T., and Y. Ogiba. 1961. Conditioned orientation reflex audiometry. Arch. Otolaryng. 74:192–198.

Suzuki, T., and K. Origuchi. 1969. Averaged evoked response audiometry (ERA) in young children during sleep. Acta Otolaryng. (Suppl.) 252: 19–28.

Suzuki, T., and I. Sato. 1961. Free field startle response audiometry: A quantitative method for determining hearing threshold of infant children. Ann. Oto. Rhin. & Laryng. 70:997–1007.

Suzuki, T., and K. Taguchi. 1968. Cerebral evoked response to auditory stimuli in young children during sleep. Ann. Oto. Rhin. & Laryng. 77:102–110.

Suzuki, T., Y. Tanaka, and T. Arayama. 1966. Detection of hearing disorders in children under three years of age. Int. Audiol. 5:74–76.

Swigart, E. 1974. A comparison of behavioral and standard audiometric examinations at three age levels. Presented at ASHA, Las Vegas.

Symmes, D., and K. V. Anderson. 1967. Reticular modulation of higher auditory centers in monkeys. Exper. Neurol. 18:161–176.

Symmes, D., and J. D. Newman. 1974. Discrimination of isolation peep variants by squirrel monkeys. Exper. Brain Res. 19:365–376.

Szentágothai, J., and M. A. Arbib (eds.). 1974. Conceptual model of neural organization. Neurosci. Res. Program Bull. Vol. 12.

Taguchi, K., W. S. Goodman, and W. M. Brummitt. 1970. Evoked response audiometry in mentally retarded subjects. Acta Otolaryng. 70: 190–196.

Taguchi, K., T. W. Picton, J. A. Orpin, and W. S. Goodman. 1969. Evoked response audiometry in newborn infants. Acta Otolaryng. (Suppl.) 252:5–17.

Takahara, S. 1965. Evaluation of electroencephalographic reflex audiometry as a practical test of hearing for infants. Otolaryngology (Tokyo) 37:325–328.

Tallal, P. 1974. Developmental dysphasia: A defect of perception not language? Presented at the Acoustical Society of America, New York.

Tallal, P., and M. Piercy. 1973a. Defects of non-verbal auditory perception in children with developmental aphasia. Nature 241:468–469.

Tallal, P., and M. Piercy. 1973b. Developmental aphasia: Impaired rate of non-verbal processing as a function of sensory modality. Neuropsychologia 11:389–398.

Tallal, P., and M. Piercy. 1974. Developmental aphasia: Rate of auditory processing and selective impairment of consonant perception. Neuropsychologia 12:83–94.

Tanaka, Y., and T. Arayama. 1969. Fetal responses to acoustic stimuli. Pract. Otorhinolaryng. 31:269–273.

Tanner, J. M. 1971. Education and Physical Growth. International Universities Press, New York.

Tax, S. 1964. Horizons of Anthropology. Aldine, Chicago.

Taylor, D. J., and G. T. Mencher. 1972. Neonate response: the effect of infant state and auditory stimuli. Arch. Otolaryng. 95:119–124.

Taylor-Jones, L. 1927. A study of the behavior of the newborn. Am. J. Med. Sci. 174:357–362.

Teas, D. C. 1966. Interactions between synchronous neural response to paired acoustic signals. J. Acoust. Soc. Am. 39:1077–1085.

Teas, D. C., and G. B. Henry. 1969. Auditory nerve responses as a function of repetition rate and background noise. Int. Audiol. 8:147–163.

Teilhard de Chardin, P. 1965. The Phenomenon of Man. Harper & Row Publishers, New York.

Thalman, R., J. Kusakari, and T. Miyoshi. 1973. Dysfunctions of energy releasing and consuming processes of the cochlea. Laryngoscope 83: 1690–1712.

Thomas, J. E., and E. H. Lambert. 1958. Conduction velocity of motor fibers of peripheral nerves in infants and children. Electroencephalog. & Clin. Neurophysiol. 10:577–578.

Thompson, C. L., D. S. Samson, J. K. Cullen, and L. F. Hughes. 1973. The effect of varied bandwidth, signal-to-noise ratio, and intensity on the perception of consonant-vowels in a dichotic context. Presented at the Acoustical Society of America, Los Angeles, Calif.

Thompson, G., and B. A. Weber. 1974. Responses of infants and young children to behavior observation audiometry (BOA). J. Speech & Hearing Dis. 39:140–147.

Thompson, K. R., and L. M. Herman. 1975. Underwater frequency discrimination in the bottlenosed dolphin (1–140 kHz) and the human (1–8 kHz). J. Acoust. Soc. Am. 57:943–948.

Thompson, R. F., and M. M. Patterson (eds.). 1974. Bioelectric Recording Techniques. Academic Press, Inc., New York.

Thompson, R. F., and H. E. Smith. 1967. Effects of association area lesions on auditory frequency discrimination in cat. Psychonom. Sci. 8:123–124.

Thompson, R. F., and W. A. Spencer. 1966. Habituation: A model phenomenon for the study of neuronal substrates of behavior. Psychol. Rev. 73:16–43.

Thorpe, W. H. 1968. Perceptual basis for group organization in social vertebrates, especially birds. Nature 220:124–128.

Thorpe, W. H., and M. E. W. North. 1965. Origin and significance of the power of vocal imitation: With special reference to the antiphonal singing of birds. Nature 208:219–222.

Timmons, N. A., and J. P. Boudreau. 1972. Auditory feedback as a major factor in stuttering. J. Speech & Hearing Dis. 37:476–484.

Tobin, H., and J. T. Graham. 1968. Late responses to speech stimuli as demonstrated by EEG utilizing a summing computer technique. Unpublished paper, Purdue University, Lafayette, Indiana.

Todd, G. A., and B. Palmer. 1968. Social reinforcement of infant babbling. Child Develop. 39:591–596.

Tolman, C. 1967. The effects of tapping sounds upon feeding behavior of domestic chicks. Anim. Behav. 15:145–148.

Toriyama, M., T. Matsuzaki, and H. Hayashi. 1966. Some observations on auditory average responses in man. Int. Audiol. 5:234–237.

Trehub, S. E. 1973a. Auditory-Linguistic Sensitivity in Infants. Ph.D. thesis, McGill University, Montreal.

Trehub, S. E. 1973b. Infants' sensitivity to vowel and tonal contrasts. Develop. Psychol. 9:91–96.

Trehub, S. E., and M. S. Rabinovitch. 1972. Auditory-linguistic sensitivity in early infancy. Develop. Psychol. 6:74–77.

Truby, H. M. 1959. Acoustico-cineradiographic analysis considerations, with especial reference to certain consonantal complexes. Acta Radiologica Suppl. 182 (Stockholm).

Tsuchtani, C., and J. C. Boudreau. 1967. Encoding of stimulus frequency and intensity by cat superior olive-S-segment cells. J. Acoust. Soc. Am. 42:794–805.

Tsunoda, T. 1969. Contralateral shift of cerebral dominance for nonverbal sounds during speech perception. J. Aud. Res. 9:221–229.

Tsunoda, T. 1971. The difference of the cerebral dominance of vowel sounds among different languages. J. Aud. Res. 11:305–314.

Tulkin, S. R. 1973. Social class differences in infants' reactions to mother's and stranger's voices. Develop. Psychol. 8:137.

Tulloch, J. D., B. S. Brown, H. L. Jacobs, D. G. Prugh, and W. A. Greene. 1964. Normal heartbeat sound and the behavior of newborn infants—A replication study. Psychom. Med., Heartbeat and Behav. 26:661–669.

Turkewitz, G., H. G. Birch, and K. K. Cooper. 1972a. Responsiveness to simple and complex auditory stimuli in the human newborn. Develop. Psychobiol. 5:7–19.

Turkewitz, G., H. G. Birch, and K. K. Cooper. 1972b. Patterns of response to different auditory stimuli in the human newborn. Develop. Med. Child Neurol. 14:487–491.

Turkewitz, G., S. Fleischer, T. Moreau, H. G. Birch, and L. Levy. 1966b. Relationship between feeding condition and organization of flexor-extensor movements in the human neonate. J. Comp. & Physiol. Psychol. 61:461–463.

Turkewitz, G., T. Moreau, and H. G. Birch. 1966. Head position and receptor organization in the human neonate. J. Exper. Child. Psychol. 4:169–177.

Turkewitz, G., T. Moreau, L. Levy, and A. C. Cornwell. 1966a. Effect of intensity of auditory stimulation on directional eye movements in the human neonate. Anim. Behav. 14:93–101.

Turnure, C. 1971. Response to voice of mother and stranger by babies in the first year. Develop. Psychol. 4:182–190.

Tyberghein, J., and G. Forrez. 1969. Cortical audiometry in normal hearing subjects. Acta Otolaryng. 67:24–32.

Ulett, G., R. S. Dow, and O. Larsell. 1944. The inception of conductivity in the corpus callosum and the cortico-ponto-cerebellar pathway of young rabbits, with reference to myelination. J. Comp. Neurol. 80:1–10.

Vallbona, C., M. M. Desmond, A. J. Rudolph, L. F. Pap, R. M. Hill, R. R.

Franklin, and J. B. Rush. 1963. Cardiodynamic studies in the newborn. II. Regulation of the heart rate. Biol. Neonat. 5:159−199.

Vallbona, C., A. J. Rudolph, and M. M. Desmond. 1965. Cardiodynamic studies in the newborn. IV. Heart rate patterns in the nondistressed premature infant. Pediatrics 36:560−564.

van Bergeijk, W. A. 1964. Directional and nondirectional hearing in fish. *In* Symposium on Marine Bioacoustics, Bimini, Bahamas, 1963, pp. 281−299. Pergamon Press, Ltd., New York.

Van Hoesen, G. W., D. N. Pandya, and N. Butters. 1972. Cortical afferents to the entorhinal cortex of the Rhesus monkey. Science 175: 1471−1473.

Van Lancker, D., and V. A. Fromkin. 1973. Hemispheric specialization for pitch and "tone": Evidence from Thai. J. Phonetics 1:101−109.

Vasilu, D. C. 1969. Contributions to the morphophysiological study of the auditory apparatus. Rev. Roum. Physiol. 6:159−167.

Vassella, F., and B. Karlsson. 1962. Asymmetric tonic neck reflex. Develop. Med. Child Neurol. 4:363−369.

Veit, P., and G. Bizaguet. 1968. Auditory reactions in the neonate. Rev. Laryng. 89:433−438.

Velden, M. 1974. An empirical test of Sokolov's entropy model of the orienting response. Psychophysiology 11:682−691.

Wagner, I. F. 1937. The establishment of a criterion of depth of sleep in the newborn infant. J. Genetic Psychol. 51:17−59.

Walden, E. F. 1963. The baby cry test: A new audiometric technique for testing very young children. ASHA 5:795.

Walden, E. F. 1972. Audio-reflexometry in testing hearing of very young children. Audiology 12:14−20.

Walter, W. G. 1964. The convergence and interaction of visual, auditory, and tactile responses in human nonspecific cortex. Ann. N. Y. Acad. Sci. 112:320−361.

Walter, W. G., R. Cooper, C. McCallum, and J. Cohen. 1964. The origin and significance of the contingent negative variation or "expectancy wave." Electroencephalog. & Clin. Neurophysiol 18:720.

Warfield, D., R. J. Ruben, and R. Glackin. 1966. Word discrimination in cats. J. Aud. Res. 6:97−119.

Warren, J. M. 1965. The comparative psychology of learning. Ann. Rev. Psychol. 16:95−118.

Warren, R. M., and C. J. Obusek. 1972. Identification of temporal order within auditory sequences. Percept. & Psychophys. 12:86−90.

Warren, R. M., C. J. Obusek, and J. M. Ackroff. 1972. Auditory induction: Perceptual synthesis of absent sounds. Science 176:1149−1151.

Warren, R. M., C. J. Obusek, R. M. Farmer, and R. P. Warren. 1969. Auditory sequence: Confusion of patterns other than speech or music. Science 164:586−588.

Washburn, S. L. 1963. Classification and Human Evolution. Aldine, Chicago.

Watanabe, T., K. Yanagisawa, J. Kanzaki, and Y. Katsuki. 1966. Cortical efferent flow influencing unit responses of medial geniculate body to sound stimulation. Exper. Brain Res. 2:302−317.

Water, W. F., and D. G. McDonald. 1974. Effects of "below-zero" habituation on spontaneous recovery and dishabituation of the orienting response. Psychophysiology 11:548–558.

Weber, B. A. 1972. Short-term habituation of the averaged electroencephalographic response in infants. J. Speech & Hearing Res. 15:757–762.

Webster, D. B. 1966. Ear structure and function in modern mammals. Am. Zool. 6:451–466.

Webster, J. C., M. M. Woodhead, and A. Carpenter. 1970. Perceptual constancy in complex sound identification. J. Psychol. 61:481–489.

Webster, R. L. 1964. Infant vocalizations as a function of environmental language stimulation. Ph.D. thesis, Louisiana State University, New Orleans.

Webster, R. L. 1969. Selective suppression of infants' vocal responses by classes of phonemic stimulation. Develop. Psychol. 1:410–414.

Webster, R. L., H. F. O'Neil, Jr., and D. W. Jacobowitz. 1966. Infants' vocal response changes as a function of self-produced auditory stimulation. Presented at Southeastern Psychological Association.

Webster, R. L., M. H. Steinhardt, and M. G. Senter. 1972. Changes in infants' vocalizations as a function of differential acoustic stimulation. Develop. Psychol. 7:39–43.

Wedenberg, E. 1956. Auditory tests in newborn infants. Acta Otolaryng. 46:446–461.

Wegener, J. G. 1964. Auditory discrimination behavior of brain-damaged monkeys. J. Aud. Res. 4:227–254.

Wegener, J. G. 1974a. Role of the caudal medial geniculate nucleus and its cortical projection in the discrimination of temporally organized visual and auditory patterns. Presented at the Acoustical Society of America, New York.

Wegener, J. G. 1974b. Some variables in the learning of auditory pattern discriminations by animals. Presented at the Acoustical Society of America, New York.

Weiner, B. 1966. Effects of motivation on the availability and retrieval of memory traces. Psychol. Bull. 65:24–37.

Weir, C. 1975. Frequency discrimination in the neonate: A signal detection analysis. J. Exper. Child Psychol. (In press).

Weisberg, P. 1963. Social and nonsocial conditioning of infant vocalizations. Child Develop. 34:377–388.

Weiss, L. A. 1934. Differential variations in the amount of activity of newborn infants under continuous light and sound stimulation. Univ. Iowa Stud. Child Welf. 9, No. 4.

Weitzman, E., W. Fishbein, and L. J. Graziani. 1965. Auditory evoked responses obtained from the scalp electroencephalogram of the full-term human neonate during sleep. Pediatrics 35:458–462.

Weitzman, E., and L. J. Graziani. 1968. Maturation and topography of the auditory evoked response of the prematurely born infant. Develop. Psychobiol. 1:79–89.

Weller, G. M., and R. Q. Bell. 1965. Basal skin resistance and neonatal state. Child Develop. 36:647–657.

Wertheimer, M. 1961. Psychomotor coordination of auditory and visual space at birth. Science 134:1692.

Wever, E. G. 1971. The mechanics of hair-cell stimulation. Ann. Otol. Rhin. & Laryng. 80:786–804.

Wever, E. G., J. G. McCormick, J. Palin, and S. H. Ridgeway. 1971. The cochlea of the dolphin, Tursiops Truncatus: Hair cells and ganglion cells. Proc. Nat. Acad. Sci. 68:2908–2912.

White, B. K., P. Castle, and R. Held. 1964. Observations on the development of visually directed reaching. Child Develop. 35:349–364.

Whitfield, I. C. 1967. The auditory pathway. The Williams & Wilkins Company, Baltimore.

Whitfield, I. C. 1971. Auditory cortex: Tonal, temporal, or topical? In M. B. Sachs (ed.), Physiology of the Auditory System, pp. 289–298. National Educational Consultants, Baltimore.

Whitfield, I. C., and E. F. Evans. 1965. Response of auditory cortical neurons to stimuli of changing frequency. J. Neurol. Physiol. 28:655–672.

Wickelgren, B. G. 1971. Superior colliculus: Some receptive field properties of bimodally responsive cells. Science 173:69–72.

Wickens, D. D. 1970. Encoding categories in short-term memory. Psychol. Rev. 77:1–15.

Wiederhold, M. L., and N. Y-S. Kiang. 1970. Effects of electric stimulation of the crossed olivocochlear bundle on single auditory-nerve fibers in the cat. J. Acoust. Soc. Am. 48:950–965.

Wiederhold, M. L., and W. T. Peake. 1966. Efferent inhibition of auditory-nerve responses: Dependence on acoustic-stimulus parameters. J. Acoust. Soc. Am. 40:1427–1430.

Wiener, N., and J. P. Schadé (eds.). 1965. Cybernetics of the Nervous System. Elsevier Press, Inc., New York.

Wilder, J. 1957. The law of initial value in neurology and psychiatry. J. Nerv. Ment. Dis. 125:73–86.

Wilder, J. 1958. Modern psychophysiology and the law of initial value. Am. J. Psychother. 12:199–221.

Wilson, R. H., D. D. Dirks, and E. C. Careterette. 1968. Effects of ear preferences and order bias on the reception of verbal materials. J. Speech & Hearing Res. 11:509–522.

Windle, W. F. 1970. Development of neural elements in human embryos of four to seven weeks gestation. Exper. Neurol. (Suppl.) 5:44–83.

Winick, M., and R. E. Greenberg. 1965. Appearance and localization of a nerve growth-promoting protein during development. Pediatrics 35:221–228.

Winter, P., and H. H. Funkenstein. 1973. The effect of species-specific vocalization on the discharge of auditory cortical cells in the awake squirrel monkey (Saimiri sciureus). Exper. Brain Res. 18:489–504.

Wisdom, S. S., and B. Z. Friedlander. 1971. Pre-verbal infants' selective operant responses for different levels of auditory complexity and language redundancy. Presented at The Eastern Psychological Association.

Witelson, S. F., and W. Paillie. 1973. Left hemisphere specialization for language in the newborn: Neuroanatomical evidence of asymmetry. Brain 96:641–646.

Wolf, W. (ed.). 1962. Rhythmic Functions in the Living System. Ann. N. Y. Acad. Sci, No. 98.

Wolff, P. H. 1959. Observations on newborn infants. Psychosom. Med. 21:110–118.

Wolff, P. H. 1965. The development of attention in young infants. Ann. N. Y. Acad. Sci. 118:815–830.

Wolff, P. H. 1966. The causes, controls, and organization of behavior in the neonate. Psychol. Issues 5 (Monograph No. 17).

Wolff, P. H. 1967. The role of biological rhythms in early psychological development. Bull. Menninger Clin. 31:197.

Wollberg, Z., and J. D. Newman. 1972. Auditory cortex of squirrel monkey: Response patterns of single cells to species-specific vocalizations. Science 175:212–214.

Wood, C. C. 1973. Levels of processing in speech perception: Neurophysiological and information process analysis. Ph.D. thesis, Yale University, New Haven.

Wood, C. C. 1974. Parallel processing of auditory and phonetic information in speech and discrimination. Percept. & Psychophys. 15:501–508.

Wood, C. C. 1975. A normative model for redundancy gains in speeded classification: Application to auditory and phonetic dimensions in speech discrimination. In F. Restle, R. M. Shiffrin, J. N. Castellan, H. Lindman, and D. B. Pisoni (eds.), Cognitive Theory, Vol. I. Erlbaum Association, Potomac, Md. (In press).

Wood, C. C., W. R. Goff, and R. S. Day. 1971. Auditory evoked potentials during speech perception. Science 173:1248–1251.

Woodcock, J. M. 1971. Terminology and methodology related to the use of heart rate responsivity in infant research. J. Exper. Child Psychol. 11:76–92.

Worden, F. G. 1971. Hearing and the neural detection of acoustic patterns. Behav. Sci. 16:20–30.

Worden, F. G., and R. Galambos. 1972. Auditory processing of biologically significant sounds. Neursci. Res. Prog. Bull. No. 10 (whole).

Wormith, S. J. 1971. Pure tone discrimination in infants. M.A. thesis, Carleton University, Ottawa.

Wormith, S. J., D. Pankhurst, and A. R. Moffitt. 1975. Frequency discrimination by young infants. Child Develop. 46:272–275.

Yang, D. C. 1962. Neurologic status of newborn infants on first and third day of life. Neurology 12:72–77.

Yang, R. K., and D. H. Crowell. 1967. Classical conditioning in the human neonate with the probe technique. Presented at the Society for Research in Child Development, New York.

Yang, R. K., and T. C. Douthitt. 1974. Newborn responses to threshold tactile stimulation. Child Develop. 45:237–242.

Yeni-Komshian, G., R. A. Chase, and R. L. Mobley. 1968. The development of auditory feedback monitoring. II. Delayed auditory feedback studies on the speech of children between two and three years of age. J. Speech & Hearing Res. 11:307–315.

Yeni-Komshian, G., M. S. Preston, and P. J. Benson. 1968. A study of voicing in initial stop consonants: Lebanese arabic, pp. 5–32. Annual Report of the Johns Hopkins Neurocommunications Laboratory.

Yunker, M. P., and L. M. Herman. 1974. Discrimination of auditory temporal differences by the bottlenose dolphin and by the human. J. Acoust. Soc. Am. 56:1870–1875.

Zaidel, E. 1974. Language, dichotic listening, and the disconnected hemispheres. Presented at the Conference on Human Brain Function, University of California, at Los Angeles, Los Angeles. (To be published by BRI.)

Zurif, E. B., and M. Mendelsohn. 1972. Hemispheric specialization for the perception of speech sounds: The influence of intonation and structure. Percept. & Psychophys. 11:329–332.

Zwislocki, J. J., and W. G. Sokolich. 1973. Velocity and displacement responses in auditory-nerve fibers. Science 182:62–64.

APPENDIX A:
Glossary

ABX PROCEDURE

An experimental technique that has yielded most of the data relative to "categorical perception" of speech sounds during adult life. It involves trials with three stimuli, two of which (A and B) always differ from each other and one of which (X) is similar either to A or to B. In speech perception experiments, A and B are drawn from different phonemic categories and the task of the subject is to report which of the two the X most closely resembles. The set induced by instructions accordingly exerts significant effects (Lane, 1965 and 1968) and the procedures tend to confound memory processes with perceptual processes (Fujisaki and Kawashima, 1969, 1970, and 1971).

ACTIVATION (ENERGY MOBILIZATION) THEORY

A set of postulates based upon the commonly accepted idea that activation is some function of bombardment by the reticular activating system (RAS). The theory, used by many investigators to explain relations between an organism's level of arousal and his behavioral efficiency (Berlyne, 1960; Cromwell, Baumeister, and Hawkins, 1963; Duffy, 1957 and 1962; Hebb, 1955; Lindsley, 1951; Malmo, 1962; Malmo and Bélanger, 1967; Semmel, 1963) assumes that: (1) behavior is mediated by both organized neural activity and tonic background activity; and (2) there is some optimal amount of background activity (activation level) which best supports the organized activity. (See also inverted U hypothesis and state.)

ACOUSTIC NERVE

The eighth cranial nerve, which is composed of an auditory portion and a vestibular portion that serves in the maintenance of equilibrium.

ADAPTION

Peripheral or local changes in the sensitivity of cells or cellular assemblies as a function of repeated stimulation (Stevens, 1951; p. 1180).

ALLOPHONES

In psycholinguistics (Greenberg, 1966), perceptual variants of a given phonemic unit that are consequent upon its sound environment, for example, *ta* vs. *ti*. Allophenes, on the other hand, are sound combinations involving identical phonemic types, for instance ta vs. at. Wickelgren has suggested that "concept-sensitive allophones" may constitute minimal perceptual units (Gilbert, 1972; pp. 187–262).

ALPHA RHYTHM

In adult EEG records, waves of 8–13 Hz, ranging in amplitude between 10 and 150 μv, that are present in occipital and parietal areas when subjects are relaxed and have their eyes closed. Such waves are blocked by arousal, particularly by visual stimuli. While there is some disagreement as to the developmental time table for alpha frequency activity, it is generally accepted that it first appears over the occiput at 3–4 months post-term with a frequency of 4/sec, increasing in frequency thereafter until late childhood or early adolescence (Eichorn, 1970; pp. 244–252; and Thompson and Patterson, 1974; pp. 85–98).

ANENCEPHALY (HYDRANENCEPHALY)

Congenital absence of all or part of the cerebral hemispheres in the presence of an intact cranium.

APGAR SCORE

Named after the physician who devised it (Apgar, 1953), the Apgar scoring system is a 10-point rating scale that is used routinely at many hospitals and commonly accepted as an index of newborn viability. It is based upon five equally weighted indices, one of which (HR) can be measured, and the others of which (the cry pattern, muscle tone, reflex response, and color) must be judged. A total score of 10 indicates an infant to be in optimum condition; a total score of 4 or less indicates an immediate need for special resuscitative measures. About 70% of all infants born obtain Apgar scores of 7 or better (Barrie, 1962).

BAND WIDTH

The number of cycles per second, expressed in Hertz (Hz), denoting the lower and upper frequency limits of any signal transmission system. The band width of a *white noise* signal, containing equal energy at all component frequencies (specified as 20–20,000 Hz for many generators), is limited by the earphone or loudspeaker (transducer) through which the signal is transmitted; and it rarely exceeds 100–8,000 Hz. In audiometric test systems, the band width of *speech noise* (usually 500–2,000 Hz) is specified. In typical telephone systems, the transmission band width seldom exceeds 300–3,500 Hz.

For frequencies above 500 Hz or so, bands narrower than 70 Hz, although perceived as sounding much like the pure tones around which they center, differ substantially from pure tones because amplitude and phase variations are random rather than periodic (Moore, 1973). (See also *pure tone*.)

BEST FREQUENCIES

In electrophysiologic studies (Kiang, 1965; Kiang, Sachs, and Peake, 1967; and Tsuchtani and Boudreau, 1967), those characteristic frequencies to which single cells or nerve fibers are most responsive, or "tuned."

BIT

The basic (binary) unit of information both in computer and in CNS processing.

BRADYCARDIA

Decrease in heart rate.

BRAIN STEM

Those portions of the brain not derived from prosencephalon, that is, the pons, medulla, and midbrain.

CARRIER (CARRIER FREQUENCIES)

Generally speaking, any wave that can be modulated to convey information is termed a carrier. In reference to verbal communication, the carrier frequencies for speech are determined by the basic (fundamental) rate of vibration of the vocal cords and linguistic information is conveyed by the formants, or modulation frequencies, that alter the amplitude of these fundamental carrier frequencies. (See *formants*.)

CATEGORICAL PERCEPTION

The phenomenon whereby listeners can discriminate among the members in a given class of sounds only those they can identify (label) as being different from each other, as opposed to continuous perception, whereby they can discriminate many more members of the class than they can identify. Putting this another way, in categorical perception, the boundaries for perceptual discrimination and the boundaries for labeling are more or less equivalent; whereas, in continuous perception, the perceptual boundaries seem to be more sharply demarcated than the labeling boundaries. Recent studies (Baumrin, 1974; Harris and Siegel, 1975; and Siegel and Sopo, 1975) strongly suggest that the phenomenon, once considered unique to speech, in fact may relate to other acoustic continua as well. Although many experiments in speech perception undertaken by the Haskins Laboratory group (Studdert-Kennedy, in press) have yielded data suggesting that consonants are perceived categorically and vowels continuously, these findings lately have been questioned on procedural or other grounds (Fujisaki and Kawashima, 1969, 1970, and 1971; and Locke and Kellar, 1973). There currently is reason to suppose that differences in vowel and consonantal perception may relate in part to the manner in which acoustic information is stored (Dorman, 1974; Pisoni, 1971 and 1973; and Pisoni and Lazarus, 1974). Whether or not this is the case, data relative to differences among speechlike sounds or other patterned signals have to be evaluated cautiously, particularly in terms of the effects of task variables and the relative dimensions of component parameters such as duration and the rate of frequency change over time (Divenyi and Hirsh, 1974).

CINERADIOGRAPHY

A motion picture technique used extensively in cleft palate and related research whereby, through the use of radioactive substances, actions of the speech apparatus can be visualized.

CLICK

An acoustic stimulus which represents a very brief (transient) change in sound pressure, usually generated by a square wave electrical pulse. The maximum pulse duration which produces a clean click is about 1 msec.

COCHLEAR NUCLEUS (CN)

The cellular masses in the medulla (near the restiform body) which, divided into a larger dorsal and smaller ventral portion, constitute the first central relays for the auditory nerve (Moore and Cashin, 1974). The ventral nucleus seems to be more simply organized than the dorsal nucleus (Moushegian, Rupert, and Galambos, 1962) and its cellular activities more closely resemble the response characteristics of cochlear nerve fibers. In addition, there are differences in the frequency response and activity patterns of cells within the two nuclei, although so far as presently is known, no cells in either of them show any real specialization for feature detection (Sachs, 1971, pp. 159–223). Whether or not such specilization exists, it seems increasingly clear that the cochlear nuclei are not merely relay stations, as once was thought, but centers for sensory integration and recoding as well (Moushegian, Rupert, and Whitcomb, 1964a). There are about 90,000 cells in the dorsal cochlear nucleus alone and, given physiologic evidence that each auditory nerve fiber synapses with 75 or more cells, there obviously is great convergence.

Postsynaptic fibers from the CN pursue complicated paths, going in small part to the superior olivary nucleus (SON) on the same side and in larger part, as the trapezoid body, to the SON on the opposite side. In addition, some fibers feed into the brain stem reticular formation.

CODING

The process whereby information units are organized. In reference to verbal communication, *decoding* constitutes the process whereby the eighth nerve (auditory) system transforms environmental sound into suitable form for processing by the CNS while *encoding* constitutes the process whereby internal events are transformed into action.

CONCEPTIONAL AGE

A classification, distinct from *gestational age* (intrauterine time) or *chronological age* (extrauterine time), sometimes used in specifying the developmental status of premature infants during earliest life. It usually is computed with reference to the elapsed time from the first day of the last menstrual period to delivery. For example, an infant with a calculated gestational age of 30 weeks, studied 10 weeks after birth, would have a conceptional age of 40 weeks (Falkner, 1966, pp. 255–256; Parmalee et al., 1964; Schulman, 1970a and 1970b; and Silverman et al., 1967).

CONTINGENT NEGATIVE VARIATION (CNV)

A term coined by Walter (1964; Walter et al., 1964) to designate a "protracted, widespread negative potential" ($\bar{x}$ amplitude, 20 μv) that is seen in the EEG record at about 300 msec following stimulus onset and found most prominently in recordings from prefrontal electrode derivations (F_1 and F_2). The CNV, which is associated with conditioning phenomena and attentional behavior of one kind or another (Hillyard, 1969; Poon et al., 1974), has been studied most extensively in adults (see Price and Smith, 1974, for extended bibliography).

COUPLING

Any connection between related systems such that effects in one system produce effects in the other. In psychoacoustics and related areas, a *coupler* is a standardized electronic device simulating the physical characteristics of the external ear canal and, as routinely employed for calibration purposes, it accordingly is termed an *artificial ear*.

CROSSED OLIVOCOCHLEAR BUNDLE (COCB)

An efferent tract of nerve fibers (Wiederhold and Kiang, 1970; and Wiederhold and Peake, 1966) originating in the accessory nucleus of the superior olivary complex and forming synaptic junctions at the base of the hair cells of the contralateral cochlea (Konishi and Slepian, 1971a and 1971b). Release of a transmitter substance, acetylcholine, by the COCB nerve endings is thought to be one mechanism for inhibiting hair cell activity (Bobbin and Konishi, 1974; and Maw, 1974). (See also *haircells*.)

CUE FUNCTION

The inverted U curve describing the relation between activation and behavioral efficiency (Hebb, 1955; and Suchman and Trabasso, 1966).

DAMPING

The decrease in amplitude of any vibrating system because of energy loss (due to friction, absorption, or other factors). Vibrations that decay slowly are said to be lightly damped; those that decay quickly are termed heavily damped.

DECIBEL (dB)

The basic unit of measurement for sound intensity, which represents a ratio between two energies. In practice, sound usually is calibrated in terms of sound pressures referenced to 0.0002 dynes/cm (0.0002 μbar, or, in new terminology, μNewton).

DELAYED AUDITORY FEEDBACK (DAF)

An experimental technique whereby self-monitoring of speech output can be studied. A subject, reading aloud, has his own utterance fed back to him (usually via earphones) at various delay times until dysfluency or other forms of aberrant verbal behavior can be provoked. For a majority of normal listeners, delays of 170–200 msec between utterance and auditory feedback prove effective in disrupting speech performance (Sullivan et al., 1973).

DICHOTIC

In studies of auditory function, procedures involving the simultaneous presentation of a different signal to each ear, as opposed to *binaural*, or simultaneous presentation of the same signal to each ear (Katz, 1972, pp. 280–312).

DISTINCTIVE FEATURES

In psycholinguistics, the acoustic and/or articulatory characteristics by which components of spoken language can be distinguished from each other (Cole, Sales, and Haber, 1969; and Eimas, 1975). (See also *VOT*.)

DUTY-CYCLE

The relative percentage of time during which a pulsed signal is *on:* when *on* time and *off* time are equal, the cycle is termed *even-duty;* when only one of the values remains constant, it is termed *variable-duty*. In dealing operationally with the effects of *repetition rate* upon auditory behavior, then, four factors must be defined: (1) critical *on* time, or the duration below which a reciprocal relation with intensity becomes demonstrable (energy integration); (2) critical *off* time, or the physiologic interval below which responsivity to longer than critical pulses is reduced; (3) optimal repetition rate, or the combination of predetermined *on* and *off* times that maximizes response; and (4) optimal presentation time, or that duration above which response to a given pulsed envelope cannot be increased.

From adult studies (Eisenberg, 1956): (1) critical *on* time lies somewhere between 150 and 200 msec; (2) critical *off* time probably is about 140 msec; (3) optimal repetition rate for pulses shorter than about 150–200 msec may be 2.5/sec; and (4) 5 sec may represent optimal presentation time. Whether these values apply in early life is unknown.

ELECTROMYOGRAPHY (EMG)

An electronic technique by which the electrical response of muscle units can be visualized on an *electromyogram*. Action potentials obtained from a muscle site may be recorded on a paper tracing, photographed from an oscilloscope trace, or made audible through a loudspeaker.

ELECTROOCULOGRAPHY (EOG)

An electronic technique by which ocular movement patterns can be visualized on an *electrooculogram*. Using the forehead as a ground, corneoretinal potentials, obtained from surface electrodes attached at the outer canthus of each eye, can be analyzed with reference to changes in ocular movement as a function of auditory stimulation of alternative experimental manipulations (McFarland and Kirksey, 1973). Similarly, the *electroretinogram (ERG)* is a record obtained by placing an active electrode over the cornea. (Armington, 1974).

ENVELOPE

The physical wrapper of a sound, within which is included all of its specifiable physical dimensions.

EPOCH

A term commonly used in mathematics and related fields to describe any defined interval (or period) of time during which a function is analyzed.

FEATURE DETECTOR

In perceptual theory and in other contexts as well, any mechanism specially adapted to code a given parameter or attribute. Thus, a visual neuron responding only to lateral movement or an auditory cell responding only to rate of change over time can be considered a feature detector. Cells of this kind in a sense can be considered passive filters, however, and some investigators (Abbs and Sussman, 1971) accordingly have defined feature detectors more narrowly, as mechanisms capable of response to several stimulus attributes at the same time.

FONTANEL

A membranous space between the cranial bones that normally exists during fetal life and infancy. Six fontanels are present in newborns and they close, at various rates, as the skull ossifies during the first 2 years of life. The most prominent of these is the anterior fontanel (just above the forehead) which constitutes the point of union of the frontal, sagittal, and coronal sutures and closes during the second year.

FORMANTS (FORMANT FREQUENCIES)

Localized bands of energy concentration which reflect the natural resonant modes of a given vocal tract and which, displayed visually with the aid of a sound spectrograph, are seen as relatively dark bars. The fundamental frequency of a given utterance, or its lowest component, depends largely upon the size of the speaker's vocal apparatus; the formant structure of that utterance, designated numerically with reference to a low to high frequency continuum (F_1, F_2, and so on), depends upon the positioning of his articulators. In terms of acoustic cues for speech perception, it is fundamental frequency that distinguishes male from female voices while it is formant structure, or the relation between major energy bands, that distinguishes one speech sound from another. Most English speech sounds are characterized by three or four formants. (See also *transition*.)

FOVEA CENTRALIS

A small area on the retina of the eye (opposite the visual axis) at which vision is most distinct.

HABITUATION

A systematic waning of response activity that occurs during repeated bombardment with a given stimulus and is specific to that stimulus (Harris, 1943). The process, which is distinguishable from receptor fatigue or adaptation because the initial pattern of response activity can be reinstated (*dishabituated*) by any just noticeable change in stimulus parameters, may be measured in terms of response strength, latency, or mode as well as changes in arousal level. Many investigators consider the habituation process to be a primitive form of discrimination learning that is centrally mediated (Thompson and Spencer, 1966).

Neural substrates of habituation have been studied in infrahumans as a function of stimulus variables (Dunlop et al., 1964; and Parker, et al., 1974) and at several sites along the auditory pathway (Dunlop, Webster, and Day, 1964; Dunlop, Webster, and Rodger, 1966; Humphrey and Buchwald, 1972; Marsh and Worden, 1964; and Sharpless and Jasper, 1956). Moreover, since habituation measures lend themselves to any number of research questions (Leibrecht, 1974), behavioral and electrophysiologic data on human infants are relatively abundant (Graham, 1973; Jeffrey and Cohen, 1971; Kessen, Haith, and Salapatek, 1970; and Olson, 1975; Appendix B). (For related information, see also *negative perception, orienting response*, and *stimulus satiation theory*.)

HAIR CELLS
The specialized end-organ receptors that convert sound pressure waves to electrical energy for transmission of acoustic information. Receptor mechanisms for hearing consist of these cells and accessory structures of the *organ of Corti* (Johnsson, 1971; and Kimura, 1966), particularly structures of the *basilar membrane*, which support the hair cells and also serve to distribute and filter incoming stimuli.

In humans and other vertebrates, the hair cells lack axonal segments and the transmission of acoustic information results from graded activity rather than all-or-none impulses (as in nerves). An acoustic stimulus acts to deform the uppermost portion of the hair cell, thus generating local electrical processes at the lowermost, or presynaptic, region of the cell body (Wever, 1971). This lowest portion is surrounded by nerve endings, the axonal components of which are myelinated and the dendritic portions of which are unmyelinated. Chemical transmitter substances (Thalman, Kusakari, and Miyoshi, 1973), diffused through the synaptic gap between the hair cell body and the dendritic endings of associated nerve fibers, set up a generator potential which, conducted to the nerve fibers, in turn sets up propogated neural spikes (Kaneko and Daly, 1968).

In physiologic studies, the electrical events associated with end-organ transmission are differentiated as *cochlear microphonics* (AC potentials reflecting displacements along the basilar membrane) and DC *summating potentials* (those reflecting the nature of the stimulus envelope (Dallos, 1972; and Sachs, 1971; pp. 25–29, 57–67).

HEART RATE (HR)
A measure of heart beats per unit time (commonly 1 min), usually determined with reference to the R wave, or most prominent component in the electrocardiogram (EKG) record, and most easily obtained with a *cardiotachometer*. The time between successive heart beats (tau), known as the *heart period*, interbeat interval, or R-R interval, is measured in msec and reciprocally related to HR. Thus, the formula HR = 60/tau permits conversion between HR and heart period data (Brown, 1967; Eisenberg, 1975b; Lewis, 1974; and Woodcock, 1971).

HR is generally thought to be regulated by a complex of sympathetic and parasympathetic influences in the autonomic nervous system, or ANS (Schachter et al., 1971). However, recent evidence (Reis et al., 1973) suggests that the cerebellum also may play a part. Various theories have been advanced to account for the lability of infant heart rates under steady-state conditions and for the effects of sensory or other stimuli. Vallbona and his colleagues (1963; and Vallbona, Rudolph, and Desmond, 1965) have postulated a servomechanism that works under cybernetic principles and implicates the reticular formation. Schulman (1970*a* and 1970*b*) and her colleagues (Schulman and Kreiter, 1970) have suggested that HR responses to sound reflect a loop between the eighth nerve, midbrain, and heart which "can have little to do with cognitive function." Graham and her colleagues, in an enormously influential series of papers (1966, 1968, and 1970), have related the direction of sensory evoked HR responses to orienting (decelerative) and defense (accelerative) reflexes. Yang and Douthitt (1974), on the other hand, have suggested that different rules may apply to proximal and distal senses.

INFERIOR COLLICULUS (IC)

An extremely complicated nucleus in the brain stem that, as a major auditory way station, receives both ipsilateral and contralateral post-synaptic fibers from the lateral lemniscus, the cochlear nuclei, and the superior olivary nucleus. Each IC which may be "biased towards the reception of contralateral sounds" (Barrett, 1973), is connected to its counterpart in the opposite hemisphere by way of the inferior collicular commisure and strands of intercollicular gray matter. Single cell studies (Gershuni et al., 1969) have shown that five or perhaps more patterns of unit activity are present and that units can be classed in two distinct groups according to their frequency thresholds and temporal characteristics.

INVERTED U HYPOTHESIS

The notion that vigilance and related performance improves with arousal (as measured by behavioral state and/or various physiologic indices of internal arousal) up to some moderate level of activation and declines as that level is exceeded. In other words, past some optimal level, arousal is apt to become a disorganizing factor (Buckner and McGrath, 1963; Hebb, 1955; Malmo, 1962; and Lindsley, 1951). An inverted U function has been found to describe the relation between preference and stimulus complexity (Berlyne, 1960; and Jeffrey, 1968) and also between long-term retention in memory and autonomic measures of arousal (Weiner, 1966).

K COMPLEX

A triphasic disturbance of the recorded EEG pattern that is indicative of arousal and nonspecific, that is, it may appear in the absence of external sensory stimulation (Ellingson, 1964; Johnson and Karpan, 1968; and Metcalf, Mondale, and Butler, 1972) or as a consequence of stimulating any modality (Johnson and Lubin, 1967).

LANUGO

A fine textured hair, present on the body of the newborn infant, usually on the back, that most often is shed within the first week of life.

LATERAL LEMNISCUS

The bundle of fibers leaving the superior olivary nucleus which synapses in the nucleus of that bundle. Little is known about the nucleus, probably because it is so difficult to study: the orderly spatial arrangement found elsewhere in the auditory system at the brain stem level is lacking, the nucleus being composed of scattered groups of cells. However, Suga and Shimozawa (1974) have reported data suggesting that it may serve importantly in attenuating self-produced sound. If indeed this is the case, it well may play a role in the monitoring of vocal behavior in man.

LAW OF INITIAL VALUES (LIV or WILDER'S LAW)

A hypothesis, first advanced by Wilder (1957 and 1958) and since modified by the Laceys (1970) and others (Elliott, 1972), stating that the magnitude and direction of change elicited in a particular behavior or physiologic index is inversely related to the prestimulus value of that behavior or index. For example, a given sound introduced when an infant is fast asleep will tend to raise his HR and elicit large motor responses, whereas the same sound, introduced when he is wide awake, will tend to lower his HR and elicit small motor responses (Bench, 1970; Hutt and Hutt, 1970; Schmidt, Rose, and Bridger, 1974; and Wolf, 1962; pp. 1211–1315).

LIMBIC SYSTEM

A ringlike group of structures (septal area, cingulate gyrus, entorhinal cortex, part of the amygdala) derived from a portion of the old brain, connected in a network of well-defined pathways, and widely viewed as the neural substrate for emotion. All of the structures have extensive connections with sensory-motor areas of the brain, with the reticular formation at various levels, and with the autonomic nervous system (McCleary and Moore, 1956; pp. 109–135; and Isaacson, 1974).

MARASMUS

One of two distinct types of severe (grade III) malnutrition. Usually occurring early during the first year of life, it is associated with the change from breast feeding to a weanling diet that is deficient in both protein and calories. Clinical signs include general wasting due to utilization of body tissue stores as well as retarded growth and development. *Kwashiorkor*, the second type of grade III malnutrition, differs from marasmus in several ways: it generally occurs later in infancy, following cessation of adequate breast feeding; it results from long-term ingestion of a weanling diet that, although deficient in protein, contains a moderate amount of calories; it routinely is manifest in edema (pot-belly, and so on) rather than wasting, and often is precipitated by stress factors such as low environmental temperatures or infection (Cravioto, Hambraeus, and Vahlquist, 1974).

MEDIAL FOREBRAIN BUNDLE (MFB)

An extremely important neural tract that is considerably larger in lower vertebrates than it is in man. Located in the hypothalamic region, it contains diffusely spread fibers that serve to interconnect the reticular system, the lateral hypothalamus, and the rhinencephalon.

MEDIAL GENICULATE BODY (MG)

A cellular mass springing from the ventral surface of the pulvinar (posterior tubercle of the thalamus) that receives fibers from lower auditory centers via the lateral lemniscus and projects, by way of radiating fibers (geniculotemporal tract or auditory radiations), to auditory cortex. Single unit studies (Aitkin and Webster, 1972) suggest that about 30% of the cells within each densely packed ventral portion of the MG respond to both contralateral and ipsilateral stimulation while the remainder may be more sensitive to stimulation from the opposite ear.

MESENCHYME

Embryonic connective tissue from which middle ear structures derive (Dayal, Farkashidy, and Kokshanian, 1973; and McLellan et al., 1964). Mesenchymal tissue is present in the middle ear at birth, particularly in the area around the ossicles (Igarashi, personal communication). It has been thought until recently that perhaps as long as 4–6 weeks might be required for complete absorption of this tissue, but new data, derived from middle ear compliance measurements (Keith, in press), suggest this may not be the case.

MIDDLE EAR (tympanic cavity)

Middle ear structures derive embryologically from endoderm (the brachial arches), as opposed to inner ear structures, which derive from ectoderm (Anson, Harper, and Hanson, 1962; Kakizaki and Altmann, 1970; McLellan et al., 1964; McLellan and Struck, 1965; and Strickland et al., 1962). Situated between the outer ear canal and the labyrinth of the inner ear (Curthoys, Markham, and Blank, 1970) and separated from each by a thin membrane, the middle ear is delimited by six walls. Within this so-called tympanic cavity are the three ossicles, the malleus (hammer), incus (anvil), and stapes (stirrup), each of which is held in place by minute ligaments and muscles and covered by mucous membrane that is continuous with the eardrum (tympanic membrane). Sound waves impinging upon the eardrum cause it to vibrate, and this vibration, conducted through the ossicular chain, is transmitted to the oval window which, vibrating in its turn, sets up fluid perturbations in the inner ear. In addition to their conductive function, the eardrum and ossicles, working in tandem as it were, constitute a mechanism for amplifying sound by about 30 dB (Kobrak, 1959).

MORO REFLEX

A bilaterally symmetrical reaction of early life involving strong movements of the upper extremities and considerably weaker movements of the lower extremities. It can be self-induced as well as elicited by sound or various forms of vestibular stimulation and differs from the similar startle (or fright) reaction in two major ways: (1) movements are extensor rather than flexor in nature; and (2) it wanes during development, normally disappearing by 5–6 months of age, as opposed to the startle reflex, which persists into adult life. The Moro reflex is commonly seen during the newborn period and is thought by some (Prechtl, 1953) to represent a phylogenetic relic of clinging behavior in infrahuman species (Peiper, 1963).

MOTOR THEORY OF SPEECH PERCEPTION

The long held and very influential notion that speech perception results from an active matching between articulatory "neural motor commands" and the speech output (Allport, 1924; Lane, 1965 and 1968; and Liberman et al., 1963 and 1967). Although some investigators (Lenneberg, 1967; and McCaffrey, 1971) have postulated that developmental changes in the ability to perceive phonemic categories would parallel changes in the ability to produce those categories, mounting evidence relative to the perception of speechlike sounds by human infants and some primates (Kavanagh and Cutting, in press; Morse and Snowden, 1975; and Sinnott, 1974) suggest that the theory no longer is tenable.

NEGATIVE PRECEPTION (NP)

The attenuation of a noxious stimulus such as shock, an unpleasant or loud sound, etc., by some preceding or preparatory signal. According to the *preception hypothesis*, habituation and NP are complementary mechanisms for reducing the impact of aversive or disruptive stimuli, but preception involves attention and awareness, whereas habituation is an automatic process (Epstein, Boudreau, and Kling, 1975; and Lykken and Tellegen, 1974)

NEOTENY

A relatively prolonged retention of fetal or neonatal characteristics manifest in the persistence of early reflex patterns such as rooting, sucking, and the like (Hulse, 1963; pp. 86–88). It has been suggested (Mason, 1968) that maturation rates for simple, nonsocial behaviors vary among species according to the amount of directly supportive behavior given by the mother, for example, physical contact during nursing. Other investigators (Ehrlich, 1974) view this notion as highly disputable, however.

ORIENTING RESPONSE (OR)

First described by Pavlov as the investigatory or "what is it?" reflex, the OR was defined as a response to novel stimulation by which an organism orients its receptors in order to acquire information about its environment. Sharpless and Jasper (1956) first distinguished between phasic and tonic components of the OR, relating them to control mechanisms in the brain stem reticular formation (tonic) and thalamic projection system (phasic) according to their differential properties: the tonic component is characterized by long latency, long response duration, and rapid habituation; the phasic component is characterized by short latency, short response duration, and greater resistance to habituation.

In recent years, largely as a result of Sokolov's work (1963), the OR has come to be viewed as a generalized response system (Brackbill and Fitzgerald, 1969; and Lynn, 1966) that is independent of stimulus quality, sensitive to any change in stimulation, and characterized by specific skeletal, autonomic, and EEG properties that distinguish it from defense and adaptation responses: (1) it can be elicited by both stimulus onset and stimulus offset; (2) it most easily is elicited by weak stimuli; (3) it induces peripheral vasoconstriction together with cerebral vasodilation and desynchronization of the EEG alpha rhythm, these changes serving to sensitize sensory analyzers so that information intake increases and environmental changes acquire greater salience; and (4) it habituates quickly when a given stimulus is repeated and dishabituates when that stimulus is changed because the neuronal model acquired by function of the OR acts as a selective filter, a match between the neuronal model and the incoming stimulus resulting in inhibitory influences upon the RAS and a mismatch resulting in activating influences upon it.

Data supporting the OR properties specified by Sokolov are equivocal in some cases and modifications of his concepts already have been suggested (Bernstein, 1969; Edwards, 1974; Graham and Clifton, 1966; Graham and Jackson, 1970; Leavy and Geer, 1967; Moreau, Birch, and Turkewitz, 1970; Smith and Strawbridge, 1969; Velden, 1974; and Water and McDonald, 1974). Since most of these data were acquired with adult subjects, it is likely that further modifications will become apparent as the properties of ORs during early life are explored more widely.

PACER SIGNAL

A stimulus at some level of complexity just enough above an organism's level of complexity that he can deal with it and, by doing so, proceed to a higher level of functional organization (Dember and Earl, 1957; and Sackett, 1966).

PARALLEL TRANSMISSION

In speech perception theory, that process by which a single acoustic cue carries information about a sequence of phonemes, for instance, the distinction between /di/ and /du/ is based upon a second formant transition which characterizes both the vowel and the consonantal elements (Liberman, 1970; and Wood, 1974 and in press).

PARIETAL HUMPS

In EEG work, low voltage diphasic waves, appearing in central derivations, that are bilateral, synchronous, and indicative of drowsy states. They are poorly defined in the term infant, become prominent at about 3 months, and reach maximum amplitude at about 3 years, declining thereafter.

PHONE

A segment of speech, for example, a vowel, a consonant, or a syllable, that, although meaningless, can be distinguished by the ear and/or produced by the speech apparatus as a discrete unit.

PRAGMATICS

A term coined by Cherry (1961) that refers to the significance of signals to communicants. The study of pragmatics now is subsumed under the relatively new science of *semiotics* (Marler, 1961), which also includes *syntactics* (the study of signals as physical phenomena) and *semantics* (the study of the meaning of signs).

PREPOTENT STIMULUS

As originally conceived, that particular stimulus which, under naturally occurring conditions of competing stimulation, determines an organism's reflex action. As more recently viewed (Jane, Masterton, and Diamond, 1965), that signal in a given stimulus hierarchy to which the organism is tuned by virtue of some underlying neural selection process.

PURE TONE

An acoustic signal in which sound pressure level changes, as a function of time, assume a sine wave form. With the exception of speech hearing measures, all standardized audiometric tests of threshold sensitivity are based upon the use of pure tones at the octave intervals between 125–8,000 Hz.

The manner in which pure tones are perceived depends mainly upon frequency but judgments of *pitch* are affected significantly by such factors as duration and intensity. As the duration of pure tones is increased in the range between 2–200 msec, there is a progressive change in the quality of sensation from (1) click alone through (2) click-pitch and (3) tone-pitch to (4) tone alone (Eisenberg, 1956).

RESPIRATORY CENTER

Two groups of nerve cells situated in the reticular formation of the medulla that, by way of the phrenic and intercostal nerves, discharge impulses for inspiration and expiration to muscles of the diaphragm and thorax. Breathing patterns are regulated by the so-called Hering-Breuer reflex, the afferent component of which is supplied by vagus nerve fibers in the lung tissue.

RETICULAR ACTIVATING SYSTEM (RAS)

A phylogenetically old system that constitutes the bulk of the CNS in primitive organisms and, in higher vertebrates, is thought to constitute a kind of master control mechanism for nervous activity. In man, the RAS is centrally located in brain stem and thalamic areas, surrounded by complex masses of fiber tracts and nuclei that afford connections with most, if not all, portions of the nervous system, including the cerebellum. Available neurophysiologic data indicate that reticular cells are extremely versatile. Stimuli applied to almost any conductor or receptor mechanism, including auditory neurons, will evoke responses in the reticular formation, and single cells within the formation are capable of exerting influences bilaterally. Connecting upward toward the brain, reticular fibers convey arousing information; connecting downward toward the spinal cord, they mediate visceral motor functions; connecting laterally with sensory and other channels, they filter environmental information so that some incoming signals will be perceived and others rejected (Beritoff, 1965; pp. 276–292; Evans and Mulholland, 1969; French, 1960; Kilmer and McCulloch, 1969; and McCleary and Moore, 1956; pp. 72–89).

SCHEMA

In psychologic and particularly in Piagetan theory (Flavell, 1963), an internal representation of a stimulus that develops as a result of exposure to and experience with that stimulus.

SCLERA

The outer membrane of the eyeball or, in popular parlance, the white of the eye.

SINUS ARRHYTHMIA

A periodic waxing and waning in HR, usually synchronous with respiration rate, that is mediated by the vagus nerve. A sinus arrhythmia pattern is easily visible on neonatal HR records (Lipton et al., 1964) and characteristically is found on the records of adults who smoke (unpublished Bioacoustic Laboratory data).

SLEEP SPINDLES

In EEG work, short runs or bursts of 12- to 16-Hz activity seen during light to moderate sleep and having maximum amplitude in central derivations. Spindles may be present in rudimentary form from birth, but they are hard to discern in early infancy since they lack consistent symmetry and synchrony. They are reasonably prominent by 11−12 months and their voltage and duration increase with age (Curzi-Dascalova, Pajot, and Dreyfus-Brisac, 1974; and Metcalf, 1970).

SOUND SPECTROGRAPH

An electronic device which shows (on a spectrogram) the distribution of acoustic energy within a frequency range (shown on the ordinate) over time (the abscissa).

SPEECH CUE

A specific acoustic event that carries linguistic information, for example, the difference in VOT that distinguishes voiced from voiceless sounds.

SPIRAL GANGLION

The cluster of nerve cell bodies within the inner ear giving rise to the cochlear (auditory) branch of the eighth nerve system. Axons terminate centrally in the dorsal and ventral cochlear nuclei; dendrites terminate in the hair cells. Most of the ganglion cells are unipolar, but a small percentage of multipolar cells, which possibly may exert parasympathetic influences upon inner ear structures (Ross and Burkel, 1973), also has been identified.

SQUARE WAVE

A term describing the physical shape of a periodic wave encompassing a range of harmonically related frequencies that can be analyzed into a series of sine and cosine components. A square wave of 250 Hz, for instance, has a fundamental of 250 Hz, a third harmonic at 750 Hz, and a fifth harmonic at 1,250 Hz, but no energy at the intervening frequencies of 500 and 1,000 Hz. In general, the sharper the corners of a square wave, the greater the range of frequencies required to express it.

Square waves and sine waves (pure tones) differ from each other physically in specific ways and any valid comparison between the functional effects of these signals must take the differences into account. As an example, if a pure tone and a square wave are equated for an SPL of 60 dB, conditions for response are weighted in favor of the latter because the fundamental of the square wave is 4/pi more intense.

STATE (ACTIVITY STATE; AROUSAL LEVEL)

That activation level which results from the interaction between stimuli arising within an organism and stimuli arising within his external environment. The "state" obtaining at any given moment can be ordered on a defined scale referable to a given measurement index. For instance, overt activity can be quantified with reference to the continuum between sleep and wakefulness while brain wave and cardiac activity can be quantified with reference to the relative distribution of given frequency bands and heart rates (Prechtl, 1974; and Prechtl, Weimann, and Akiyama, 1969). The term, *basal state*, frequently is used to distinguish measures obtained before experimental stimulation is introduced from measures obtained after stimulation has begun.

Numerous studies of neonatal performance and function have shown that the nature of reflex behavior varies according to state and the modality stimulated (Lenard, Bernuth, and Prechtl, 1968; Lewis, Bartels, and Goldberg, 1967; Martinius and Papousek, 1970; Papousek, 1961; Prechtl et al., 1967; Weller and Bell, 1965; and Wolff, 1966).

STEADY STATE

In control systems, that state in which the variables in a feedback loop remain more or less constant over the time required for the loop to be traversed. As applied in this volume, any state of the organism that can be measured or scored subsequent to adaptation in a constant physical environment.

STIMULUS SATIATION THEORY

The notion that repeated exposure to environmental stimuli results in the build up of some hypothetic quantity which reduces the potency of such stimuli during subsequent exposures (Glanzer, 1953). Since this quantity is presumed to dissipate spontaneously over time, it follows that the rate of exposure to external stimuli can alter the characteristics of response behavior.

SUBCEPTION

A term coined by Lazarus and McCleary (1951) to describe that "process by which some kind of discrimination is made when the subject is unable to make a correct conscious discrimination." In terms of formal network theory (Powers, 1973), a subception can be viewed as a first-order perception in that it bears a direct relation to some physical phenomenon just outside the nervous system.

SUPERIOR OLIVARY NUCLEUS (SON)

That portion of a complex of cells in the medulla (near the facial nerve) receiving postsynaptic fibers from the cochlear nuclei, and the first point along the auditory pathway to receive input from both ears. The SON, which is believed to mediate auditory reflexes relating to movements of the middle ear muscles (Campbell, 1965), is variously implicated in binaural hearing (Harrison and Beecher, 1967) and in inhibition of cochlear activity (Dayal, 1972; Moushegian, Rupert, and Whitcomb, 1964b; Raab, 1971; and Rasmussen, 1964). (See also *crossed olivocochlear bundle.*)

TACHYCARDIA

Increase in heart rate.

TRACÉ ALTERNANT

In EEG records, bursts of irregular slow electrical activity mixed with 4–6/sec waves with superimposed faster low voltage activity and alternating with electrical silence, that characterize quiet sleep during late gestation and the earliest months of infancy (Dreyfus-Brisac, 1966; and Engel and Milstein, 1971).

TRANSIENT

In a general sense, a transient is any very short-duration change that reflects underlying readjustments and constitutes an acoustic cue. In electronics, the audible click, or *switching transient*, produced when a circuit is activated, almost instantaneously results from momentary current fluctuations.

TRANSITION

In speech perception, the time-dependent shift, or transition, in formant structure permitting discrimination of speech sounds results from rapid articulatory adjustments: the duration of the first formant transition affords cues as to whether consonants are voiced or unvoiced while the direction of frequency change over time for the second and third formant trnasitions affords information on place of articulation (i.e., whether alveolar as in /da/, bilabial as in /ba/, or velar, as in /ga/. (See also *formant* and *VOT.*)

VERNIX CASEOSA

A waxy oil, overlaying the skin of the newborn infant and lining his external auditory canal, that usually disappears within a few postnatal days (Keith, in press; and Sprunt and Redman, 1964).

VERTEX (V) POTENTIAL

A change in the ongoing EEG pattern recorded from an electrode placed on the vertex of the scalp (i.e, at the crown of the head). The vertex placement is commonly used for clinical measures of the sound-evoked response, but since it is nonspecific, this slow diffuse change in the EEG patterns can be elicited by many other sensory stimuli as well (Davis et al., 1966; and Davis, and Zerlin, 1966).

VOICE ONSET TIME (VOT)

The time between the release burst of energy from the articulators and the onset of voicing (laryngeal activity) that, in English and other languages as well, permits hearers to differentiate voiced from voiceless consonants. From the standpoint of speech production, this difference relates to the source of the acoustic energy. For voiced sounds, the energy is generated at the level of the larynx and the rate at which the vocal cords open and close, together with the tension of the laryngeal muscles, determines the fundamental frequency. For unvoiced sounds, the energy may be generated at more peripheral sites (for instance, the lips, as in /p/, or the teeth, as in /s/) and the turbulence resulting from constriction at these sites determines the acoustic character of the utterance. Thus, voiced syllables such as /ba/ or /da/ are characterized by a very short lag between consonant and vowel whereas their voiceless counterparts, /pa/ and /ta/, are characterized by a relatively longer lag (Lisker and Abramson, 1964). From a processing standpoint, then, the ability to differentiate consonant-vowel (CV) combinations depends upon the ability of the auditory system to deal with very short units of time.

Various experiments with adult subjects support the idea, which can be related to physiologic evidence of short-time constant mechanisms in the auditory system (Gersuni, 1971), that duration in the neighborhood of 20 msec is a critical determinant of auditory processing operations (Stevens and Klatt, 1974). Acoustic variations occurring within 20–25 msec are processed as a single event while sounds separated from each other by intervals larger than this are perceived as successive events (Hirsh, 1959; and Hirsh and Sherrick, 1961).

Stevens and Klatt (1974), in an interesting paper, have suggested that the distinction between voiced and voiceless consonants involves a processing strategy whereby: (1) the cue for the presence of a consonant is rapid spectral change at a point of abrupt SPL increase; (2) the completion of spectral change within 20-odd msec signifies a voiced consonant; and (3) the persistence of spectral change beyond this time signifies an unvoiced consonant. Such a strategy applies as well to current thinking about parallel processing as it does to theories of categorical perception.

APPENDIX B:
An Alphabetical and Chronological Listing of Studies Relative to the Effects of Sound on Human Subjects Under the Age of Three Years

Sound stimuli are used by so many investigators of infant function for such varied purposes that locating information pertinent to one's interests is a time consuming and all too often fruitless task. The purpose of this Appendix, therefore, is to provide a selective guide to clinical and research material that is scattered throughout journal literature and dissertation files of many disciplines and a number of geographic areas in addition to the United States.

The guide may not include every study ever undertaken in which sound was used as a stimulus in subjects under the age of 3 years, but it is as complete as many years of effort at the Bioacoustic Laboratory can make it, and is organized in a manner that should make it variously useful to students or specialists in many fields of study. It is divided chronologically into four sections according to year of publication or, in the case of unpublished or in-press work, year of informal or prepublication report:

(I) before 1960; (II) 1960–1969; (III) 1970–1975; (IV) in press, as of 1975. Where the number of reports is relatively large, as in Sections II and III, each section is subdivided by year. Citations are listed alphabetically in all cases and four general kinds of information are provided about each report listed: (1) the kind(s) of signal(s) employed (column 2); (2) the acoustic parameter(s) and/or the phenomena investigated (columns 3 and 4); (3) characteristics of the study population (columns 5 and 6); and (4) the kinds of measures employed (final columns).

Except where it would be misleading to specify stimuli in any fashion except that described by the author(s), signals in column 2 are shown under nine general categories as: *clicks*, however generated; *noisemakers*, which refer to any sounds generated by toys, environmental objects, or other unstandardized devices; noises generated by standardized electronic equipment, which are specified as *white noise, band noise* (restricted band widths of any dimensions), or *square waves* (bands in which the frequency components are harmonically related); *pure tones,* which refer to sine wave signals of any frequency, whether continuous or interrupted; *music*, which refers both to instrumental sounds and singing voice; speech, which is differentiated according to whether an utterance was generated naturally by *live voice* or by computer, as *synthetic speech.*

Columns 3 and 4 are designed to complement one another and they are handled similarly to column 2 in that specific descriptors are used only where it would be misleading to employ general descriptors. To provide adequate information about each report, all major parameters and/or phenomena considered in a particular paper are noted. In column 3, which refers to physical attributes of sound, conventional acoustic terminology is used wherever possible. In column 4, which refers essentially to the conceptual basis of experiments, generic terms serve to specify major issues. Thus, (1) a blank space in column 3 may mean that physical parameters of the signal(s) were held constant, not specified, considered indeterminable on the basis of the information provided, or irrelevant to the purposes of the report. (2) A blank space in column 3, in conjunction with a "responsivity" listing in column 4, indicates that the purpose of the study was merely to determine whether sound per se could evoke some form of response activity (shown in the final columns). (3) A sound pressure level listing in column 3, in conjunction with responsivity in column 4, indicates a concern with threshold definition whereas the same sound pressure level listing, in conjunction with stimulus differentiation in column 4, connotes a concern with loudness function. (4) A column 4 listing such as conditioning or habituation may apply to an experiment designed to show whether the phenomenon could be demonstrated at a given developmental stage (column 5) or, alternatively, to one designed to show whether the nature of the phenomenon differed according to factors shown in other columns. In the same way, a listing of individual differences applies to any study designed to differentiate among subject groups on the basis of physiologic status or any factors other than age. The latter factor is considered specifically under the heading, "maturational change."

Experiments relating to auditory screening of infant or preschool-aged groups are not shown separately. However, it can be assumed that a "responsivity" heading, combined with a substantial N in column 6, refers to studies of this kind. By the same token, longitudinal studies are not specified, though they can be determined from study of columns 4 and 5.

It must be pointed out that this guide is selective only in the sense that it permits users to pick out particular reports that bear upon their interests. No papers have been excluded on a qualitative basis or because they represent redundant reporting on a single experiment. It is important to recognize that redundant reporting is commonplace, however, and the number of papers found in the listings, therefore, is a specious index of the amount of work relating to hearing in infancy. The number of investigators whose names recur over the years probably is a more valid index of this, and, as one considers such names in the context of the volume of reports each year, a disconcerting trend becomes evident: despite substantial gains in information during the past decade or so, research relative to developmental auditory processing clearly is declining rather than accelerating (see Figure B-1, p. 244). This is reflected in the sharply reduced number of current reports.

The pattern seen in Figure B-1 can be related quite directly to changing patterns of support for basic research: the years of heavy reporting reflect a period of substantial government funding for developmental studies of all kinds; the years of diminished reporting represent mainly the final fruits of earlier support. Unless matters change, then, the optimistic forecast for progress in the area of developmental communicative behavior (Chapter 7) surely will have to be revised. In research, as in all things, lost momentum cannot be regained without increased expenditure of effort.

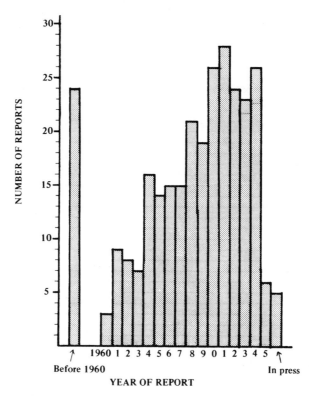

Figure B-1. Studies bearing upon auditory competence in early life by year of report (1910–1975).

Appendix B Abbreviations

BW	band width
Cond.	conditioning
DAF	delayed auditory feedback
Dif. rf.	differential reinforcement
Dim.	dimensionality
Dur.	duration
EEG	electroencephalography
EMG	electromyography
EOG	electrooculography
ERG	electroretinography
F	frequency
Form. str.	formant structure
Hab.	habituation
HR	heart rate
Ind. d.	individual differences
ISI	interstimulus interval
LIV	law of initial values
Loc.	localization
Mat. ch.	maturational change
OR	orienting response
Ov. beh.	overt behavior
Pac.	pacification (soothing)
Rep. r.	repetition rate
Resp. rt.	respiration rate
Resp.	responsivity
Rise t.	rise time
R+D t.	rise and decay time
Skin res.	skin resistance (EMF; GSR; PGSR)
SPL	sound pressure level
Stab.	stabilimeter
Stim. dif.	stimulus differentiation
Suck.	sucking
Unspec.	unspecified

SECTION I. Studies Undertaken Before 1960

Author(s)	Information Available			Subjects		Measures Employed							
	Stimuli Employed	Parameters	Phenomena	Age Range	N	EEG	HR	Ov. Beh.	Resp. Rt.	Skin Res.	Stab.	Suck.	Other
Aldrich (1928)	Noisemaker	–	Resp.	3 mos	1	–	–	X	–	–	–	–	–
Bryan (1930)	Noisemakers	–	Mat. ch.; resp.; stim. dif.	1–10 days	75	–	–	X	–	–	–	–	–
Canestrini (1913)	Live voice; noisemakers	–	Resp.	Newborns (unspec.)	70	–	–	–	X	–	–	–	Pulse rate
Clarke (1939)	Noisemaker	–	Resp.	>14 hrs– 20 wks	14	–	–	X	–	–	–	–	-
Dearborn (1910)	Music; noisemaker	F	Mat. ch.; resp.	6–67 days	1	–	–	X	–	–	–	–	–
Eichorn (1951)	Clicks; noisemakers	Rep. rt.	Resp.; stim. dif.	7–81 days	38	X	X	–	X	X	–	–	–
Ewing and Ewing (1944)	Live voice noisemakers	Dim.	Mat. ch.; stim. dif.	1–59 mos	(Unspec.)	–	–	X	–	–	–	–	–
Froeschels and Beebe (1946)	Noisemakers; pure tones	SPL	Stim. dif.	12 hrs– 9 days	33	–	–	X	–	–	–	–	–
Haller (1932)	Pure tones	F; SPL	Resp.; stim. dif.	2–5 wks	30	–	–	X	–	–	–	–	–
Hardy, J. B. et al. (1959)	Live voice; noisemakers	F; SPL	Mat. ch.; resp.; stim. dif.	4 hrs– 52 wks	481	–	–	X	–	–	–	–	–
Hardy, W. G. and Bordley (1951)	Pure tones	F; SPL	Resp.; stim. dif.	7 mos–6 yrs	500	–	–	–	–	X	–	–	–
Irwin (1932)	Pure tone	–	Reaction time	15 hrs– 15 days	12	–	–	–	–	–	X	–	–
Kasatkin (1957)	Noisemaker	SPL	Cond.	27–55 days	2	–	–	–	–	–	–	X	–
Kasatkin and Levikova (1935)	Noisemakers; pure tones	F	Cond.; stim. dif.	11–28 days	3	–	–	–	–	–	–	X	–

Author(s)	Stimuli Employed	Parameters	Phenomena	Age Range	N	EEG	HR	Ov. Beh.	Resp. Rt.	Skin Res.	Stab.	Suck.	Other
Marquis (1931)	Noisemaker	—	Cond.	24 hrs–10 days	8	—	—	—	—	—	—	×	—
Pratt (1934)	Pure tones	ISI	Sequence effects	2–11 days	28	—	—	×	—	—	—	—	—
Pratt et al. (1930)	Noisemakers; pure tones	Dim.; SPL	Resp.	24 hrs–10 days	50	—	—	—	—	—	×	—	—
Richmond et al. (1953)	Noisemakers	—	Resp.	30 min–8 days	46	—	—	×	—	—	—	—	—
Stubbs (1934)	Pure tones	Dur.; F; SPL	Stim. dif.	1–10 days	75	—	—	×	×	—	×	—	—
Stubbs and Irwin (1934)	Pure tones	—	Reaction time	1–10 days	6	—	—	—	×	—	×	—	—
Taylor-Jones (1927)	Noisemakers	—	Resp.; state effects	<24 hrs	55	—	—	×	—	—	—	—	—
Wagner (1937)	Pure tones	F	State effects; stim. dif.	3 hrs–11 days	69	—	—	×	×	—	—	—	—
Wedenberg (1956)	Noise pulse	F; SPL	Resp.	1–10 days	21	—	—	×	—	—	—	—	—
Wolff (1959)	Live voice; noisemakers	SPL	State effects; stim. dif.	1–5 days	4	—	—	×	—	—	—	—	—

SECTION II. Studies Undertaken from 1960 to 1969

		Information Available		Subjects		Measures Employed							
Author(s)	Stimuli Employed	Parameters	Phenomena	Age Range	N	EEG	HR	Ov. Beh.	Resp. Rt.	Skin Res.	Stab.	Suck.	Other
1960													
Chun et al.	Buzzer	—	Loc.; mat. ch.	2–49 wks	26	—	—	×	—	—	—	—	—
Frodig	Noisemakers; pure tones	—	Resp.	Newborns >30 min	2,000	—	—	×	—	—	—	—	—

(continued)

Author(s)	Stimuli Employed	Information Available		Subjects		Measures Employed							
		Parameters	Phenomena	Age Range	N	EEG	HR	Ov. Beh.	Resp. Rt.	Skin Res.	Stab.	Suck.	Other
Salk	Heartbeats	—	Pac.	Newborns (unspec.)	214	—	—	—	—	—	—	—	Food intake; recorded cries; weight change
1961													
Bridger	Pure tones	Dur.; F; ISI	Hab.; stim. dif.	1–5 days	50	—	X	X	—	—	—	—	—
DiCarlo and Bradley	Music; noisemakers; white noise	Dim.	Resp.; stim. dif.	10 mos–3 yrs	50	—	—	X	—	—	—	—	—
Dougherty and Cohen	Noisemakers	—	Resp.	4–28 wks	300	—	—	X	—	—	—	—	—
Eagles et al.	Pure tones	F; SPL	Resp.	2–3 yrs	67	—	—	—	—	—	—	—	Audiometric testing
Engel	Noisemakers; pure tones	—	Ind. d.	Newborns (unspec.)	Unspec.	X	—	X	—	—	—	—	—
Salk	Heartbeats	—	Pac.	Newborns (unspec.)	214	—	—	—	—	—	—	—	Food intake; recorded cries; weight change
Suzuki and Ogiba	Pure tones	F; SPL	Resp.	1–3 yrs	250	—	—	X	—	—	—	—	—
Suzuki and Sato	Noisemakers	SPL	Resp.	18–42 mos	181	—	—	X	—	—	—	—	—
Wertheimer	Noisemaker	—	Resp.	3–10 min	1	—	—	X	—	—	—	—	—
1962													
Bartoshuk (a)	Clicks	ISI	Ind. dif.; mat. ch.; resp.; sequence effects	1–4 days	120	—	X	—	—	—	—	—	—

Study	Stimulus	Parameters	Procedure/Measure	Age	N										Remarks
Bartoshuk (b)	Clicks; square waves	F; ISI; SPL	Hab.	48–96 hrs	80	—	X	—	—	—	—	—	—	—	—
Beadle and Crowell	Pure tones	F; SPL	Resp.; stim. dif.	41 hrs	1	—	X	—	—	—	—	—	—	—	—
Bridger (a)	Pure tones	Dur.; F; ISI	Hab.	5 days	43	—	X	X	—	—	—	—	—	—	—
Hardy et al.	Live voice; noisemakers	F; SPL	Predictive value of neonatal tests	4–12 mos	1,388	—	—	X	—	—	—	—	—	—	—
Parr	Pure tones	SPL	Resp.	24 hrs–6 days	140	—	—	X	—	—	—	—	—	—	—
Salk	Heartbeats; metronome; music	—	Pac.	1 day–37 mos	127	—	—	X	—	—	—	—	—	—	Food intake; recorded cries; weight change
Suzuki et al.	Pure tones	SPL	Mat. ch.	1–23 yrs	92	X	—	—	—	—	—	—	—	—	—
1963															
Bordley et al.	Live voice; noisemakers	F; SPL	Predictive value of neonatal tests; resp.	4–12 mos	1,077	—	—	X	—	—	—	—	—	—	—
Goldstein and Kendell	Pure tones	SPL	Mat. ch.; resp.	9–59 mos	34	X	—	—	—	—	—	—	—	—	—
Kaye and Levin	Pure tones	—	Cond.	<5 days	70	—	—	—	—	X	—	—	—	—	—
Lipton et al.	White noise	SPL	Stim. dif.	2–5 days	9	—	X	X	—	—	—	—	—	—	—
Miller et al.	Noisemakers	F; SPL	Mat. ch.; resp.; stim. dif.	3–5 mos	54	—	—	X	—	—	—	—	—	—	—
Walden	Baby cry; pure tones	Dim.	Resp.; stim. dif.	1 mo–3 yrs	185	—	—	X	—	—	—	—	—	—	—
Weisberg	Live voice; noisemakers	—	Dif.; ref.; stim. dif.	3 mos	33	—	—	—	—	—	—	—	—	—	Recorded vocalizations

(continued)

SECTION II (*continued*)

Author(s)	Stimuli Employed	Parameters	Phenomena	Age Range	N	EEG	HR	Ov. Beh.	Resp. Rt.	Skin Res.	Stab.	Suck.	Other
		Information Available		Subjects		Measures Employed							
				1964									
Appleby	Clicks; pure tones	SPL	Resp.; stim. dif.	2–10 days	40	X	–	–	–	–	–	–	–
Bartoshuk	Pure tones	SPL	Stim. dif.	24–100 hrs	30	X	X	–	X	–	X	–	–
Boehm and Haynes	Clicks	–	Resp.	1 day–2 mos	30	–	X	–	!	–	–	X	–
Downs and Sterritt	Band noise; white noise	–	Resp.; stim. dif.	<7 days	117	–	–	X	–	–	–	–	–
Eisenberg et al.	Noisemakers	BW; dur.; F	Mat. ch.; resp.; sequence effects; state effects; stim. dif.	3–200 hrs	170	–	–	X	–	–	–	–	–
Goodman et al.	Pure tones	F; ISI; SPL	Resp.	2–10 days	50	X	–	–	–	–	–	–	–
Keen	Pure tones	Dur.; F	Stim. dif.	3–5 days	48	–	–	–	–	–	–	X	–
Leventhal and Lipsitt	Square waves	F	Stim. dif.	21–118 hrs	94	–	–	X	X	–	X	–	–
Lewis et al.	Live voice; music; pure tones	–	Stim. dif.	24 wks	32	–	X	X	–	–	–	–	–
Lipsitt and Kaye	Square wave	–	Cond.	3–4 days	20	–	–	–	–	–	–	X	–
Mukhina-Korotova	Pure tones	F	Cond.	6 mos–2 yrs	(Unspec.)	–	–	X	–	–	–	–	–
Parmalee	Noisemaker	–	Resp.	1 day–12 wks	7	–	–	X	–	–	–	–	–
Simons	Music	–	Stim. dif.	9–31 mos	24	–	–	X	–	–	–	–	–
Suzuki et al.	Pure tones	F; SPL	Resp.	5–7 days	45	–	–	X	–	–	–	–	–

Study	Stimulus	Parameters	Procedure	Age	N						Recorded cries; weight change	Phonetic analyses
Tulloch et al.	Heartbeat	—	Pac.	1–4 days	119	—	—	X	—	—	—	—
Webster	Live voice	—	Feedback effects; stim. dif.	6–9 mos	5	—	—	—	—	—	—	—
1965												
Barnet and Goodwin	Clicks	SPL	Resp.	2–5 days	18	X	—	X	—	—	—	—
Birns	Pure tones	F: SPL	Pac.; stim. dif.	2–5 days	30	—	X	X	—	—	—	—
Birns et al.	Pure tones	F	Pac.; stim. dif.	36–96 hrs	20	—	—	X	—	—	—	—
Bridger et al.	Pure tones	—	Ind. d.	2–5 days	20	X	X	X	—	—	—	—
Chase	Noisemaker	—	Hab.	36–90 hrs	20	—	X	X	X	—	—	—
Crowell et al.	Pure tones	—	Resp.	20–40 hrs	10	—	—	—	—	X	—	—
Eisenberg (a)	Band noise; pure tones; white noise	BW; dur.; F; ISI; SPL	Resp.; stim. dif.	<5 days	32	X	X	X	—	—	—	—
Frey and Relke	Noisemakers	—	Resp.	<1 hr	Unspec.	—	—	—	—	—	—	—
Kagan and Lewis	Live voice; music; pure tones	—	Mat. ch.; stim. dif.	24 wks–13 mos	32	X	X	X	—	—	—	Vocal utterance
Keen et al.	Buzz	Dur.	Hab.	42–66 hrs	40	X	X	—	—	—	—	—
Maezawa	Pure tones; "social sounds"	SPL	Stim. dif.	13–33 mos	51	—	X	X	—	—	—	—
Solomons et al.	Pure tones; square waves	—	Resp.	48–72 hrs	10	—	—	—	—	—	X	—
Takahara	Live voice; noisemakers; pure tones	SPL	Resp.; stim. dif.	6 mos–6 yrs	36	X	X	X	—	—	—	—

(continued)

SECTION II (*continued*)

Author(s)	Stimuli Employed	Parameters	Phenomena	Age Range	N	EEG	HR	Ov. Beh.	Resp. Rt.	Skin Res.	Stab.	Suck.	Other
		Information Available		Subjects		Measures Employed							
Weitzman et al.	Clicks	–	Resp.; state effects	1.5 hrs–15 days	16	X	–	–	–	–	–	–	–
				1966									
Barnet et al.	Clicks	–	Ind. d.; resp.	3 days–3.5 mos	1	X	–	X	–	–	–	–	ERG
Barnet and Lodge	Clicks; pure tones	F; SPL	Mat. ch.	1–8 mos	22	X	–	–	–	–	–	–	–
Birns et al.	Pure tones	–	Pac.	2–3 days	35	–	X	X	–	–	–	–	–
Brackbill et al.	Heartbeat; metronome; music	–	Pac.; stim. dif.	48 hrs–38 mos	65	X	X	X	X	–	X	–	–
Eisenberg et al.	Tonal sequences	–	Hab.; ind. d.	16 hrs–7 days	13	–	–	X	–	–	–	X	–
Gottlieb and Simner	Pure tones	SPL	Cond.	25–68 days	9	X	X	–	–	–	–	X	–
Kaye	Pure tones	SPL	Cond.	47–110 hrs	120	–	–	X	–	X	–	X	–
Polikanina	"Rhythmic sound"	–	Mat. ch.	<2 weeks	(Unspec.)	X	X	–	X	–	–	–	–
Schachter et al.	Pure tones	Dur.	Resp.	2–4 days	17	–	X	X	X	X	–	–	–
Steinschneider et al.	White noise	SPL	Stim. dif.	2–5 days	9	–	X	X	–	–	–	–	–
Suzuki et al.	Pure tones	SPL	Resp.	<3 mos	(Unspec.)	X	–	–	–	–	–	–	–
Toriyama et al.	Pure tones	F; SPL	Resp.	3 hrs–8 days	(Unspec.)	X	–	–	–	–	–	–	–
Turkewitz et al. (*a*)	White noise	SPL	Loc.; stim. dif.	23–72 hrs	53	–	–	–	–	–	–	–	Eye movements

Turkewitz et al. (b)	White noise	–	Loc.	40	32–70 hrs	–	–	–	–	–	–	Eye movements
Webster et al.	Self-produced vocalization	–	Feedback effects	4	7 mos	–	–	–	–	–	–	Spectro-graphic analyses
1967												
Barnet and Lodge (a)	Clicks; pure tones	F; SPL	Ind. d.; resp.	22	1–8 mos	X	–	X	X	–	–	Biochemical analyses
Barnet and Lodge (b)	Clicks	–	Resp.	70	<14 mos	–	–	X	–	–	–	ERG
Bronshtein and Petrova	Pure tones	F	Cond.	30	2 hrs–5 mos	–	–	–	–	–	X	–
Cody et al.	Pure tones	SPL	Resp.	5	2 mos–2 yrs	X	–	–	X	–	–	–
Field et al.	Band noise	SPL	Resp.	45	1–65 days	–	–	X	–	–	–	–
Fitzgerald et al.	Pure tones	–	Cond.	32	26–86 days	–	–	–	–	–	–	Pupil diameter
Groth et al.	Pure tones	F	Resp.	40	2 days	–	X	X	X	–	–	EMG
Lewis and Spaulding	Live voice; pure tones	–	Cross-modal (audiovisual) effects; stim. dif.	24	24 wks	–	X	X	X	–	–	–
Lintz et al.	Pure tones	–	Cond.	20	2–3 mos	–	–	–	–	–	–	Blink reflex
McCandless	Live voice; noisemakers; pure tones	SPL	Resp.	79	3 days–4 years	X	–	X	X	–	–	–
Polikanina and Sergeeva	"Rhythmic sound"	–	Mat. ch.	13	1–10 days	X	–	–	X	–	–	–
Rapin and Graziani	Clicks; pure tones	F; SPL	Mat. ch.	61	1 wk–3 yrs	X	–	X	–	–	–	–
Reddell and Calvert	Pure tones	F; SPL	Resp.; stim. dif.	20	15–47 mos	–	–	X	–	–	–	–
Roberts and Campbell	Heart beats; pulse tones	SPL	Puc.	50	24–48 hrs	–	X	–	X	X	–	–

(continued)

253

Author(s)	Information Available			Subjects		Measures Employed							
	Stimuli Employed	Parameters	Phenomena	Age Range	N	EEG	HR	Ov. Beh.	Resp. Rt.	Skin Res.	Stab.	Suck.	Other
Yang and Crowell	Pure tones	–	Cond.	45–56 hrs	20	–	×	–	×	–	×	–	–
				1968									
Clifton et al.	Buzz	Dur.	Resp.; sequence effects	42–65 hrs	100	–	×	–	×	–	–	–	–
Cullen et al.	Self-produced vocalization	–	DAF	24–68 hrs	16	–	–	–	–	–	–	–	Recorded utterance patterns
Friedlander	Live voice; music	Dim.	Stim. dif.	11–15 mos	3	–	–	×	–	–	–	–	Listening time
Graham et al.	Band noise	–	Hab.; mat. ch.	37–129 hrs	26	–	×	×	×	–	–	–	–
Gray and Crowell	Clicks	–	Resp.	2 days–11 wks	36	–	×	–	–	–	–	–	–
Graziani et al.	Clicks	–	Resp.	<1 mo	31	×	–	×	–	–	–	–	–
Hutt et al. (a)	Live voice; pure tones; square waves	Dim.	Hab.; stim. dif.	4–8 days	10	×	×	×	×	–	–	–	EMG; ERG
Hutt et al. (b)	Live voice; pure tone; square waves	Dim.; F	Stim. dif.	3–8 days	12	×	×	×	×	–	–	–	EMG; ERG
Korner	Noisemaker	–	State effects	45–88 hrs	32	–	–	×	–	–	–	–	–
Lumio and Laukola	Pure tones	F; SPL	Resp.	3–7 days	158	–	–	×	–	–	–	–	–
Matkin et al.	Pure tones	F; SPL	Resp.	11 mos–5 yrs	100	–	–	×	–	–	–	–	Audiometric testing

Author	Stimulus	Measure	Variable	Age	N									Notes
Mendel	Band noise; noisemakers; pure tones; white noise	BW	Stim. dif.	4–11 mos	30	—	—	—	×	—	—	—	—	—
Moncur	Live voice; music; pure tones	SPL	Observer reliability	30–34 wks	8	—	—	—	×	—	—	—	—	—
O'Doherty	Live voice	—	Pac.	Unspec.	Unspec.	—	—	×	×	—	—	—	—	—
Semb and Lipsitt	Square waves	F	Stim. dif.	37–117 hrs	30	—	—	×	—	×	×	—	×	—
Steinschneider	White noise	SPL	Stim. dif.	2–5 days	9	—	×	×	×	—	×	—	—	—
Suzuki and Taguchi	Clicks	SPL	Mat. ch.; resp.	16 days–5 yrs	55	×	—	—	×	—	—	—	—	—
Todd and Palmer	Live voice	—	Social reinforcement	75–100 days	16	—	—	—	—	—	—	—	—	Recorded vocalizations
Veit and Bizaguet	Band noise; white noise	Dur.; F; SPL	Stim. dif.	<8 days	Unspec.	—	—	×	×	—	—	—	—	—
Wietzman and Graziani	Clicks	—	Mat. ch.	Prematures	25	×	—	—	—	—	—	—	—	—
Yeni-Komshian et al.	Self-produced vocalization	—	DAF	21–59 mos	15	—	—	—	—	—	—	—	—	Phonation time
1969														
Akiyama et al.	Clicks	SPL	Resp.	<1 wk	17	×	—	—	—	—	—	—	—	—
Bench (*a*)	Pure tones	F; SPL	Hab.; state effects; stim. dif.	2–6 days	93	—	×	×	×	×	×	—	—	—
Bench (*b*)	Band noise; pure tones	F	Pac.	2–6 days	50	×	×	×	×	—	—	—	—	—
Clifton and Meyers	Buzz	—	Mat. ch.	4 mos	14	—	×	×	×	—	—	—	—	—

(continued)

SECTION II (*continued*)

Author(s)	Stimuli Employed	Information Available		Subjects		Measures Employed							
		Parameters	Phenomena	Age Range	N	EEG	HR	Ov. Beh.	Resp. Rt.	Skin Res.	Stab.	Suck.	Other
Connolly and Stratton	White noise	—	Cond.	50–90 hrs	12	—	—	X	X	—	—	—	—
Davis and Onishi	Pure tones	—	Mat. ch.	<1 yr	Unspec.	X	—	—	—	—	—	—	—
Downs and Hemenway	Band noise	—	Resp.	Newborns (unspec.)	17,000	—	—	X	—	—	—	—	—
Engel and Young	Pure tones	F; SPL	Resp.	3 days	138	X	—	—	—	—	—	—	—
Hoversten and Moncur	Live voice; music; pure tones; white noise	Dim.; F; SPL	Mat. ch.; stim. dif.	3–8 mos	43	—	—	X	X	—	—	—	—
Lenard et al.	Band noise; pure tones; square waves	Dim.; F	Stim. dif.	4–8 days	14	X	X	—	—	—	—	—	—
Lidén and Kankkunen	Pure tones	F; SPL	Resp.	3 mos–6 yrs	120	—	—	X	—	—	—	—	—
Ornitz et al.	Pure tones	—	Mat. ch.; state effects	6–12 mos	12	X	—	—	—	—	—	—	—
Papousek	Noisemakers	F	Cond.	<6 mos	Unspec.	—	—	X	—	—	—	—	—
Reddell and Calvert	Band noise; pure tones	F; SPL	Ind. d.; resp.	<1 wk	3,200	—	—	X	X	—	—	—	—
Routh	Live voice	—	Cond.; stim. dif.	2–7 mos	30	—	—	X	—	—	—	—	—
Simner and Reilly	Infant cries (recorded)	—	Feedback effects	2–5 days	75	—	X	X	X	—	X	—	—
Suzuki and Origuchi	Pure tones	F; SPL	Mat. ch.	4 mos–5 yrs	180	X	—	X	—	—	—	—	—
Taguchi et al.	Pure tones	F; SPL	Resp.	6 hrs–12 days	250	X	—	—	—	—	—	—	—
Webster	Live voice	—	Cond.; stim. dif.	6 mos	4	—	—	—	—	—	—	—	Phonetic analyses

Author(s)	Stimuli Employed	Parameters	Phenomena	Age Range	N	EEG	HR	Ov. Beh.	Resp. Rt.	Skin Res.	Stab.	Suck.	Other
		Information Available		Subjects		Measures Employed							
				1970									
Ando and Hattori	Aircraft noise	—	Stress effects	<1 yr	188	—	—	—	—	—	—	—	Maternal report (questionaire)
Bench	Band noise	—	LIV	3–5 days	12	—	X	X	—	—	—	—	—
Brackbill	Clicks; white noise	—	Pac.; stim. dif.	1 mo	18	X	X	X	X	—	X	—	—
Friedlander and Whitten	Live voice; music	F; SPL	Resp.; stim. dif.	18 mos	1	—	—	—	—	—	—	—	Listening time
Graham et al.	Pure tones	Dur.; R+D t.; SPL	Mat. ch.	30 hrs–16 wks	60	—	X	X	—	—	—	—	—
Hutt and Hutt	Square waves	F	LIV	3–7 days	6	X	X	X	X	—	—	—	EMG
Kaplan	Live voice	Intonation contours	Hab.; stim. dif.	4–8 mos	40	.	—	X	—	—	—	—	—
Kopp	Live voice; noisemakers; white noise	—	Pac.; stim. dif.	1–3 mos	10	—	—	X	—	—	—	—	—
League and Bzoch	Live voice	—	Affect	1–15 mos	16	—	—	X	—	—	—	—	—
Lesak	Band noise; live voice; music; white noise	F; SPL	Resp.	4 mos–12 yrs	62	—	—	X	—	—	—	—	—
Ling et al.	Pure tones	—	Observer bias	Newborns (unspec.)	144	—	—	X	—	—	—	—	—

(continued)

257

SECTION III (continued)

Author(s)	Information Available			Subjects		Measures Employed								
	Stimuli Employed	Parameters	Phenomena	Age Range	N	EEG	HR	Ov. Beh.	Resp. Rt.	Skin Res.	Stab.	Suck.	Other
McCall and Melson	Tonal sequences	–	Hab.	5.5 mos	27	–	X	–	–	–	–	–	–
Miller and Rabinowitz	Pure tones	F; SPL	Resp.	2–3 yrs	183	–	–	X	–	–	–	–	–
Moreau et al.	White noise	–	Cross-modal (auditory somasthetic) effects; hab.	24–71 hrs	35	–	X	X	–	–	–	–	Eye movements
Motta et al.	Pure tones	F; SPL	Resp.	1–4 yrs	130	–	–	X	–	–	–	–	–
Rapin et al.	Pure tones	F; SPL	Mat. ch.; resp.	1–12 mos	27	X	–	–	–	–	–	–	–
Rosenblith	Noisemakers	SPL	Predictive value of neonatal screening	5 days–4 yrs	802	–	–	X	–	–	–	–	Psychological testing
Sameroff	Pure tones	Duty cycle; SPL	Hab.	16–54 hrs	12	–	–	–	X	–	–	X	–
Schulman (a)	Buzzer	–	Hab.; ind. d.	Prematures	15	–	X	X	–	–	–	–	–
Schulman (b)	Buzzer	–	Mat. ch.	Prematures	35	–	X	X	X	–	–	–	–
Schulman and Kreiter	Band noise; pure tones; white noise	BW; F; SPL	Resp.; stim. dif.	2 days	35	–	X	–	–	–	–	–	–
Schulman and Wade	Band noise	SPL	Mat. ch.	6 wks–9 mos	30	–	X	–	–	–	–	–	–
Schulman et al.	Band noise; pure tones	SPL	Mat. ch.	3 wks–8 yrs	24	X	X	X	–	–	–	–	–
Simner	Infant cries	–	Feedback effects	2–5 days	120	–	X	X	–	–	–	–	–
Stratton	Band noise	F; SPL	Hab.	3–5 days	24	–	X	–	X	–	X	–	–
Taguchi et al.	Pure tones	SPL	Resp.	<5 yrs	98	X	–	–	–	–	–	–	–

1971

Study		Stimulus	Method	Age	N							
Altman and Shenhav	—	Noisemakers	Mat. ch.; resp.	7–10 mos	10,000	—	—	X	—	—	—	—
Aronson and Rosenbloom	—	Live voice	Cross-modal (audiovisual) effects	30–55 days	8	—	—	X	—	—	—	—
Ashton (b)	F	Square waves	Resp.; state effects	3–5 days	17	X	—	X	—	—	—	—
Barnet	SPL	Clicks; pure tones	Mat. ch.	<3 yrs	241	X	—	—	—	—	—	—
Barnet et al.	—	Clicks	Mat. ch.; hab.; ind. d.	8 days–13 mos	98	X	—	X	—	—	—	—
Bench and Parker	—	Noise bands	Ind. d.; resp.	1–3 wks	40	—	—	X	—	—	—	—
Berg et al.	Rise time; SPL	Pure tone	Mat. ch.; state effects; stim. dif.	109–119 days	24	—	X	X	—	—	—	—
Brackbill (a)	SPL	White noise	Hab.; ind. d.	3–5 mos	1	—	—	X	—	—	—	—
Brackbill (b)	—	Heartbeat	Pac.	1 mo	24	—	X	X	X	—	—	—
Campos and Brackbill	—	White noise	Hab.; state effects	1–4 wks	39	—	X	X	—	—	—	—
Clifton	—	Square wave	Cond.	27–103 hrs	14	X	—	—	—	—	X	—
Eimas et al.	Form. str.	Synthetic speech	Stim. dif.	1–4 mos	52	—	X	—	—	—	X	—
Engel and Milstein	—	Clicks	Resp.; state effects	1–3 days	7	X	—	—	—	—	—	—
Jackson et al.	Rise time; SPL	Pure tones	Stim. dif.	30–62 hrs	48	—	X	—	—	—	—	—
Lamper and Eisdorfer	SPL	Pure tones	Resp.; state effects	8–72 hrs	40	—	—	X	—	—	—	—
Lewis	—	Music	Hab.; mat. ch.	12–52 wks	62	X	—	—	—	—	—	—
Lentz and McCandless	F; SPL	Live voice; noisemakers; pure tones	Ind. d.; mat. ch.	1–12 mos	13	X	—	X	—	—	—	—

(continued)

259

Author(s)	Stimuli Employed	Parameters	Phenomena	Age Range	N	EEG	HR	Ov. Beh.	Resp. Rt.	Skin Res.	Stab.	Suck.	Other
		Information Available		Subjects		Measures Employed							
Ling et al.	Band noise	F	Resp.	24 hrs–24 days	400	–	–	×	–	–	–	–	–
McCaffrey	Live voice	–	Stim. dif.	11–28 wks	20	–	×	×	–	–	–	–	–
Moffitt	Synthetic speech	Form. str.	Hab.; stim. dif.	20–24 wks	37	–	×	–	–	–	–	–	–
Monod and Garma	Clicks	–	Mat. ch.	Prematures	10	×	×	×	×	–	–	–	EMG
Prather et al.	Live voice	–	Stim. dif.	27–38 mos	42	–	–	×	–	–	–	–	–
Robson	Live voice; noisemakers; pure tones	BW; F; SPL	Resp.; stim. dif.	9 mos	378	–	–	×	–	–	–	–	–
Schachter et al.	Clicks	–	OR	2–3 days	6	×	×	×	–	–	–	–	EMG; ERG
Simner	Infant cries	–	Feedback effects	2–5 days	75	–	×	×	×	–	×	–	–
Turnure	Live voice	–	Mat. ch.; stim. dif.	3–9 mos	11	–	–	×	–	–	–	–	Filmed movement
Wisdom and Friedlander	Music; live voice	Dim.	Stim. dif.	9–18 mos	16	–	–	–	–	–	–	–	Listening time
Wormith	Pure tones	F; SPL	Stim. dif.	16–60 days	40	–	–	–	–	–	–	×	–
1972													
Arnold and Porges	Pure tones	–	Hab.; mat. ch.	24–48 hrs	32	–	×	–	–	–	–	–	–
Bench et al.	Noisemakers	–	Stim. dif.	1–5 days	12	–	–	×	–	–	–	–	–
Berg	Tonal patterns	Duty cycle; F	Hab.; stim. dif.	15–17 wks	32	–	×	×	–	–	–	–	–
Bergman and Schultz	Synthetic speech	Form. str.	Stim. dif.	4.5–19.5 wks	8	–	–	×	–	–	–	×	–
Butterfield and Siperstein	Band noise; music	–	Stim. dif.	20–47 hrs	60	–	–	–	–	–	–	×	–

Study	Stimuli			Age	N									
Fior	Band noise; live voice; pure tones	Dim.; SPL	Mat. ch.	3–13 yrs	70	—	—	—	—	—	—	—	—	Audiometric testing
Haugan and McIntire	Live voice	—	Vocal reinforcement effects	3–6 mos	24	—	X	—	—	—	—	—	—	Vocalization time
Horowitz	Tonal sequence	—	Hab.	6 mos	32	—	X	—	—	—	—	—	—	—
Khachaturian et al.	Clicks	—	Resp.	2 days	1	—	—	—	—	—	—	—	—	—
Ling (a)	Pure tones	Dur.; F	Resp.	1–7 days	120	—	—	X	—	—	—	—	—	—
Ling (b)	Band noise	Dur.; F; rep. r.	Resp.	1–14 days	160	—	—	X	—	—	—	—	—	—
Molfese	Live voice; noisemakers	Dim.	Hemispheric asymmetry; mat. ch.; stim. dif.	7 days–10 mos	10	X	—	—	—	—	—	—	—	—
Morse	Synthetic speech	Form. str.	Stim. dif.	40–54 days	25	—	—	—	—	X	—	—	—	—
Ohlrich and Barnet	Clicks	—	Mat. ch.	24 hrs–12 mos	45	X	—	—	—	—	—	—	—	—
Ricciuti and Poresky	Buzzer	—	Affect	3–12 mos	32	—	—	X	—	—	—	—	—	—
Segall	Live voice; white noise	—	Ind. d.; state effects; stim. dif.	Prematures	60	—	X	X	—	—	—	—	—	—
Sohmer et al.	Clicks	SPL	Resp.	4–31 mos	31	X	—	X	—	—	—	—	—	—
Taylor and Mencher	Band noise	BW	Resp.; state effects	2–124 hrs	225	—	—	X	—	—	—	—	—	—
Trehub and Rabinovitch	Live voice; synthetic speech	Form. str.	Stim. dif.	4–17 wks	60	—	—	—	—	X	—	—	—	—
Turkewitz et al. (a)	Pure tones white noise	BW; F; SPL	Resp.; stim. dif.	24–72 hrs	45	—	X	X	—	—	—	—	—	Eye movements
Turkewitz et al. (b)	Pure tones; tonal sequences	Dim.; dur.	Resp.; stim. dif.	24–72 hrs	45	X	X	X	—	—	—	—	—	Eye movements

(continued)

261

Author(s)	Stimuli Employed	Information Available		Subjects		Measures Employed							
		Parameters	Phenomena	Age Range	N	EEG	HR	Ov. Beh.	Resp. Rt.	Skin Res.	Stab.	Suck.	Other
Walden	Baby cries	–	Resp.	4 wks–2 yrs	124	–	–	×	–	–	–	–	–
Weber	Pure tone; square wave; synthetic speech	BW; F; dim.	Hab.; stim. dif.	14–18 wks	12	×	–	–	–	–	–	–	–
Webster et al.	Live voice; pure tones	F	Stim. dif.	7 mos	12	–	–	×	–	–	–	–	Spectrographic analyses
1973													
Anderson	Band noise; synthetic speech	Dim.	Hab.; stim. dif.	14–18 wks	16	×	–	×	–	–	–	–	–
Ashton	Square waves	SPL	Resp.; state effects	3 days	35	–	×	×	–	–	–	–	–
Cody and Townsend	Pure tones	–	Ind. d.; mat. ch.	2 mos–5 yrs	38	×	–	–	–	–	–	–	–
Dorman and Hoffman	Synthetic speech	–	Hab.	10–14 wks	6	×	–	–	–	–	–	–	–
Eisenberg et al.	Synthetic speech	–	Mat. ch.; resp.; state effects	13 hrs–27 yrs	60	×	×	×	–	–	–	–	–
Fargo et al.	Self-produced vocalization	–	DAF	6–9 mos	28	–	–	–	–	–	–	–	Spectrographic analyses
Godovikova	Live noise; music; noisemakers	–	Stim. dif.	<1 yr	15	–	–	×	–	–	–	–	–
Goldstein et al.	Clicks	Rep. r.	Resp.	12–18 hrs	10	×	–	–	–	–	–	–	–
Kearsley	Band noise; pure tones	F; R+D t.; SPL	Cross-modal (audiovisual) effects	12–84 hrs	48	–	×	×	–	–	–	–	–
Keith	Pure tones	SPL	Middle ear compliance	36–51 hrs	40	–	–	–	–	–	–	–	Tympanograms

Study	Stimuli	Parameters	Confounds/effects	Age	N							
Langford and Bench	Pure tones	–	Observer bias	Newborns (unspec.)	2	–	–	–	–	–	–	–
McRandle and Smith	Clicks	–	Resp.	12–18 hrs	32	X	–	–	–	–	–	–
Moffitt	Pure tones	SPL	Stim. dif.	20–24 wks	28	–	X	X	–	–	–	–
Pomerleau-Malcuit and Clifton	Square waves	–	Cross-modal (audiotactile) effects; state effects	38–88 hrs	65	–	X	X	–	–	–	–
Porges et al.	Pure tone	ISI	On and off effects	24–72 hrs	24	–	X	–	X	–	–	–
Rewey	Pure tones	Dim.; dur.	Mat. ch.; state effects	6–12 wks	29	–	X	X	X	–	–	–
Roberts and Watson	Live voice; noisemakers; pure tones	SPL	Resp.	7–8 mos	20	X	–	X	X	–	–	–
Schulman	Band noise; pure tones; white noise	BW; F; rep. r.; SPL	Ind. d.; resp.; state effects	24–110 hrs	185	–	X	X	X	–	–	–
Shriner et al.	Pure tones; synthetic speech	Dim.	Ind. d.; resp.; state effects	6–14 wks	3	–	–	–	–	–	X	–
Stratton and Connolly	Band noise; pure tones	Dur.; F; SPL	Sequence effects	3–5 days	21	–	X	X	X	X	–	–
Suzuki	Clicks	–	Sedation effects	<4 yrs	355	X	–	'	X	–	–	–
Trehub (a)	Live voice; pure tones; square waves; synthetic speech	Dim.; form. str.; F; syllable length	Stim. dif.	4–17 wks	306	–	X	X	–	–	X	–
Trehub (b)	Live voice; pure tones; square waves	Dim.; F	Stim. dif.	4–17 wks	182	–	–	–	–	–	X	–

(continued)

Author(s)	Stimuli Employed	Parameters	Phenomena	Age Range	N	EEG	IIR	Ov. Beh.	Resp. Rt.	Skin Res.	Stab.	Suck.	Other
		Information Available		Subjects		Measures Employed							
				1974									
Barnet et al.	Clicks; live voice	Dim.	Hemispheric asymmetry; ind. d.	5–12 mos	14	X	–	X	–	–	–	–	–
Barrager	Live voice; synthetic speech	SPL	Resp.; stim. dif.	4–12 wks	48	–	X	X	–	–	–	–	–
Berkson et al.	Noisemaker	–	Ind. d.; mat. ch.	Prematures	20	–	X	–	–	–	–	–	–
Clifton (*b*)	Square wave	–	Cond.	27–103 hrs	21	–	X	–	–	–	–	X	–
Cohen	Live voice	–	Cross-modal (audiovisual) relations	5–8 mos	48	–	–	X	–	–	–	–	–
Collyer et al.	Band noise	Dur.	Observer reliability	2–8 days	10	–	–	X	–	–	–	–	–
Condon and Sander	Live voice	–	Sensorimotor synchrony	Newborns (unspec.)	11	–	–	X	–	–	–	–	–
Eisele and Berry	Pure tones	F; SPL	Resp.	52 hrs	100	–	–	–	–	–	–	X	–
Eisenberg et al. (*a*)	Synthetic speech	–	Mat. ch.; resp.; state effects	13 hrs–3 mos	8	–	X	X	–	–	–	–	–
Eisenberg et al. (*b*)	Synthetic speech	–	Ind. d.	7 days–27 yrs	4	–	X	X	–	–	–	–	–
Eisenberg et al. (*c*)	Synthetic speech	–	Mat. ch.; resp.; state effects	13 hrs–27 yrs	29	X	X	X	–	–	–	–	–
Ellingson et al.	Pure tones	–	State effects	2–5 days	6	X	–	X	X	–	–	–	EMG; EOG
Harker and Van Wagoner	Pure tones	–	Middle ear impedance	<2 yrs	35	–	–	–	–	–	–	–	Tympano-grams
Hecox and Galambos	Clicks	SPL	Mat. ch.; resp.	3 wks–3 yrs	35	X	–	–	–	–	–	–	–

	Stimulus	Parameter	Measure	Age	N							Acoustic reflex
Jerger et al.	Pure tones	—	Middle ear impedance	3–71 mos	398	—	—	—	—	—	—	—
McGurk and Lewis	Live voice	—	Cross-modal (audiovisual) relations	1–7 mos	35	—	—	X	—	—	—	—
Meyer and Wolfe	Band noise	—	Resp.	Newborns (unspec.)	450	—	—	X	—	—	—	—
Mills and Melhuish	Live voice	—	Stim. dif.	20–30 days	48	—	—	—	—	—	X	—
Morse	Synthetic speech	Form. str.	Ind. d.; stim. dif.	8 weeks	60	—	—	—	—	—	X	—
Porges	Pure tones	ISI	Cond.; ind. d.; mat. ch.; on and off effects	24–75 hrs	44	—	X	—	—	—	—	—
Russ and Simmons	Clicks; pure tones	SPL	Resp.	1–5 days	40	X	—	—	↓	—	—	—
Shallop	Pure tones	—	Loc.	6 mos	1	—	—	X	—	—	—	—
Shapiro	Band noise	—	Resp.	<1 wk	4,141	—	—	X	—	—	—	—
Simmons and Russ	Band noise; pure tones	—	Resp.	<5 days	6,000	—	—	—	—	X	—	—
Swigart	Live voice; noisemakers; pure tones; white noise	F; SPL	Loc.; resp.	2.5–3.5 yrs	232	—	—	X	—	—	—	Audio-metric testing
Thompson and Weber	Band noise; live voice	SPL	Mat. ch.; resp.	3–59 mos	190	—	—	X	—	—	—	—
1975												
Eilers and Minifie	Live voice	Form. str.	Hab.; stim. dif.	4–17 wks	84	—	—	X	—	—	X	—
Eisele et al.	Pure tones	F; SPL	Resp.	24–108 hrs	105	—	—	X	—	—	X	—
Mencher et al.	Band noise; warble tone; white noise	BW; rep. r.	"Sensitization;" state effects	<5 days	450	—	—	X	—	—	—	—

(continued)

SECTION III (continued)

Author(s)	Information Available				Subjects		Measures Employed							
	Stimuli Employed	Parameters	Phenomena		Age Range	N	EEG	HR	Ov. Beh.	Resp. Rt.	Skin Res.	Stab.	Suck.	Other
Moore et al.	Noise bands	–	Reinforcement methods; resp.		12–18 mos	48	–	–	×	–	–	–	–	–
Palmqvist	Heartbeat	Rep. r.	–		<6 days	175	–	–	–	–	–	–	–	Weight change
Wormith et al.	Pure tones	F	Stim. dif.		16–60 days	40	–	–	–	–	–	–	×	–

SECTION IV. Reports in Press as of 1975

Author(s)	Information Available				Subjects		Measures Employed							
	Stimuli Employed	Parameters	Phenomena		Age Range	N	EEG	HR	Ov. Beh.	Resp. Rt.	Skin Res.	Stab.	Suck.	Other
Barnet et al.	Clicks	–	Mat. ch.		10 days–37 mos	140	×	–	×	–	–	–	–	–
Berg	Pure tones	Rep. r.	Hab.; mat. ch.		5.5–17 wks	50	–	×	×	–	–	–	–	–
Keith	Pure tones	SPL	Middle ear compliance		2.5–20 hrs	20	–	–	–	–	–	–	–	Tympanogram
Stamps and Porges	Pure tones	ISI	Cond.		40–75 hrs	47	–	–	–	–	–	×	×	–
Weir	Pure tones; square waves	Dim.; I	Stim. dif.		3–8 days	6	–	–	–	–	–	–	–	EMG

APPENDIX C:
Some Helpful Hints on Tools, Techniques, and Instrumentation for Developmental Studies in Audition

SECTION I. MATERIAL RELEVANT TO BEHAVIORAL OBSERVATION AND THE TREATMENT OF STRIP CHART DATA   *Rita B. Eisenberg*

Judgments of Behavioral State

Laboratory criteria for judgments of behavioral state during newborn life and early infancy are shown in Table I.1. They are criteria commonly used by investigators of infant performance. However, since "state" refers to a constellation of behavioral and electrophysiologic events that may vary among individual babies and within given babies over time, it must be recognized that rigid adherence to some complex of specified criteria is unrealistic. Not all of the events listed in the table will be or need to be present simultaneously, and the ability to judge behavioral state with a high degree of consistency and reliability (as measured by agreement among independent observers) depends heavily upon experience with an infant population. There is no substitute for such experience, and the criteria shown in the table merely serve to provide clues which, in the context of experience, may permit reasonable judgments.

Table I.1. Criteria for Judgments of Behavioral State During Early Infancy[a]

State	Index				
	Bodily Activity	Visual Activity	Respiration	Other Remarks	Electrophysiologic Concommitants
I. Deep Sleep	Little except for spontaneous startles at 2–3 min intervals	Eyes closed; no signs of either slow or rapid eye movements beneath lids	Deep; regular (about 30–40/min)	Low muscle tonus	HR relatively slow (in the neighborhood of 100 bpm) and regular, with abrupt jumps during startle intervals. Tracé alternant pattern in EEG
II. Light or Irregular Sleep	Some movements, including writhing, but few spontaneous startles; small twitches of extremities, but little limb displacement	Eyes mostly closed, but occasional fluttering of lids and bursts of rapid eye movements beneath them	Periods of rapid shallow breathing alternating with slow deep excursions	Occasional sighs or "friction" sounds; periods of spontaneous sucking; skin may appear mottled	Increased wave amplitude (as compared with I) in EEG, with irregular slow voltage pattern
III. Doze	Considerable movement and intermittent spontaneous startles (6–8 min intervals)	Intermittent opening and closing of eyes, with "glassy" look; occasional blinking	Fairly regular	Occasional vocalizations; periods of spontaneous sucking and grimacing	Sporadic theta-like (5–6 Hz) activity in EEG, primarily at central and parietal sites

268

IV. Awake-Quiet	Considerable movement of head and extremities	Eyes open and fairly bright	Mostly regular but not consistently so	Face relaxed	Relatively nonrhythmic low voltage EEG activity with some rhythmic activity in the delta (2–4 Hz) range at central sites
V. Awake-Alert	Little motor activity	Eyes wide open and shiny-looking; visual scanning of environment	Occasional "breath holding"	Seldom observed in the absence of "focus" stimulation	EEG "flattening" during focus episodes
VI. Awake-Active	Much movement, including gross body activity	Eyes open and moving	Irregular	Intermittent whimpering and related utterance	Motor overlay in EEG pattern
VII. Awake-Excited	Much mass movement	Concomitant with facial and vocal activity	Irregular	Loud and prolonged crying; tonic muscle activity	Very rapid HRs, sometimes in the range above 200 bpm; EEG pattern literally obliterated by motor activity

[a] In early laboratory work (see Figure 1 in text), where a four-point activity state continuum was employed, states I and II were subsumed under I; state III was scored as II; states IV and V were subsumed under III; and states VI and VII were scored as IV.

On-the-Spot Notation of Behavioral Events

As discussed in Chapter 2, three general kinds of stimulus-bound activity (motor, visual, and RAS-dependent responses) can be related to the communicative process. This activity can be broken down into a number of subsets, depending upon investigator interests. When on-the-spot observers are very highly trained over prolonged periods of time, as in the Bioacoustic Laboratory situation, the number of subsets can become very large and notation of response events, according to some strictly defined coding system, becomes increasingly difficult. Thus, over the years, procedures have evolved whereby individual observers score experimental events in any hieroglyphics of their choice and code them into standardized form for computer processing after study sessions have been concluded. Although such procedures appreciably increase the amount of paper work, they also serve to increase the amount of observational data available for analysis.

Table I.2 shows the standardized work sheet on which behavioral observations are noted. As can be seen, it includes identifying information that permits correlation with other findings, ancillary data whereby procedural factors can be considered, pre- and post-test times and ratings from which various kinds of information can be extrapolated, and trial-by-trial columns for the recording of observed events. In essence, then, the work sheet constitutes a sort of log which details the nurse-observer's activities during the entire period between a subject's arrival at and departure from the laboratory.

As can be seen from the arrangement of the *observations* columns, provision is made for noting any artifacts that may invalidate individual trials. Each signal presentation is accompanied not only by response descriptors, but also by a pre-trial state rating and, where possible, a post-trial respiration count as well.

To assure that all scoring tasks have been considered, no columns are left blank in on-the-spot scoring. Behavioral state is indicated according to the number scale shown in Table I.1. The absence of response is designated either by an "NR" or "9→" notation in the first *observations* column, and, similarly, the absence of artifact is shown by an "N.A." or "9→" notation in the second *observations* column. Where respiration rate data are obtained, the two-digit count is given; where they are not, the appropriate column is scored as zero.

To guard against faulty recollection or other sources of error in transforming the raw work sheet data into standardized form, the observer routinely codes the behavioral findings onto a *comment card* work sheet (Table I.3) immediately after a subject's departure from the laboratory.

Furthermore, where time and circumstances permit, the coded observations are checked and proofread with another member of the staff.

Treatment of Electrophysiologic Strip Chart Data

Inasmuch as both EEG and HR data derived from strip chart recordings can be analyzed at leisure, standardized work sheets for notation of these observations are not required. However, in preliminary work with these measures—where we were concerned with the incidence of single trial responses and their variability over time—we have had recourse to forms similar to that shown in Table I.2.

Data extracted from the EEG strip chart tracings for purposes of analysis, coded directly onto the comment card (Table I.3), are the following: (1) real time, as indicated by the IRIG B time code channel on each record; (2) state ratings, as indicated by wave forms during the 10-sec period immediately preceding stimulus onset; (3) the nature of wave form events considered to be responses; and (4) artifacts that may invalidate individual trials. The only important information for purposes of correlating study findings is that obtained from the time code channel. It provides a mechanism whereby behavioral response events can be related to stimulus onset and to other indicators of auditory processing.

Data extracted from the HR strip chart tracings for purposes of analysis other than preliminary eyeballing have had to do solely with artifacts, that is, with delineating time periods that should be ruled out during computer analysis.

Comment Card Work Sheets and Number Codes
for Recording Behavioral and EEG Strip Chart Observations

The standardized work sheet for coding behavioral and EEG observations on auditory behavior is shown as Table I.3, and instructions for its use are provided in Tables I.4 and I.5. Each of the numbered lines on the work sheet form refers to a single IBM card (80 x 9), and the entire series of comment card entries encompasses a period of real time beginning 5 to 10 min before the first sound presentation and ending 5 to 10 min after the final sound presentation (as indicated by the pre- and post-stimulus entries on the form labeled Table I.2). Ancillary information noted below the double line marking off the last comment card entry on each work sheet relates to the quality of correlative HR data, as determined from visual inspection of strip chart records. These data, as noted earlier, only relate to specialized computer treatments discussed in Chapter 5.

Number codes now used for recording the EEG and behavioral obser-vations on the work sheet form are presented as Table I.6 (stimulus-bound events) and Table I.7 (non-stimulus events and artifactual behavior).

The system outlined here has been found to work very well for studies of the kind considered in this book. Keypunchers at outside facilities seem to have no difficulty with it. In addition, the number code system developed, which permits efficient computer treatment of on-the-spot behavioral observations, appreciably reduces the time required for analysis of study findings.

Table I.2. Form for Nurse-Observer's Test Chamber Work Sheet

SUBJECT _____ M F   Tape No. _____   Date of Test _____
            (last name, inits) (circle 1)

PRESTIMULUS INFORMATION: Resp. Rate _____   Basal State _____
  (T_0−5−10 min)
                                  Room Temp. _____   Prep. Time _____

Other _____
      (observed physical anomalies, incidental information, etc.)

EXPERIMENTAL INFORMATION FOR CODING

	OBSERVATIONS						OBSERVATIONS			
T	State			Resp.		T	State			Resp.
No	(Pre)	Response	Artifact	(Post)		No	(Pre)	Response	Artifact	(Post)
1	___	___	___	___		16	___	___	___	___
2	___	___	___	___		17	___	___	___	___
3	___	___	___	___		18	___	___	___	___
4	___	___	___	___		19	___	___	___	___
5	___	___	___	___		20	___	___	___	___
6	___	___	___	___		21	___	___	___	___
7	___	___	___	___		22	___	___	___	___
8	___	___	___	___		23	___	___	___	___
9	___	___	___	___		24	___	___	___	___
10	___	___	___	___		25	___	___	___	___
11	___	___	___	___		26	___	___	___	___
12	___	___	___	___		27	___	___	___	___
13	___	___	___	___		28	___	___	___	___
14	___	___	___	___		29	___	___	___	___
15	___	___	___	___		30	___	___	___	___

POST-STIMULUS INFORMATION: Resp. Rate _____   Post Experimen-
  (T_{30} + _____ min)   Room Temp. _____   tal State _____
      (note to nearest min.)
1. Arrived Test Chamber with Parent _____   5. Finished Prep. _____
2. Began Feeding: a. Time _____   6. Began Recorded Basal Run _____
                  b. Formula & amt. _____   7. End of Test Tape _____
3. Finished Feeding _____   8. Left Lab. _____
4. Began Prep.

Table I.3. Comment Card Information Work Sheet (for Transfer to Keypuncher)

PUNCH COLS:→(1-8)	10 11	13	15	18 (20-38)	41 (43-61)	64 65	(68-79)
INDEX: TIME		STATE		STIMULUS-BOUND EVENTS			
CD No : HR:MI:SE	TR NO	EEG ( )	BEH ( )	EEG RECORDING ( ) NO:KIND(S) & SEQ.	BEHAVIORAL OBS ( ) NO:KIND(S) & SEQ.	RESP RATE	NON-STIM AND ART EVENTS
1							
2							
3							
4							
5							
6							
7							
8							
9							
10							
11							
12							
13							
14							
15							
16							
17							
18							

19
20
21
22
23
24
25
26
27
28
29
30
31
32
33
34
35
36
37
38
39
40

Summary: Sanborn Rating:
(for lab staff only)

Pre-Stim. ___
Post-Stim. ___

G ___

G ___   NG ___
G ___   NG ___

NG ___   ? ___
NG ___   ? ___

(trials classified as NG and ? must be listed by No)

Trials.
NO. S →

Table I.4. Comment Card Format Relative to Table I.3 Work Sheet Form

Index	Type of Information Coded	Column Assignments		Code for No Stimulus or No Information Obtained	Blank Spaces
		Sub-column(s)	Range		
Time	hr, min, sec		1–8	–	9
Trial No.	01–99		10–11	00	12
State[a]					
EEG	1, 3, or 5		13	9	14
Behavior	1–7		15	9	16 + 17
EEG Events[a]					
No.	1–8		18	9	19
Kind	4-no. code (class; subclass; specifier; modifier)		(20–38)	9	
Event 1		20–23		9	24
2		25–28		9	29
3		30–33		9	34
4		35–38		9	39 + 40

			41 (43–61)	9	
Behavioral Events[a]					
No.					
Kind	1–8	4-no. code (as shown for EEG events, above)		9	
Event 1		43–46			47
2		48–51			52
3		53–56			57
4		58–61			62 + 63
Respiration Rate	2 numbers (as measured)		64–65	00	66–67
Nonstimulus and Artifactual Events[a]	2-no. codes (01–99)		68–79	00	

[a]See specific instructions in Tables I.5, I.6, and I.7.

Table I.5. Instructions for Using Comment Card Work Sheet, Table I.3 (Based on 80 Entry Spaces Containing 9 Bins Each)

A. Time (Columns 1–8)
   All events coded on the comment card must be associated with a time of occurrence (hr, min, sec): these can be determined exactly from the IRIG-B code of the EEG strip chart

B. Trial No. (Columns 10–11)
   If an observation is not associated with a trial, as with artifacts or pre- and post-trial events, columns 10–11 should be coded as 00. If an observation is associated with a trial, specify in two digits as 01, 02, and so on.

C. State (Column 13 for EEG and Column 15 for Behavior)

EEG (13)[a]	Code No.	Behavior (15)
Sleep, undifferentiated	1	Deep sleep
	2	Irregular sleep
Doze	3	Doze
	4	Awake and quiet
Awake, undifferentiated	5	Awake and alert
	6	Awake and hyperactive or irritable
	7	Awake and screaming

D. Stimulus-Bound Events
   1. No. of events (column 18 for EEG and column 41 for behavior)
      a. The number of events observed is coded in exactly the same way for both measures.
      b. For coding purposes, *number* refers not only to the count of events observed but also to *their time relations with each other*, as shown on the next page and a half

(continued)

Table I.5 (*continued*)

Code No.	Events and Examples
1	1 event only, e.g. TNR
2	2 events that occurred simultaneously, e.g., Moro + TNR
3	2 events that occurred sequentially, e.g., Moro → TNR
4	3 events, two that occurred together and one that preceded or followed, e.g., Moro + TNR → Cry, or CPR → body movement + behavioral arousal
5	3 events that occurred sequentially, e.g., Moro → TNR → Cry
6	4 events, only two that occurred sequentially, e.g., Moro + TNR → opened eyes + whimpered
7	4 events, three that occurred sequentially and one that preceded or followed, e.g., Moro + TNR → opened eyes → whimpered
8	4 events that occurred sequentially, e.g., Moro → TNR → opened eyes → whimpered
9	Not scored or no response

2. Kind(s) of stimulus-bound behavior (columns 20–38 and 43–61)
   a. "No response" should be coded as 99999.
   b. Each event of stimulus-bound behavior must be represented by 4 characters as follows:

(1)	General class of response	space 1
(2)	Subcategory within this class	2
(3)	Specific descriptor number within subcategory	3
(4)	Modifier indicating relation between this event and any subsequent event(s)	4

(continued)

Table I.5 (*continued*)

c. Items (1), (2), and (3) are specified exactly on the attached code listings.
d. Only three modifiers (0 - 5 - 9) are required as follows:
   (1) 0 indicates that the particular event recorded occurred *in conjunction with* (+) the next event recorded
   (2) 5 indicates that the event recorded wa:: followed by (→) the next event recorded
   (3) 9 indicates that the event recorded was not followed by any other events, i.e., specifying completion of the stimulus-bound activity observed
e. There is no modifier for *latent* responses, but these should be considered as follows:
   (1) If a response is scored as L, code the first four event columns as 9999 and record the observation(s) in the second four event columns
   (2) If a response is scored as LL, follow the same procedures, coding the first *two* event columns as 9999 and recording the observation(s) in the third-event columns (and fourth, if it falls in number code 2 or 3 categories)

E. Respiration Rate (Columns 64–65)
If there is no count associated with observation, code columns 64–65 as 00.

F. Nonstimulus and Artifactual Events (Columns 68–79)
1. Events should be noted in these columns under the following conditions:
    a. They occurred immediately around the signal presentation period, preventing us from obtaining valid (responsive) data.
    b. The events noted occurred in association with a push of the artifact button during the intersignal period.
    c. Something occurred which resulted in a procedural change.
2. If no events in this category were noted, code columns 68 and 69 as 00.
3. See attached code listings (Table I.7) for specific artifacts.
4. If an artifact occurs repeatedly during trials (e.g., hiccups or similar problems), note it repeatedly.
5. If a number of related events occurred, code them in order (as and if you can), using a colon (:) to separate your entries.

[a]N.B. to EEG Technician. State ratings should be noted according to the 1–7 behavioral scale (to the extent this is possible).

Table I.6. Code Assignments for Scoring Stimulus-Bound Behavior on IBM Cards

STIMULUS-BOUND EVENT (columns 20–38 and 43–61)	CODE LISTING
Motor Behavior (General Class 1)	
Articulatory precursors	11
Extremity movements	12
Head and neck movements	13
Lower face activity	14
Upper face activity	15
Visual musculature	16
Whole body movements	17
Arousal Behavior (General Class 2)	
Articulatory precursors	21
Body movements	22
Brain wave activity	23
Facial movements	24
Respiratory activity	25
Visual activity	26
Vocal activity	27
Orienting and Orienting-Quiet (General Class 3)	
Articulatory precursors	31
Attentive behavior	32
Body movements	33
Brain wave activity	34
Facial activity	35
Respiratory activity	36
Visual activity	37
Vocal activity	38

(continued)

Table I.6 (*continued*)

	Specific Code No.	
Stimulus-Bound Event	EEG Events	Behavior

MOTOR BEHAVIOR (General Class 1)
  ARTICULATORY PRECURSORS (11)
   1   Starts to suck — 111 / 111
   2   Undifferentiated lip movements — / 112
   3   Utterance associated with movements or physiologic state — / 113
   4   Swallow — 114 / 114

Stimulus-Bound Event	EEG Events	Behavior
MOTOR BEHAVIOR (General Class 1)		
ARTICULATORY PRECURSORS (11)		
1 Starts to suck	111	111
2 Undifferentiated lip movements		112
3 Utterance associated with movements or physiologic state		113
4 Swallow	114	114
5		
6		
7		
8		
EXTREMITY MOVEMENTS (12)		
1 Fingers only, one side only		121
2 Hand movements, one side only		122
3 Foot movements, one side only		123
4 Hand and foot movements, one side only		124
5 Hand movements, both right and left sides		125
6 Foot movements, both right and left sides		126
7		
8		
HEAD AND NECK MOVEMENTS (13)		
1 Tonic neck reflex (TNR)	131	131
2 Nondirectional head movements, without startle	132	132
3		
4		

(continued)

Table I.6 (*continued*)

Stimulus Bound Event	Specific Code No. EEG Events	Behavior
5		
6		
7		
8		
LOWER FACE ACTIVITY (14)		
1 Grimaces or frowns		141
2 Undifferentiated lower face movements		142
3		
4		
5		
6		
7		
8		
UPPER FACE ACTIVITY (15)		
1 Wrinkles brows or forehead	151	151
2 Undifferentiated upper face activity		152
3		
4		
5		
6		
7		
8		
VISUAL MUSCULATURE (16)		
1 Closes eyes	161	161
2 Cochleopalpebral reflex (CPR)		162

(continued)

Table I.6 (*continued*)

Stimulus Bound Event	Specific Code No.	
	EEG Events	Behavior
3 Eyelids droop		163
4 Eyelids tremble		164
5 Eyeslit narrows		165
6 Rapid eye movements (REM), with closed eyes	166	166
7 Rolls eyeballs backwards		167
8		
WHOLE BODY MOVEMENTS (17)		
1 Movements of Moro- or startle-like intensity	171	171
2 Body movements less intense than above	172	172
3 Minimal whole body movements		173
4 Mild movements of upper torso only		174
5 Mild movements of lower torso only		175
6		
7		
8		
Arousal Behavior (General Class 2)		
ARTICULATORY PRECURSORS (21)		
1 Starts to suck, with arousal	211	211
2 Sucks more vigorously	212	212
3		
4		
5		
6		
7		
8		
BODY MOVEMENTS (22)		
1 Generalized stirring, with arousal	221	221
2 Increased amount of bodily activity	222	222

(continued)

Table I.6 (*continued*)

Stimulus Bound Event	Specific Code No.	
	EEG Events	Behavior
3		
4		
5		
6		
7		
8		
BRAIN WAVE ACTIVITY (23)		
1 K-Complex in *one lead* only	231	
2 K-Complex in several, but *not all* leads	232	
3 K-Complex in *all leads*	233	
4 Generalized brain wave arousal in *all leads*	234	
5		
6		
7		
8		
FACIAL MOVEMENTS (24)		
1 Puckers as if to cry		
2 Squints		
3		
4		
5		
6		
7		
8		
RESPIRATORY ACTIVITY (25)		
1 Increases respiration rate noticeably		251
2		
3		
4		

(continued)

Table I.6 (*continued*)

Stimulus Bound Event	Specific Code No. EEG Events	Behavior
5		
6		
7		
8		
VISUAL ACTIVITY (26)		
1 Moves eyelids up and/or down, with arousal		261
2 Opens eyes, with arousal		262
3 Pupillary contraction		263
4		
5		
6		
7		
8		
VOCAL ACTIVITY (27)		
1 Displeasure utterance other than cry (grunt, whimper, etc.)		271
2 Increases intensity of above, when ongoing		272
3 Starts to cry or otherwise vocalize loudly	273	273
4 Cries more lustily (usually with increase in general brain wave activity)	274	274
5 Becomes grossly upset and screaming	275	275
7		
8		

Orienting (Older Subjects) and Orienting-Quiet (Infants) (General Class 3)

	EEG Events	Behavior
ARTICULATORY PRECURSORS (31)		
1 Sucks less vigorously		311
2 Stops sucking entirely, momentarily	312	312
3 Stops sucking entirely, more than momentarily	313	313
4		
5		
6		
7		
8		
ATTENTIONAL BEHAVIOR (32)		
1 Apparent attentional behavior of undifferentiated kind		321
2 Obvious "listening" behavior of undifferentiated kind		322
3 Starts to cry immediately before signal onset		323
4 Starts to suck immediately before signal onset		324
5 Turns or moves directionally toward sound source		325

(continued)

Table I.6 (*continued*)

	Stimulus Bound Event	Specific Code No.	
		EEG Events	Behavior
6			
7			
8			
BODY MOVEMENTS (33)			
1	Decreases amount of ongoing body activity markedly		331
2	Stops moving entirely, momentarily	332	332
3	Stops moving entirely, more than momentarily	333	333
4	Orients whole body toward sound source		334
5			
6			
7			
8			
BRAIN WAVE ACTIVITY (34)			
1	Flattening or quieting in *one lead*	341	
2	Flattening or quieting in several but *not all* leads	342	
3	Flattening or quieting in *all leads*	343	
4	Alpha-blocking	344	
5[a]	Anticipatory changes involving Excitation	345	
6[a]	Anticipatory changes involving blocking or flattening	346	
7			
8			
FACIAL ACTIVITY (35)			
1	Undifferentiated expression suggesting pleasure		351
2	Definite smile of pleasure		352
3			
4			
5			
6			
7			
8			

(continued)

Table I.6 (*continued*)

Stimulus Bound Event	Specific Code No.	
	EEG Events	Behavior
RESPIRATORY ACTIVITY (36)		
1 Decreased respiration rate markedly		361
2 Holds breath momentarily		362
3 Changes respiratory pattern markedly (responsively)		363
4 Stopped snoring		364
5		
6		
7		
8		
VISUAL ACTIVITY (37)		
1 Moves eyes directionally, seeking sound source		371
2 Pupillary dilatation		372
3 Widens eyes as if to "see" or "hear" better		373
4 Definite "What-was-that?" look		374
5		
6		
7		
8		
VOCAL ACTIVITY (38)		
1 Decrease in ongoing vocal activity other than crying		381
2 Ceases above utterance, momentarily		382
3 Ceases above utterance, more than momentarily		383
4 Decreases intensity of ongoing crying	384	384
5 Stops crying entirely, momentarily	385	385
6 Stops crying entirely, more than momentarily	386	386
7		
8		

[a]These code numbers should be used only to indicate presignal (anticipatory) chan associated with stimulus presentation.

Table I.7 Code Assignments for Nonstimulus Events and Artifactual Behavior on IBM Cards

Behavioral Interference (01–09)
- 01   Possible responses to nontest object or event
- 02   Subject fixated on nontest object or event
- 03   Subject generally uncooperative (older subjects)
- 04   Subject fussy (infants)
- 05   Subject talking
- 06   Subject moving
- 07   Subject yawning
- 08
- 09

Electrical Problems (10–19)
- 10   Loose EKG electrode
- 11   Loose EEG electrode
- 12   Radio interference noted by control room monitor
- 13   Voltage fluctuation
- 14   Subject Touching EKG electrode
- 15   Subject Touching EKG electrode
- 16
- 17
- 18
- 19

Pathologic Observations (20–29)
- 20   Interseizure pattern
- 21   Petit mal seizure
- 22   Grand mal seizure

(continued)

Table I.7 (*continued*)

===

23
24
25
26
27
28
29

Physiologic Interferences (30−44)
  30 Bowel movement
  31 Burp
  32 Hiccups
  33 Regurgitation (spits up)
  34 Sneeze
  35 Spontaneous startle
  36 Swallow
  37 Urination
  38 Flatulence
  39 Snoring
  40
  41
  42
  43
  44

Procedural Changes (45−79)
        nurse intervention without procedural stop
  45 For atmospheric problem
  46 For behavioral problem (comforting, etc.)
  47 For electrical problem

(continued)

Table I.7 (*continued*)

48	For physiologic problem (diaper change, etc.)
49	Stopped experiment temporarily for intervention
50	Intervention of technician (second person in room), with procedural halt
51	Changed EKG electrode
52	Changed EEG electrode
53	Changed EKG settings
54	Increased gain on EEG
55	Decreased gain on EEG
56	
57	Resumed experiment after intervention
58	
59	
60	Alternate signal introduced (deliberately)
61	
62	
63	Increased SPL of signal
64	Decreased SPL of signal
65	
66	
67	
68	
69	
70	Stopped experiment before completion for reasons of subject's condition
71	
72	
73	

(continued)

Table I.7 (*continued*)

74	Scrubbed test for electrical reasons
75	Scrubbed test for subject's reasons (uncooperative or untestable)
76	
77	
78	
79	

Procedural Errors (80–99)

80	Atmospheric problems (heat, high humidity, excess light, etc.)
81	Observer forgot to push artifact button
82	Observer pushed artifact button instead of response button
83	Observer pushed response button instead of artifact button
84	Observer forgot to push response button
85	Nontest signal introduced in error
86	Extraneous sound produced within test chamber
87	Transient inadvertently allowed through speaker from control room
88	Extra signal inadvertently introduced through speaker
89	
90	False trigger: signal recorded on paper (and/or tape) record, but no sound heard in test chamber
91	
92	
93	
94	
95	
96	
97	
98	Observer pushed response button inadvertently
99	Observer pushed artifact button inadvertently

SECTION II. MATERIAL RELEVANT TO CIRCUIT DESIGN AND INSTRUMENTATION *Anthony Marmarou, with Rita B. Eisenberg*

This section, which considers Bioacoustic Laboratory circuitry currently in use, is primarily directed to engineers or investigators with a reasonable background in biomedical electronics. It is hoped, however, that readers with more limited expertise will find some of the descriptive material useful as an adjunct to the information provided in Chapter 5.

Figure II.1 is a block diagram of the system used for presentation of acoustic signals and for acquisition of correlative behavioral and electrophysiologic data on auditory behavior. Each item of equipment in the circuit is identified by a number to which the discussion that follows is keyed, and commercially available gear incorporated in the system are listed in Table II.1.

Circuitry for Signal Presentation and Control

The system is designed for controlled presentation of sound from two major sources: from a function generator ① , serving for on-line presentation of pure tones, swept tones, noise bands, and clicks; and from a magnetic tape deck ② , serving for storage and playback of more complex prerecorded stimuli (live voice, synthetic speech, special log rate patterns, and so on).

The outputs of these devices are routed to an electronic switch ④ which gates the signals to the audioamplifier ⑤ and speaker ⑥ upon command of the stimulus control logic ③ , the latter being triggered by either push button or automatic timer. One purpose of the logic module ③ is to deactivate the input signal to the audioamplifier during interstimulus intervals, thus precluding tape noise. A second purpose is to provide a stimulus marker pulse that is synchronized with signal onset and routed to the event code logic ⑦ for recording on the master data tape ⑩ .

All items blocked out in Figure II.1—except the stimulus control logic, which was designed to meet special experimental needs—are commercially available (see Table II.1).

Stimulus Control Logic (SCL)

SCL circuitry, which is composed of commercially available digital and analog modules (Digital Electronics; Philbrick Analog Devices), is shown in Figure II.2. Functions of this circuitry are listed below.
1. Gate the electronic switch to *on* during presentation of sound and gate it to *off* during interstimulus intervals.

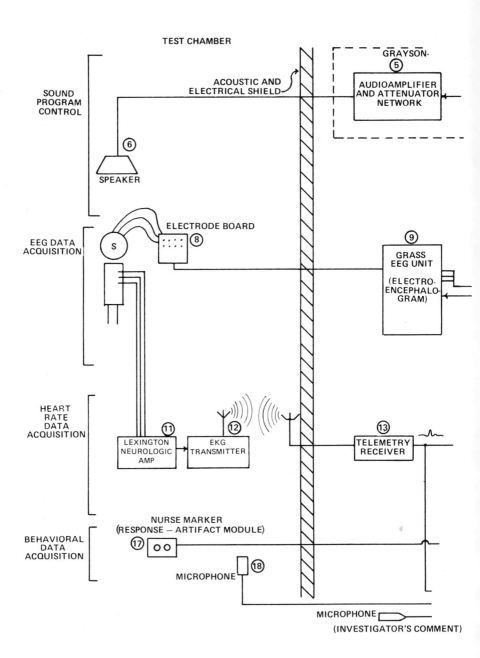

Figure II.1. Schematic of Bioacoustic Laboratory circuitry for data acquisition and storage.

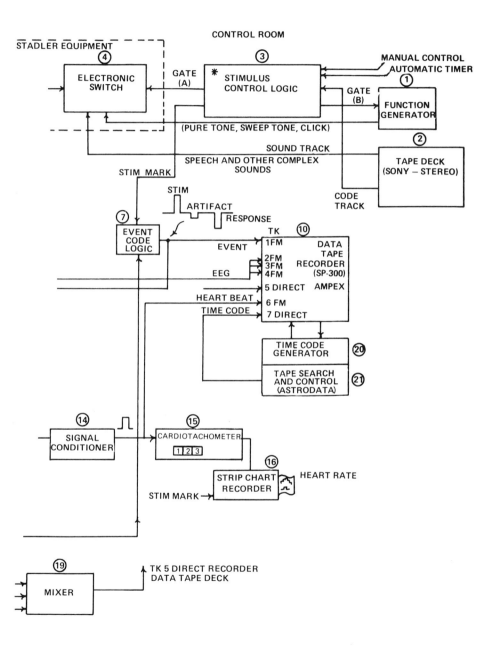

Table II.1. Equipment Items Schematized in Figure II.1

Code No.	Item	Manufacturer and Model No.
①	Function generator	Wavetek, 114[a]
②	Stereo tape deck	Sony, TC-630
③	Stimulus control logic	Laboratory design, Figure II.2
④	Electronic switch	Grason-Stadler, 829-D[a]
⑤	Audioamplifier and attenuator	Grason-Stadler, 162
⑥	Speaker	Acoustic Research, AR-4
⑦	Event code logic	Laboratory design, Figure II.2
⑧	Electrode board	Grass, 6EBN-25
⑨	Electroencephalogram	Grass, 78
⑩	7-channel tape recorder	Ampex, SP-300
⑪	Neurologic amplifier	Lexington, A103/B[a]
⑫	EKG transmitter	Laboratory design
⑬	Telemetry receiver	Sony, tuner ST-80W[a]
⑭	Signal conditioner	Laboratory design, Figure II.2
⑮	Cardiotachometer	Gilford, 121
⑯	2-channel strip chart recorder	Sanborn, 322[a]
⑰	Response-artifact logic module	Laboratory design, Figure II.6
⑱	Microphone (test chamber)	Sony, F26
⑲	Mixer	Switchcraft, part 301-TR
⑳	Time code generator	Astrodata 5400[a]
㉑	Tape search and control	Astrodata 5244[a]
	Digital logic	Data Technology Corp.
	Operational amplifiers	Philbrick

[a]Equipment found to be especially satisfactory.

2. Provide a stimulus marker synchronized with onset and offset of an acoustic signal.

3. Provide a trigger signal to the function generator upon push button command from an investigator or upon electronic command from an external timer.

4. Advance a digital counter for each signal presentation.

5. Provide visual indicator(s) of signal presentation.

6. Provide a means for gating the electronic switch from magnetic tape.

7. Provide a means for on-line generation of prerecorded stimuli according to investigator command.

SCL Operation by Manual Mode In the manual mode, push button operation (PBB in Figure II.2) is controlled by the investigator. Closure of PBB activates the logic circuit to produce a pulse at output C and initiate the internal timer (one-shot multivibrator 540). The output pulse at C is routed to the external trigger input of the function generator, which is preset for the stimulus conditions under investigation. In the case of pure tones or noise bands, the internal timer of the SCL controls stimulus duration; for clicks or tonal sweeps, duration is controlled by adjustment of the function generator.

For each command by an investigator, the SCL will generate a stimulus marker in the form of a positive 5.0-volt pulse that can be recorded on data tape and/or on stripchart (output C). Simultaneously, an indicator light (GR) will be energized, and the stimulus counter will be advanced one digit to indicate activation and proper circuit operation of one logic cycle.

SCL Operation in Automatic Mode In the automatic mode, the logic circuit is energized by electrical pulses originating either from an external timer or from magnetic tape. The electrical output of the selected device, in the form of a positive 5.0-volt pulse, is routed to the "auto mode" input A shown in Figure II.2. This positive pulse controls the onset of a stimulus, while the internal timer of the SCL controls its duration. Upon arrival of a pulse at terminal A, the operation and logic sequence are similar to that described above for manual mode. Under conditions where use of separate external timers for stimulus onset and offset is desirable, the internal timer may be bypassed by placing switch S2 in "external reset" position.

In experiments of the kind detailed in Chapter 5, where the stimulus schedule is fixed, SCL circuitry can be used both to generate a "master" program tape and, in its "auto mode," to control playback of the signals on that tape.

In generating a program, an external timer is used to control inter-stimulus interval (onset-to-onset) and the output of the function generator

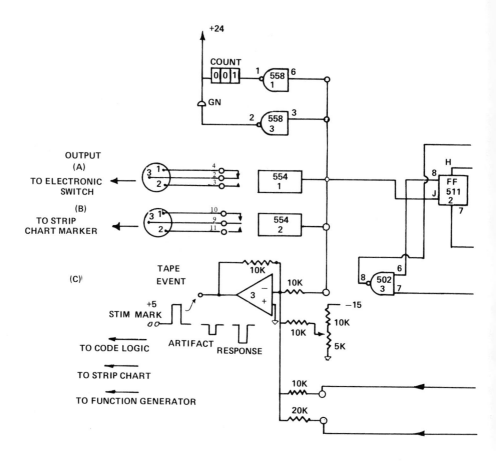

Figure II.2. Logic circuitry (SCL) for controlled presentation of acoustic stimuli.

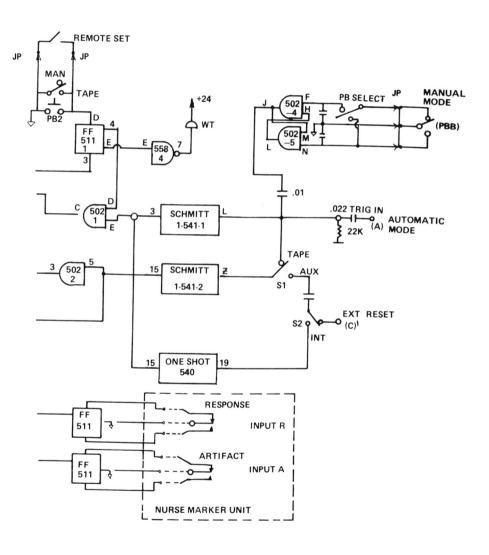

($\textcircled{1}$ in Figure II.1) is routed to one track of a stereo tape deck $\textcircled{2}$. Output C of the SCL simultaneously is recorded on the second channel, or "code track," of the stereo tape deck so that, upon playback, the latter provides a positive pulse that is synchronized with stimulus onset and a negative pulse that is synchronized with stimulus offset. This occurs as a natural consequence of the differentiation of the square output pulse of the SCL by the recording circuitry of the tape deck.

In the playback cycle, the sound track of the prerecorded tape $\textcircled{2}$ is routed to the electronic switch $\textcircled{4}$, as shown in Figure II.1, while the code track is routed to terminal A of the SCL circuitry for automatic triggering of the normal logic cycle.

SCL Operation for On-Line Generation of Complex Acoustic Signals One important feature of the SCL circuitry diagramed in Figure II.2 is that it permits presentation of highly complex acoustic stimuli such as synthetic CV syllables or other speechlike sounds at random intervals that are subject to investigator control. Such a feature is particularly useful when, for instance, an experimental protocol specifies stimulus presentation only under conditions where the subject is in some predetermined behavioral state or when his heart rate or brain wave patterns meet certain predetermined criteria.

In this application, experimental signals are prerecorded on one channel of a 90-min magnetic tape in serial fashion, with a 5-msec separation between successive stimuli. A second track on the tape recorder contains bipolar pulses synchronized with onset and offset of the test signals. A two-channel "stacked" tape of this kind can be produced easily at Haskins Laboratories or other facilities similarly equipped with the sophisticated gear required for generation of synthetic speech sounds.

Upon playback through the circuitry diagrammed in Figure II.1, the sound track $\textcircled{2}$ containing the sequential acoustic stimuli is routed to the electronic switch $\textcircled{4}$, as shown in Figure II.2, thus blocking any input to the speaker $\textcircled{6}$ until a "gate" signal is received from the SCL. In this application, the function of the SCL circuitry is to select a stimulus from the stacked tape in response to the investigator's push button command. This function is effected by placing switch S1 of the SCL in "auxiliary" position, switch S2 in "external reset," and switch S3 in "manual" position so that the "code track" of the prerecorded tape is routed to the "automatic mode" input terminal of the SCL.

Whenever stimulus presentation is required by the experimental protocol, the investigator need only depress push button PB2 on the SCL panel. This places the logic circuit in "standby" condition, and the first positive pulse, identifying the onset of the sound envelope, is fed to the SCL by the code track which, in turn, initiates the logic cycle and triggers the electronic switch. The subsequent negative pulse, identified by the code track as signal offset, automatically resets the logic, thus preventing further sound from being processed. Given this arrangement, the maximum possible time delay from investigator command to signal presentation is equal to stimulus duration plus 5 msec.

Acquisition of Electroencephalographic (EEG) Data

Given well controlled experimental procedures, the acquisition of EEG data is quite straightforward because all signal conditioning, amplification, and calibration equipment required for proper recording of electrical activity is obtainable within commercially available units (Beckman, Grass, and the like).

As noted in Chapter 5, Bioacoustic Laboratory procedures involve the use of gold disc electrodes attached with bentonite paste. These electrodes are connected to a standard 10-20 electrode board ⑧ and routed, via a remote extension cable, to the Grass (model 78) instrument ⑨. Amplified EEG signals from external output terminals of the EEG unit then are routed directly to the FM magnetic tape recorder ⑩.

In our experience, problems encountered in routine acquisition of EEG data mainly relate to excessive noise (60-Hz interference) emanating from electrodes, the EEG instrument per se, multiple system connections, and so on. These problems may not be obvious from visual inspection of EEG strip chart recordings because the built-in 60-Hz filtering, which applies to the pen driver amplifiers, does not apply to the external output terminals (J6 on a model 78 Grass) that are routed to the tape recorder. Moreover, in a hospital environment, the level of 60-Hz interference tends to vary over time. For this reason, we have considered it necessary to check and measure the total system noise level before each experimental session.

As a start, several electrodes are mounted on a piece of 8½ X 11 inch cardboard covered with a thin layer of the bentonite paste. This "dummy" board is positioned in the same physical area as the head of a subject, and gain settings of the EEG amplifier and filter networks are adjusted to our specified experimental settings. The total system noise per channel then is measured by monitoring the "tape" output terminal (J6) of each amplifier with an oscilloscope. Experiments are initiated only when it can be demonstrated that the maximum peak-to-peak noise level is less than 50-mv. Under these conditions, a signal to noise ratio (S/N) of greater than 10:1 is provided for EEG signals averaging 25% of full scale pen deflection.

Acquisition of Heart Rate (HR) Data

As noted in Chapter 5, the potential change transmitted to the surface of the body by the activity of cardiac muscle is a complex wave form consisting of five major components. For acquisition of rate information, however, it is necessary to detect only the beat-to-beat interval. This task most frequently is accomplished with electronic gear designed to detect the leading edge of the QRS complex, or what commonly is termed the "R" wave. The processing cycle of a typical commercially available cardiotachometer is shown in Figure II.3.

As shown in the figure, the EKG signal (a), sensed by the electrodes positioned on a subject's body, has an amplitude of approximately 2.0 mv. This signal is amplified electronically and routed to a digital circuit that provides a uniform square wave pulse when the R wave potential exceeds the "trigger threshold" of the circuitry (b). The computation intervals of the cardiotachometer take place during a single interbeat interval (c), and, at the end of this interval, a voltage output proportional to heart rate is provided (d). Thus, as shown in Figure II.4, each heart rate (voltage

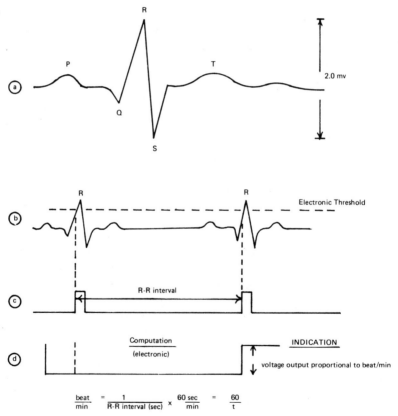

Figure II.3. Processing cycle of a cardiotachometer. (a) cardiac potential at electrode terminals; (b) position of electronic threshold relative to cardiac complex; (c) pulse output digital circuitry for measurement of R-R interval; (d) voltage output of cardiotachometer, proportional to heart rate calibrated in beats per minute.

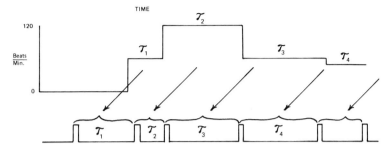

Figure II.4. Strip chart output of a cardiotachometer, showing relation between voltage output and R-R interval.

output) recorded on the strip chart is delayed in real time by the previous R-R interval, and this fact must be taken into account in data processing and analysis.

Cardiotachometer systems are designed to accept the low level EKG signal direct from the electrodes and to provide heart rate data in either digital ("Nixie") or analog (strip chart) form. Although these direct forms of recording are entirely adequate for many experimental purposes, we have found it advisable to incorporate telemetric devices into the Bio-acoustic Laboratory system. The reasons for this, noted briefly in Chapter 5, are threefold. First of all, neonates and other very young infants studied under conditions of very high excitation not infrequently may prove so hyperactive as to produce unacceptably high levels of movement artifact. Second, direction connection to a cardiotachometer system introduces a "ground loop" that can interfere with the acquisition of good EEG data. Finally, multiple ground connections to a subject introduce the possibility of electrical hazard.

The manner in which telemetry has been incorporated into the Bio-acoustic Laboratory system is shown in Figure II.1. As can be seen, cardiac electrodes are connected to a battery-operated Lexington neurologic amplifier (11) which provides suitable amplification of the EKG complex and has the additional advantage of built-in adjustable filters for the elimination of high frequency noise. The output of the Lexington (11) is routed to an FM transmitter (designed by AM) operating at a carrier frequency of 108 mHz. The FM carrier modulated by the EKG complex then is transmitted via antenna to a receiver (13) located in the control room adjoining our test chamber. The output of the receiver, in its turn, feeds into a signal conditioner (14) which converts the R wave to a uniform square pulse. This uniform positive square wave, corresponding to each R wave, is routed to the commercial tachometer (15) providing the usual "Nixie" and strip chart data. As can be determined from Figure II.1, the pulse output from the heartbeat signal conditioner is also routed to the

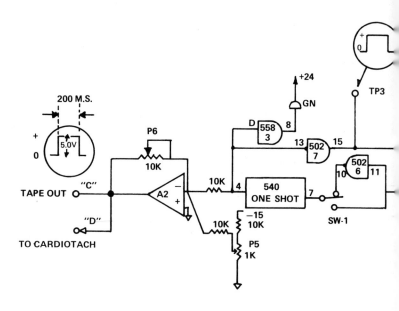

Figure II.5. Heart beat signal conditioner (module (14) in Figure II.1).

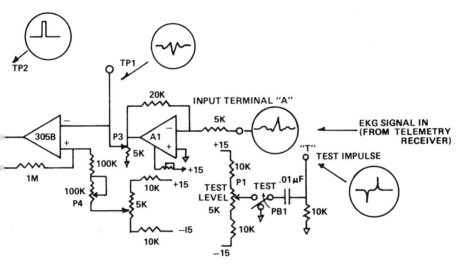

TP2

TP1

20K

INPUT TERMINAL "A"

5K

EKG SIGNAL IN
(FROM TELEMETRY
RECEIVER)

305B

P3   A1

5K

"T"   TEST IMPULSE

+15

100K

+15

1M

10K

100K

10K   +15

TEST   P1   TEST
LEVEL

.01 µF

P4

5K

5K   PB1

10K

−15

10K

10K

10K

−15

event code logic ⑦ so that the individual pulses can be recorded on magnetic tape and subjected to off-line computer analysis.

Signal Conditioning of Heart Rate Data A detailed schematic of the heart beat signal conditioner ⑭ is shown in Figure II.5. As can be determined from the diagram, the demodulated output from the FM receiver ⑬ is routed to input terminal A and amplified by module A1 (Philbrick OP-AMP P85AU). The inverted EKG pulse thus derived is routed to a comparator module (Analog Devices, model 350B) that is triggered into saturation by each R wave of the QRS complex. The threshold level of the comparator is adjusted by a 20-turn 5K potentiometer (P2) mounted on the front panel of the circuit housing. The comparator threshold is adjusted visually by connecting test point TP1 to the vertical axis of an oscilloscope and triggering the horizontal axis from the pulse output of TP2. In this mode, the precise point of trigger on the QR portion of the EKG complex can be determined by observing the scope display, and premature triggering of the P wave of the EKG pulse is precluded.

The output of the comparator is routed to a nonretriggerable multivibrator (Digital Equipment Corp., model 540) in order to stretch the pulse to a width of 200 msec and thus reduce the possibility of false triggering between heart beats.

The pulse output from the one-shot multivibrator is inverted by OP-AMP module A2. This serves to adjust the amplitude of the output pulse to +5.0 volts and provides a low impedance source for pulse recording on magnetic tape (output terminal C on the schematic).

Satisfactory operation of the entire logic cycle can be tested by connecting pulse terminal T to input terminal A and depressing push button PB1. This test pulse activates a green indicator light when circuit threshold is exceeded and all modules are operative.

Electronic Recording of Behavioral Data

The purpose of the response-artifact module ⑰ is to record onto magnetic tape the kinds of observations made by a nurse-observer in the test chamber. This is effected by a simple relay circuit that acts in combination with the event code logic module ⑦ diagrammed in Figure II.6.

The control box held by the nurse-observer contains only two buttons and a light indicator. When button PBR is depressed, the *response* relay situated on the behavioral data panel is energized, resulting in closure of relay contacts R2 and thus triggering flip-flop FFR 511 on the SCL circuit. The output of FFR 511, fed to a summing amplifier, generates a negative 2.5-volt rectangular pulse for each closure of the response relay;

and the output of the summing amplifier is recorded on magnetic tape. Similarly, when button PBA is depressed, the *artifact* relay is energized, resulting in closure of relay contacts A2 and thus activating flip-flop FFA. The output of flip-flop FFA also is routed to the summing network with an overall gain of unity. Thus, closure of the artifact relay generates a negative 5.0-volt pulse for recording on magnetic tape. The third input to the summing amplifier is the negative pulse signifying a *stimulus event,* and this results in a positive 5.0-volt pulse at the output of the amplifier network. The combined code corresponding to "response," "artifact," and "stimulus event" for recording onto a single tape channel is shown in Figure II.6 at the lower right side of the diagram. Relay contacts A-IN and R-IN prevent simultaneous activation of the response and artifact relays.

A light signal to the nurse-observer in the test chamber may be activated from the control room by depressing PB5, while visual indicators of artifact or response events observed in the chamber are signaled automatically to the control room when relays A and R are energized.

The relays considered above, in conjunction with the coded observations detailed in Section I of this Appendix, permit careful monitoring (cross-checking) of response and artifact events recorded during the course of experiments.

All sounds emanating from the test chamber, including subject utterances, are detected by a microphone ⑱ , the output of which is routed to one channel of a commercially available mixer ⑲ . Additional inputs to the mixer include the demodulated EKG pulse from the FM receiver and a hand-held microphone for identification (ID) information and other experimental commentary. The output of the mixer, monitored by a speaker located in the control room, is recorded onto one channel of the data tape ⑩ .

Storage of Experimental Data on Magnetic Tape

Bioacoustic Laboratory data of the kind discussed in Chapter 5 are recorded onto magnetic tape at a speed of 7.5 IPS according to the format shown in Table II.2.

The record-playback gain of each channel is set and maintained at a 1:1 ratio to simplify calibration procedures and to permit rapid interchange of channels should any of the record amplifiers malfunction during an experiment.

The IRIG B time code ⑳ is recorded on channel 5 in the form of a modulated 1 KC carrier that addresses the tape serially in hours, minutes, and seconds. It is generated by a commercially available unit (Astrodata) initiated, as time zero, at the start of each experiment. When used in conjunction with a "tape search and control" system ㉑ , it allows the

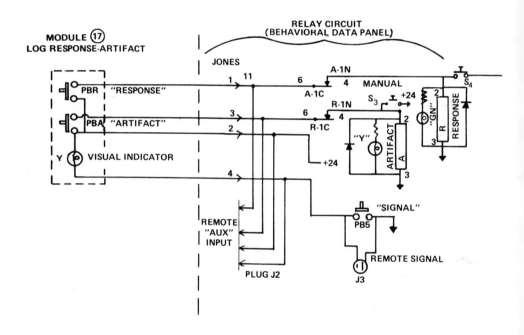

Figure II.6. Response-artifact module.

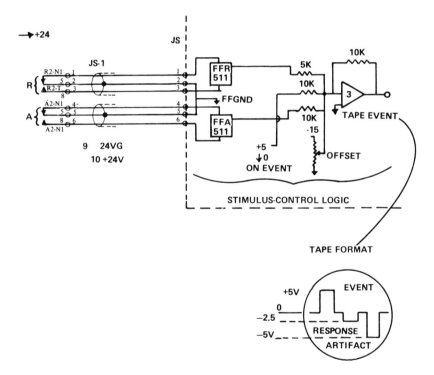

Table II.2. Bioacoustic Laboratory Format for Recording Data on a 7-Channel Magnetic Tape Recorder

Channel	Mode	Kind of Data	Source of Data (Figure II.1)
1	FM	Event Code	⑦
2	FM	EEG	⑨
3	FM	EEG	⑨
4	FM	EEG	⑨
5	Direct	Time code	⑳
6	FM	Heart beat	⑭
7	Direct	Commentary	⑲

investigator to cycle a tape automatically, with an accuracy of 1.0 sec, to any desired time period in an experiment.

In addition to recording real time on magnetic tape, the time code generator provides an auxiliary binary output that is (a) continuous and (b) reproducible on strip chart for visual decoding off-line. Given this arrangement, the onset and duration of all experimental events can be identified and tabulated (in hours, minutes, and seconds) by strip chart; and corresponding physical locations on a data tape can be located automatically for off-line data processing tasks (as, for instance, in EEG averaging).

Most of the magnetic tape recorders of instrument quality now manufactured include, as a purchase option, built-in circuitry for tape search and control. It is possible to interface a tape search system with older models, however, provided that two conditions are met. First, the speed of the fast forward and rewind modes must not exceed 60 IPS. Second, the tape must remain in continuous contact with the playback head during these modes. This interface option, which was employed during early Bioacoustic Laboratory studies utilizing an Ampex SP-300, requires revisions in internal wiring so that additional resistance can be placed in series with the control windings of the motor transport during a "search" cycle. (Investigators wishing further information and/or specifications on circuit revisions for the SP-300 may contact the Bioacoustic Laboratory for a detailed wiring diagram.)

Index